AV PVBLIC

THE GREAT DEAD BODY TEACHERS

Published in 2023 by Ultimo Press,
an imprint of Hardie Grant Publishing

Ultimo Press
Gadigal Country
7, 45 Jones Street
Ultimo, NSW 2007
ultimopress.com.au

Ultimo Press (London)
5th & 6th Floors
52–54 Southwark Street
London SE1 1UN

ultimopress

NATIONAL LIBRARY OF AUSTRALIA
A catalogue record for this book is available from the National Library of Australia

The Great Dead Body Teachers
ISBN 978 1 76115 048 7 (hardback)

10 9 8 7 6 5 4 3 2 1

Cover design Design by Committee
Typesetting Shaun Jury | Typeset in 11/15 pt Baskerville URW
Copyeditor Jocelyn Hungerford
Proofreader Jessica Friedmann

Printed in Australia by Griffin Press, an Accredited ISO AS/NZS 14001 Environmental Management System printer.

Ultimo Press acknowledges the Traditional Owners of the Country on which we work, the Gadigal People of the Eora Nation and the Wurundjeri People of the Kulin Nation, and recognises their continuing connection to the land, waters and culture. We pay our respects to their Elders past and present.

THE GREAT DEAD BODY TEACHERS

An adventure into the world of anatomy and dissection

Jackie Dent

'I was never hysterical but, as all spiritual human beings often are, very nervous and my most prominent character traits are: a sanguine temperament, strong impulsiveness, cheerful disposition, energy, determination, courage and the presence of spirit in all, even the most difficult, situations, a rare persistence in everything, and fearlessness to encounter anything; here also come fierceness and liveliness but not a truly violent temper; I should also mention: veracity, pride and healthy sensuality.'

Anna Astl-Leonhard, journalist and potential body donor, Vienna, late 19th century

'Let them never forget that without anatomy there is no physiology, no surgery, no medicine; that in a word, all the medical sciences are grafted on the anatomy.'

Jean Cruveilhier, *Traité d'Anatomie Descriptive*, 1834

'The almost fashionable success of anatomy cannot be attributed solely to scientific curiosity. It is not hard to understand; it corresponds to an attraction to certain ill-defined things at the outer limit of life and death, sexuality and pain.'

Philippe Ariès, *The Hour of Our Death*, 1977

Preface

Dissection might not be a normal topic to contemplate but when both your paternal grandparents donate their bodies to science it does intermittently cross your mind. My grandmother Ruby's body went to the University of Queensland in 1969 and my grandfather Julie's—yes, that was his name—in 1981.

So while this is book is about me finding out what have might have happened, it somehow morphed into the history of the world. By slowly crawling back in time and then quietly prancing to the present, I accidentally found myself in the middle of a massive production called WTF ANATOMY, a part drama, comedy, horror, science fiction and Marina Abramović concept piece.

It starred contemporary medicine, embalming fluid, God, art, 14th-century Italian nuns, Indian communists, sun-sized ethical dilemmas, Twitter and of course lots of dead people. I used to think of science, medicine and anatomy as relatively objective, ordered, unprejudiced, hospital-white spaces where people measured everything, made perfect findings and spoke very clearly to one another in lab coats. I now see that while they do indeed strive for objectivity, science is nonetheless a human endeavour, and parts of it are as wild as a haphazard doof festival in a sweaty jungle with rainbows and poison arrows.

I think every second person I spoke to when writing this book confused whole-body donation with organ donation. So it's very important from the outset to point out that whole-body donation is very different to organ donation.

Organ donors usually die in a hospital, and are kept alive so the parts that are needed—heart, kidney and liver for example—are still working when they are transplanted into someone else. Whole-body donation is what it sounds like and the donation occurs when the person is 100 per cent dead. To donate your whole body in Australia, you need to sign up at your local university.

Once you die, your family needs to call the university ASAP and an undertaker will collect your body within twenty-four hours. In some instances, you may not be accepted—if you have moved away from the university area or you have one of a number of disqualifying diseases. Once your body arrives, it will be used for 'medical research and education'. The university will cover the cost of cremating your body once they are finished with it.

While millions of medical professionals have dissected bodies, the intricacies, histories and realities of it were absolutely unknown to me—and I think to most people. That makes sense. Why would we need to know about it? Let's just leave it to the doctors. Also, this isn't an easy world to contemplate. Dismemberment is pretty horrible, really.

But I think this is where the problem starts—people start to imagine what happens in a dissecting hall. I know I have. And then every so often there is a terrible scandal, which taps into the worst in our imagination. In 2019, the French newspaper *L'Express* reported that 'thousands of people' who had donated their bodies to the prestigious Paris Descartes University body donation centre had been keep in shocking conditions. As they reported: 'Bodies were left to rot, eaten by mice, to the point where some had to be incinerated without being dissected. Bodies piled on top of each other, without any dignity and contrary to any ethical rule.' Families and many anatomists were left horrified, the centre was closed and the public's fears were confirmed.

The varied way people react to whole-body donation reminds me of 19th-century Irish surgeon and artist Joseph Maclise's drawing of the aortic arch.

His drawing of the arches may look like a page of half-cinnamon-donuts with little twigs coming out the side. But what I love is the different ways the arteries come off the arch. They split, curve and wander in an array of patterns. It says to me: aha—so we *are* all just a tiny bit different

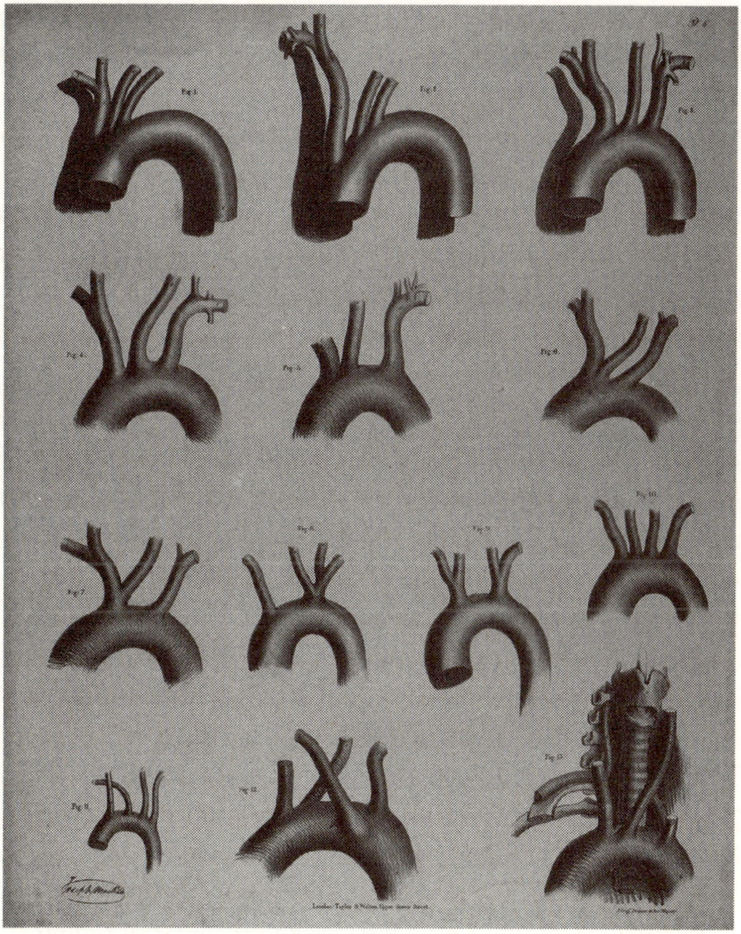

A lithograph by Joseph Maclise of circulatory system dissections of the aortic arch. Note the thirteen variations. The image is from Richard Quain's 1844 book *The Anatomy of the Arteries of the Human Body and Its Applications to Pathology and Operative Surgery. Wellcome Collection.*

on the inside. Humans are not all exactly like each other. These sorts of little variations occur absolutely everywhere in our bodies—just as we are distinct on the outside, we are unique on the inside too.

It's the same with the way we view the world—we all have our own take. I've had some people say to me *whatevs dissection, what's the big deal;*

you're dead while others have blanched, disgust in their eyes, and I feel embarrassed and wish I was writing a book about bees or something. Within the profession, responses are varied too—some anatomists are absolutely devoted to the body donor, some just go about their daily work. Some would donate, others wouldn't.

All I know is this: studying and cutting up the dead is intrinsic to contemporary medicine and surgery. It's why you can get a new implant in your knee or a cancer removed from your neck.

The ancient Greek philosopher Plato came up with the concept of the 'noble lie', in which elites tell stories to persuade the masses, like *we need to invade Iraq as Saddam Hussein has weapons of mass destruction*. A variation of this idea is applicable here. It's quite stark how as society trundles along, going about its business, it kids itself. There are things happening that we actively don't want to know about, like the assignations our governments get into, how we butcher animals so we can eat meat, or how we cut up dead bodies so we can treat the living.

Some may see all this dissection as ghoulish: a disturbing and unpleasant interest in death, but the problem is that as death is inherently unpleasant and messy, one is slapped with the ghoul label for taking even a normal, pragmatic interest in it. If we were to look more broadly at the notion of 'disturbing interest in a topic', I'd put Australian obsession with real estate on the list before death. To be able to not think about death in any way is perhaps a sign of just how affluent our society has become. You call me ghoul? I call you lucky, maybe even privileged.

But people *are* instinctively interested in bodies, particularly dead ones, and this might explain why millions and millions of people have seen Dr Gunther von Hagens' *Body Worlds* exhibition in some 150 cities across the world.

My 'normal interest' in my grandparents' decision to donate themselves to science shaped me in some way—this may sound dramatic but it's always been an unusual fact sitting on the sidelines of my life, and one that I've been reluctant to really explore, let alone write a book about. I tried ignoring dissection but it kept sidling up to me and stirring my imagination.

I've discovered that families of donors often react in a variety of ways too. Some want to donate. Some want to watch the dissection. Some are horrified. So for family members of the small cadre of donors who are upset, this book might not be for you. Or maybe it is?

Messy and dark dreams laced my sleep as I was writing it. In one dream, a beautiful friend who had died turned up to a class where surgeons were practising on dead bodies and we swapped clothes. My body and brain sank into sluggishness and anxiety as I read about Nazi dissection or 19th-century medical students mocking the dead. I had days where I hoped this book wouldn't upset Desmond Dent, my father, or my Uncle Maurie, or the families of body donors.

I winced at the technicalities of anatomical study—sawing, mould, smells and dismembering—and the confusing medical ethics I encountered. Medical ethics is about doing the right thing and oftentimes four sides of the debate can seem reasonable. I'm also squeamish and get quite sick at the sight of blood: in that way, this book has been both emotionally and physically quite hard to write. I've felt ill at times.

It makes sense. This chopping up, this dismemberment of human flesh seems so diabolical and destructive, why would we dare to even contemplate it? The historian Shane McCorristine has written about the history of dismemberment, and says it is only in the last 100 years that the practice has come to be associated with abnormal or criminal behaviour. He argues that in traditional stories and myths, 'from death and dismemberment come life and order'. I too once saw dissection as horrible. But I know now that something constructive certainly springs from the destruction that dissection entails.

Trawling through countless traditional dismemberment stories, one sees this generative quality. Take 'Mother Marge', a Papua New Guinean myth of a mother who wants her two beloved sons to live in a village with lots of people, so asks them to kill her. She tells them to put pieces of her body in the forest while her blood is thrown around a clearing. They put her head and stomach near their sleeping bags. When they rise the next morning, there is a village with men, women, children and animals. Her stomach and head have turned into two young women, who then marry the sons.

Further north, there's Sedna, the Sea Goddess for the Inuit people in the Arctic, whose story is all over gnostic corners of the internet. The gist is this: Chief Anguta, her father, kept trying to marry her off but she wasn't into any of the suitors so on a whim, she took off with a sea bird who turned out to be not particularly nice. Anguta rescued his daughter, and after killing the sea bird, their boat was surrounded by other birds seeking revenge.

The chief threw Sedna in the water to save her but she clutched on to the side of the boat. To stop her, he cut off her fingers. When she tried to grab the boat with her mutilated hand, he chopped that off too. Sedna and her dismembered parts sank in the ocean and grew into whales, seals, walruses and all sorts of sea mammals. She is now seen as the goddess of underwater life.

Anatomy's cutting casts new worlds, forces and sensations and it's quite startling to me what has been and is born from it. But it's also time to put the dissected as the leading actors in the history of medicine—whether they are body donors like my grandparents or those who didn't consent to it like Chinese rebel Wang Sun-Qing in 16 AD and Polly Chapman, a twenty-two-year-old sex worker who drowned herself in 1832. And even though her friends scraped together money for a funeral, she was still sent to the London hospital for dissection as 'an example to prevent suicide amongst unfortunate women'.

Thus, as I know parts of this may be confronting, I want to open the door as gently as possible, as if you are entering a fairytale with its dark and light moments. Here is a pot of tea. Here is a nice cup. Here are the body donors. This is what I found about cutting up the dead.

Chapter 1

We are in shorts. Little lizards squiggle and jerk along the hot footpaths and a currawong squawks. Flame trees bob gently in a breeze. It's a charming December afternoon in Sydney when my world explodes.

I'm at my parents' place and their neighbour has asked us over for a Christmas drink. The neighbour lives with her two daughters in a house built like my parents' between the wars. In a sea of renovations, neither has been touched. For three decades, they speak over the fence, collect each other's mail when on holidays, and have a drink together every now and then.

As we chat over sparkling wine, one of the daughters updates us on her new job. She's working at a university and hospital teaching facility and mentions that some of the medical students are no longer using full bodies for dissection. She also says that human arms and body parts are being shipped in from the US.

'What?' I'm stunned. 'Why aren't they dissecting full bodies? And why do they have to fly in arms?'

She isn't sure.

We finish our drinks, say 'Happy Christmas' and go home.

I turn to Mum as we walk the few steps to our place and say isn't it weird that the students aren't dissecting and they are importing body parts? Yes, it is weird, she says.

As we walk up the driveway, the mental jumble of death, medicine, gore and surgery that lives in my brain explodes.

You know:

- my grandparents donating their bodies to science and getting dissected

- effigies of saints in glass coffins on the streets of Manila that as a little girl I thought were corpses
- dead bodies on the Filipino nightly news
- Mum's nursing stories about the smell of burning body parts at the Sydney hospital she trained at
- Edgar Allan Poe's story about being buried alive
- Dr William Clowes, my great-grandfather ten times back and a barber-surgeon patching up a man with a spear through his body
- digging up my dead pet budgie Zazbut

But this dissection update is particularly rattling. *What on earth has happened to it? How could dissection be over?*

My mind buzzes, unable to recall a newspaper article or TV spot about its demise.

Over the years, I'd seen grainy sepia photos of cheerful medical students in bowler hats standing next to a tattered corpse with a cigarette in its mouth. Even though a photo like that would be absolutely forbidden today, I'd assumed that medical students still spent hours, weeks and months standing over one body and slowly cutting it up.

But now—just body parts from America? Some Australians still seem to be donating to the RSPCA and rising at dawn to watch ANZAC commemorations. But these flying limbs? Had Australians really stopped donating their whole bodies to science?

I start reasoning with myself. Perhaps anatomical software is really amazing these days and the kids can study the body online. But let's face it, we are also phasing out living bodies. We can order food, work from home, snuggle into a movie, talk to friends, get a university degree or go to a funeral online. Perhaps the transhumanists' dream that our brains can be converted into data which we will then upload to a computer is the unavoidable path we are on. We increasingly can do without other people's bodies too. The checkout operators have turned into scanners. Fighter pilots replaced by drones. As living bodies fade, perhaps dead ones have too.

But seriously? The end of dissection?

It's always been a lurking fact that Ruby and Julie donated their bodies to the university. I've long seen it as a slightly intriguing *thing*, quietly spectacular and a radical but slightly weird postscript to their lives. I mean, why would anyone do that?

When it comes to body disposal you've got limited options in Australia: burial, cremation or dissection. They chose option three for some reason. Over the years, it's been very vaguely discussed in the family but not over-analysed. Or analysed at all really.

I had never met one other person who knows someone who donated their whole body, so I'd never really had the opportunity to workshop the idea. Thus, a mysterious, figment-of-my-imagination dissection hall hovered in the distance. I saw students and teachers talking but couldn't hear them. I walked closer, tried to lean over behind them to see what's on the table but couldn't. A wall of shoulders in white coats blocked me.

Something about the conversation at Christmas got to me—perhaps there were some psychopomps resting in the jasmine bush that day watching? Traditionally, psychopomps are creatures that lead the dead to the afterlife but in this instance, the psychopomps captured me alive.

They came to me in a daydream, a group of tough young girls, hair in black bobs and dressed in elaborately carved medieval armour. They stood next to an enormous tree, which throbbed over a pool of hot vibrant red lava. They spent their time training with heavy swords, and then they would dive into the lava. I suspected they were heading to another universe and that I should follow. They would soon come to me a lot.

Relaxed by a glass of bubbles, I lay on the carpet thinking about dissection, looking at the ceiling, my toddler son watching the Wiggles. Like a match pegged at petrol, my death jumble exploded. But instead of letting the fragments burn out, my little team of psychopomps began to bang a drum. I could tell something was afoot but I absolutely did not want to go there.

***

Weeks drifted by.

No. Yes. No. No. Yes. No. The psychopomps were calling. They wanted me to dive into the inferno too. I resisted. Steer clear of dissection. Go to the beach mate. Mum told me she'd mentioned my newfound curiosity about Ruby and Julie's dissection to someone and they'd remarked: 'Why does she go on about death?' I bowed my head in shame.

But the psychopomps kept calling. They had been for years really.

I vaguely recalled that Dad hadn't been happy about his parents' bodies going to the university. He'd attended the University of Queensland in the 1950s, and as an engineering student had heard stories about what some medical students got up to.

I recalled maybe asking Dad if he'd been unhappy about his parents going to the uni and he said no, that wasn't the case. But I'm not sure. I thought he was. Did he go into the dissection hall at the University Of Queensland too? Stories fall into gullies.

Even if I were wanting to find out what happened to Ruby and Julie, I saw myself draped in a hefty metal suit of armour, and holding an enormous heavy sword, fighting the whole way, particularly against myself. Dissection is basically the mutilation of the dead. Did I really want to get into it? As a Harvard professor told the 1896 meeting of the Association of American Anatomists: 'We know only too well that dissection is an abomination to the popular mind.'

Their bodies went to the university so, so long ago, fifty years. How do I find the people who were there way back then? It also involved my dad, who didn't talk about the past much. He seemed content to be retired, watching TV, reading history books, listening to the Bee Gees, cementing pathways around the family home and having dim sum in Chatswood. Did I really want to bother him? Did I want to bother his brother Maurie too? He was relaxing on Bribie Island.

It seemed too impenetrable, too gross, too hard and I'd heard absolutely nothing about it in recent years. While stories about new gene breakthroughs or cancer treatments pop up daily, the screen is blank on a new discovery from dissecting dead bodies or innovations in embalming techniques. Even though anatomy is the basis of medical science, it seemed like one that was trundling along in the background.

I also felt worried that I wasn't scientific enough. Maybe I just wouldn't 'get it'? How to read quantitative data?

And yes, dissection was intrinsically about death. Death did not exist in Australia. I was only reminded of it when I saw a skeleton or mutilated body on the band t-shirts my partner George wore. Go to the beach. Go jogging. This was the time of our lives. There was no death.

***

So I start.

I start on a long dirt driveway, draped with trees and surrounded by bush. It's a place where we used to kill cane toads with a golf club. It is also only one of three places where I can find Julie.

His pale blue Holden with its white roof is parked and I'm in the back, playing with his electric windows, up and down, up and down. Churr. Zhurr. Stop that. You'll break the windows. Come on. Enough. Stop. Someone is saying 'stop' but I can't see if it's him. We were only allowed a certain amount of time to play with these windows. Fair enough. But there he is, on the periphery of my memories.

He is tall, slightly stooped, in a hat. His image won't hold. It's akin to the shadows I sometimes catch glimpses of out of the corner of my eye, the ones that zap in and out, the ones that some call shadow people. They are meant to be menacing but I never find them that way.

The other snippet is in the kitchen of a small Brisbane home. I'm looking at him across the table; the light is coming through a window. Stop. Hold on. Was he even there? Or did we go to the house after he died? Right. Perhaps that's what happened. We went to the house after Julie died and I stood on the kitchen linoleum, marvelling that he'd died there and I was now in the spot where he had his heart attack. Maybe? I should check that with Mum and Dad.

The third memory is the haziest. We might have been eating mud crab around a large dining table. He sits at the end of the table. Had I just played with the electric windows? The memories haul themselves to their hands and knees but can't go further. Mum says Julie was friendly but a bit quirky and something of an enigma. Lindy says she thinks he had some sort of brain injury.

I can't find Ruby anywhere. It's impossible as she died in 1969, three years before I was born. The imaginary thus kicks in, coaxed along by objects of hers that I own: an art deco clock, a bowls badge with her name, an old dining table I still eat from, now smeared with my son's Weetbix. There are of course photos of her and she is always smiling as if partly amused by something. She also always seems to be in a floral print frock. Mum says she had a great circle of friends. My Aunt Lindy recalls her as a gentle sort of person.

I study their life stories looking for clues as to why they would donate their bodies to science.

Ruby was born in Boulder in Western Australia during a gold rush. She became a pupil teacher when she was just fourteen. Next, she is twenty-three, teaching in Charleville, another town in the middle of the desert but in Queensland, surrounded by towns with names perfect for showcasing the strange way we Australians say our vowels. CoolAAAAAddi. Wyaaandra. Did you go there to die mate? Nah, I went there today mate. She was a primary school teacher all her life, cracking the world open for little kindy and Grade One kids, teaching them reading, writing, numbers. She liked the name Jacqueline, which graces my birth certificate. In my mind I'm somehow cuddling her, a loved granddaughter.

Julie's family tree—and thus mine—is littered with convicts transported from Ireland and England. He grew up in a large family without a father. As an adult, he became a clerk. He had a 'job for life' in the public service but chucked it in at some point to be a wool classer. He and Ruby met somewhere in outback Queensland. But it was soon to be the start of the 1930s Depression, a time which changed good people forever. They absolutely could not be fickle.

The Depression over, he was back at his favourite hobby, dancing, often appearing in Brisbane's *Telegraph* 'Dance news and gossip' section, and later running ping-pong tournaments for US soldiers in his backyard. Always well-dressed. Obsessed with sport. He won the lottery and the money went towards his beloved Holden. When my dad lived in London in the 1960s, Ruby and Julie used to put Chinny the dog on the phone to talk to him.

Small details, squiggles of colour here and there. Watercolours lightly wash the canvas when I need an intricate Hieronymus Bosch. They lived but I know so little about their lives, particularly what drew them to be dissected.

I soon find myself searching out dissection more broadly on the internet, drinking a cup of tea and frowning. '*You know what? What did happen?*'

Chapter 2

The young clerk Samuel Edgerly wrote in his diary on 27 January 1860 that 'after wishing for a long time', he finally managed to visit a dissection room at the College of Physicians and Surgeons in New York City. He wasn't a doctor. It was just a thing to do, like going to the art gallery or heading out for lunch with friends. Edgerly's visit was during a period in the US before the Civil War when anatomy for the middle classes was a popular pastime. Punters went to museums and lectures, bought anatomical books and even occasionally visited dissection halls like young Sam did.

It wasn't just an American pastime—the comparative anatomist Carl Bernhard Brühl held anatomy lectures for the general public every Sunday from the early 1860s to 1890 at the Institute of Zootomy in Vienna, Austria where 'the most delicate ladies held the human brain parts in their hands as courageously as any medical student'. In 1880s Paris, the police laid out unidentified bodies behind a glass case in La Morgue—they were hoping someone in the public would give names to the dead faces. Soon, Parisians were flocking to have a look. In 1899 Melbourne, young working-class kids would visit the morgue to look at people killed by fatal accidents and by their own hand. The Melbourne University magazine *Alma Mater* reported at the time that 'streams' went through the morgue to look at the head of a 'poor young girl'.

Over the next hundred years, anatomy slowly waned as a public outing, until in the 1980s, Gunther von Hagens launched the sensational *Body Worlds*, a travelling show of dissected humans and animals which turns up in major cities every year. But in the main, a lived experience of anatomy now largely lives behind a secure door, accessed only by swipe card.

Thus the closest public anatomical experience I could get in Sydney is ordering a small plastic anatomy doll from Officeworks—the Fandex Human Anatomy Model, 27 cm, 8 pieces. He's a cream-coloured man that you can basically unpack—take out his heart and lungs, and there is more anatomy inside. I study the brochure that comes with him. 'Nature is peculiar,' it says. 'The more you try to learn about nature, the more you will be excited by its unexpected surprises. Start learning about nature by looking at yourself today!' There's the *inferior vena cava*. There's the ureter. It also carries a warning that the small parts may pose a hazard to children under the age of three. I haven't properly packed the organs away and they now lie scattered across my desk; the little plastic liver is lost somewhere. The other anatomical experience option is to look at one of George's band t-shirts, like the one for Raygun Mortlock, which features an image of Tony Abbott as a reclining pig, his intestines spilling out with 'Abbottoir' written underneath. I just don't know if it is anatomically correct.

Getting a sense of where Ruby and Julie went—the colour of the anatomy lab, the daily office culture, the Christmas parties, even *the science*—felt absolutely remote. Most Australian medical schools had FAQs about body donation on their websites but there was little detail on 'what happens' except benign statements about *studying the body for anatomical purposes*. What does that even mean? Taking a tour of the dissection hall like Samuel Edgerly was likely impossible.

So I started trawling real and virtual bookstores looking for memoirs by the people in the room—the anatomists, the technicians, the administrators, the body donors before they died—but it was not a flourishing genre. The only people to pick up the pen were medical students, who tended to have backgrounds in literature and poetry, their descriptions and observations elevating the dissecting hall to a place of beauty, fable and wisdom-getting.

I became particularly drawn to Albert Howard Carter III, a comparative literature professor, who wrote *First Cut: A season in the human anatomy lab*, which was about his sixteen weeks in an anatomy lab with first-year students. His inspiration? His father, also a literature professor, who had donated his body to science. Whenever I felt ashamed or weird about my interest, I turned to Albert. We shared a curiosity.

As he wrote:

> My father willed his body for medical research. Upon his death the funeral home sent his body to a medical school some 150 miles away—and that was all we knew. What happened to his body? Whom did it serve? We assumed it was used for the education of future physicians, but never had any definite notion. I wondered for many years what had happened to his body. I'm not a strong believer in the comfort of grave sites or gravestones, but I felt a yearning to know something of 'where he ended up'. Watching these young students begin their journey into the human body, I was searching for my lost father.

Doctors were telling their stories—life in war zones, dying from brain cancer and facing mortality, or how to fast. But where were the anatomists? How did they feel about it all? What were their afternoons like? Why did people spend their lives so intimately studying the dead? Equally, on the other side, while the Dalai Lama wrote of good deeds, and every year Australians were given awards for serving the people, the body donors were silent. Perhaps there were no poets amongst them.

It was a glacial start and the image of myself curled on the couch with a nice pot of Wagh Bakri tea reading *My Life in Anatomy at the University of Queensland from 1969 to 1981* or listening to a 1970s radio interview with body donors has been parked in the pure fantasy lot. The anatomists and body donors were mute.

***

I struggled reading papers with titles likes 'Anatomy of the Anterolateral Ligament of the Knee' or 'Astrocyte–endothelial Interactions and Blood–Brain Barrier Permeability'. But then I finally stumbled across a paper written in 2014 by an anatomist named Goran Štrkalj, which at last felt like a peep into the lab window. Entitled 'Attitudes of Australian Chiropractic Students Toward Whole Body Donation: A cross-sectional study', it was a study into first-, second-, and fifth-year chiropractic students about their attitudes towards body donation.

It said that the students began anatomy classes on plastic models and later moved to 'cadaveric prosections', which is the technical term for bodies that have been cut into different parts by a professional, either an anatomy teacher or technician. At the time, the paper said they weren't dissecting as they did not have enough bodies. When I first read this, I thought *voila*! What the neighbour said was true! But one finding really stood out to me: a student's willingness to donate their own body or a family member's decreased as their years of study went by.

What was happening in the anatomy lab?

I emailed Goran, writing that I'd heard anecdotally that there was a big drop in body donation and that medical students at different universities often used body parts only for anatomy. He wrote back, using exclamation marks like I do!

He also sent me another one of his papers: 'A Global Geography of Body Acquisition for Anatomy Education: Issues, challenges and prospects', which examined the world's first global 'body donor map'. Produced by Dr Andreas Winkelmann and a team of German anatomists, it showed that out of sixty-eight countries that use cadavers for anatomy teaching, only 32 per cent got their bodies exclusively through body donation and the rest were using unclaimed bodies, particularly in the Middle East, Africa and parts of China. Even some medical schools in the US were still using the unclaimed.

I'd often associated 'unclaimed' with lost property but in this instance, it referred to people who had no friends or family to collect their bodies and give them a proper burial. I'd never heard that if you were left in a hospital morgue in some parts of the world it meant that you were fated for dissection without your consent. I found it such an awful idea, particularly as I wasn't into the idea of getting dissected, largely because

I imagined myself being cold. Yes, it's a silly line of thinking as being dead, I wouldn't feel the cold.

***

In 2011 Goran was an anatomist and biological anthropologist at Macquarie University on Sydney's leafy north shore. Like many academics, he had had a winding career path—originally from Belgrade in the former Yugoslavia, he'd come to Sydney via Johannesburg.

As Goran lectured, he wondered if the students themselves would donate their bodies or if they would support a family member who signed up for it. Some students identified as Christians. Others were Muslim. Others weren't at all interested in religion. Did faith have a role in donation? How did their ethnic backgrounds play into it? So he and his colleagues set about finding out how the students felt, sending out a questionnaire to which 223 students answered.

When the results came in, they looked reasonable and made sense—the atheists and agnostics were more willing and open to the idea of donation. But they also found that as a student progressed through their degree, the less willing they were to donate their own body or support a family member to do it. While support for a stranger donating their body to science was generally high, people from an Asian background weren't into it at all. Basically, the survey also found being exposed to a donor had some sort of emotionally negative impact.

I'd never heard that dissection, this blooding into medicine, had an impact on medical students in any way. I'd never thought that of the chiropractors, doctors, dentists and physiotherapists I'd seen over the years, some slept soundly while others woke at 3 am mulling over the day or dreading the anatomy lab. I looked at medicine—and science in general—as a place where its practitioners find systemic truths with no value judgements, and little emotion.

I originally fell into this caper because of the shock of learning that after thousands of years, human dissection is out because the kitty is empty of Australian body donors and administrators have resorted to bringing body parts from America. But when I called Goran, he quickly pricked this thought bubble I'd been carrying around for a few weeks. At the time of his study, it was true that there was a shortage as Macquarie University was in the early days of establishing its medical school and body donor program, but this was no longer the case.

'There are enough bodies for anatomical study, both undergraduate and postgraduate level,' he said. In fact, you could drape a 'gold standard' sash across Australia as our medical schools only use donated bodies, whereas in many parts of the world you have this miserable issue of the unclaimed dead being dissected.

Goran also answered my question about students studying bodies in parts. 'They do,' he said, 'but they do that not because they don't have enough bodies—it's because of the educational requirements.'

Limbs were cut off so that students could look inside the joints or manipulate them individually. Bodies were also sectioned for practical reasons, as they could be used more efficiently: a group of physiotherapy students could learn from a limb while at the same time medical students could study the visceral organs or the trunk. This was also considered more ethical as the body was *really* used. Prosection was also less costly—the parts were easier to maintain and store.

I asked: 'Is that a shift now? Like this old idea that we had of the body lying on the table and the students standing around, that doesn't happen any more?'

'It does and it doesn't,' he said. 'A large majority of medical educators and all anatomists think that the best practice in teaching anatomy is to teach it from a cadaver, from a donated body. Although there are places in the world where they don't use bodies at all, they rely on models, images and so on. But the best practice is to use the body and for obvious reasons.'

He said there was some disagreement on the best way to do it—whether through dissection or prosection.

'There are cons and pros for both approaches. Dissection is good but it's really time consuming,' he said. 'Half of your time you basically try to clean the body, take the skin off, connective tissue, fatty tissue and then get to the structure that you want to analyse. So many people think that nowadays in the crowded medical curriculum, you lose too much time doing that. It's much better to have all this already dissected, and examine them and analyse them.' He said as far as he knew, anatomy in Australia was now largely learned with prosections and only a few universities dissected, and often only at a postgraduate level.

I was still confused as to why body parts were being shipped in from the US if there were enough donated bodies in Australia. He said if a university was running a workshop for surgeons, for example, they might need specific body parts of a particular age and gender. 'These body parts might not be available,' he said. 'You have to rely on other people to get them for workshops—you need fifteen knees to try a new knee implant or something like that. Bear in mind, body parts are not commodities; you cannot buy them. So they're not buying them, you are paying for transport fees, and then they're imported to Australia.'

University of Queensland medical students in the 1930s used to pen witty ditties about dissection, like this one from their days when they were based at the Masonic Hall in Alice Street, sung to the tune of 'Clementine':

In the back street, you can see feet,
Skin and bones and intestine,
Being tangled, cut and mangled,
By the blokes in Medicine.

I later composed a more fitting contemporary ditty to the same tune:

In the air plane, are fifteen knees,
There's no need for a whole body,
With knives and scissors, they'll be cut up,
For the good of surgery.

But I soon learned there was so much more going on than just chopped-up bodies and knees in the air. Goran said there has been a 'palpable shift' in many aspects of anatomy. Part of the shift had been a practical one, encapsulated in an unusually passionate, lay-down-the-gauntlet paper written in 2002 by the American anatomists Joy S. Reidenberg and Jeffrey Laitman at the Mount Sinai School of Medicine in New York, in which they hoisted a banner emblazoned with the catchy, 'The old anatomy is dead. Long live the new anatomy.'

The pair critiqued the centuries-long tradition of teaching anatomy through hours upon hours of cadaveric dissection with factual lectures. They pointed out that 'the greater majority of average students can no longer solely respond to "cut", "read", and "listen"', and having been reared on the internet and laptops, students needed a different type of education. So not only were kids now getting a 'robust dissection experience' but they were also using the latest tech to view the bodies, such as 'minimally invasive approaches, ultrasonography, three-dimensional visualizations, multiaxial computerized image reconstructions, multiplanar magnetic resonance imaging, and plastinated prosections'.

But alongside the rise of high-tech anatomy and a cutting back on dissecting time, Goran launched into another more radical life for the dead: humane anatomy.

'Way back in the past there was a detached relationship to the cadaver, the body was seen as a specimen—nowadays, the approach to anatomy, to medicine, to dissection is much more humane if you like. So in many universities, you don't relate to bodies as cadavers or as biological specimens; we look at them as our first patient,' he said.

Goran, speaking in a strong Belgrade accent, explained that this 'first patient' ethos meant they treated the donor with respect, and it formed part of their medical education, where their relationship with the cadaver was used as a way to teach medical ethics and professionalism. It also helped temper some of the anxiety that went with dissection.

In some medical schools, students were even meeting the family of their donor. Goran said in parts of East Asia—in Thailand and Taiwan—

donating the body was seen as a good thing to do because you were useful after death and becoming a teacher. 'It's one of the biggest honours in the culture,' he said.

Universities were now also holding commemorative services for body donors, and their families were invited. 'They [the families] have a chance to talk to academic staff and students, and the students and academics can express their gratitude and tell them how important the donation is, and how valuable that is. And also to reassure them that bodies are treated with utmost respect while they are in the dissection room.'

Incredibly, sculptures and memorials to donors were now found on university campuses and in graveyards around the world. From what Goran was saying, it was a change that had to happen. 'One of the problems is our history—the history of anatomy is really dark. The way anatomists and medical men in the past obtained bodies is really ethically dubious, and at times, it was illegal,' he said, adding that the issue of using unclaimed bodies still persisted throughout the world.

'There's this ethical cloud on top of anatomy; it's still shadowing anatomy and current anatomical practices.'

I asked him if he was something of an ethical anatomy activist.

'I'm engaged,' he said. 'Reflection I think is really important and history teaches us that.' He mentioned that while there has obviously been awareness of the crimes committed by Nazi doctors, in recent years German anatomists had started investigating what their predecessors had done under the Third Reich.

'The stories are horrifying. They would receive bodies for dissection from prisons, from concentration camps,' he says. What the anatomists did under the Nazis was legal at the time and Goran said he wanted to make the point that it is important for anatomists to constantly reflect on what they are doing. 'How are we doing it? How do we get our bodies? How do we keep them?'

He described the contemporary anatomy lab as the perfect place to reflect. 'Here you have life and death. You have living people and dead people. You have ethical issues. It's an excellent starting point to reflect about your profession, the meaning of what you're doing, the meaning of life,' he declared.

I hung up, my hand sore from clutching the phone so tightly, a little startled at Goran's revelations and profound meditations on the anatomy lab. I wasn't expecting anatomy to be in the middle of a revolution, where donors were revered and memorialised. My parents had never mentioned going to a memorial for Ruby or Julie. I also wasn't expecting to hear that paupers and criminals were on the dissecting table in other parts of the world. And what was so bad about anatomy's past anyway? I knew a little about body snatching but Nazi dissection? Did I want to engage with that?

If humane anatomy was only now starting to blossom in parts of the world, it naturally got me thinking: how were the students with Ruby and Julie all those years ago? And then an unexpected sense of disappointment swept through me. If dissection was waning, was it pointless that they went there in the first place? What was it all for?

Towards the end of the conversation, Goran mentioned there was a big anatomy conference coming up in London and it would be worth me going. The conference only happened once every five years and bizarrely, I would be in London at the same time.

Chapter 3

I was at my parents' place fossicking in the food cupboard. It had always been a reliable place for finding salty chips, red jelly snakes, and an interesting range of sweet and savoury biscuits. While I had been trying to get a preliminary handle on anatomy, I still wasn't exactly clear what prompted Ruby and Julie to donate in the first place.

Dad was lying on the couch engrossed in watching Question Time in the Australian parliament so I went to speak to my mother Elizabeth, aka Mum, who was in her all-purpose room—computer, sewing machine, family history charts, spare bed. I asked her why she thought Ruby donated her body. I don't know why but I sensed it was all Ruby's idea for some reason.

'It was never a big deal really. She told us one day that she was going to donate her body to the university and that was it,' said Mum, a pragmatic and fun matriarch, looking up from her sewing machine as she pieced together a magnificent quilt.

'But do you know why?' I asked.

'To help science, probably,' she said.

'And?'

'She wanted to help people. I think she was interested in disease.' Mum sounded unfazed.

Ruby obviously felt a sense of public service, as she spent most of her life as a public primary school teacher but *dissection*?

As I was beginning my tentative steps into the darkened chambers of the past dressed in a flowing white nightie, candle in hand, I had no sense in the long history of anatomy how strange it had been for her and Julie to have donated their bodies, and how utterly naive I had been about it all these years.

I would soon learn that she and Julie stood at the beginning of a shift in Western medicine, some two thousand years in the making.

In the little I knew about my grandparents' motivations, I assumed they had done it for altruism and science—why else would you?—and that they were sort of neo-Benthamites, part of a tradition inspired by British philosopher Jeremy Bentham, the father of utilitarianism—the idea of the 'the greatest happiness of the greatest number'—and the inventor of words such as 'international', 'maximise' and 'antagonising', who very publicly willed his body in London in 1832.

At the time, Bentham saw his dissection as having a two-fold purpose:

> first to communicate curious interesting & highly important knowledge & secondly to show that the primitive horror at dissection originates in ignorance & is kept up by misconception and that the human body when dissected instead of being an object of disgust is as much more beautiful than any other piece of mechanism as it is more curious and wonderful.

So when Mum said it was 'for the science' I thought, yes, okay, that's reasonable. But if it was for 'the science', what was *the science* actually about?

***

A few weeks earlier, I'd randomly found a 1977 print of a 1901 edition of *Gray's Anatomy*, 'the doctor's bible', in a pile of books in the Ku-ring-gai Council chuck-out. (It's quite scandalous what people throw out on the North Shore. Over the few years I'd lived here, I'd found a perfectly lovely old dining room table, Le Creuset pots, boogie boards etc. It's also odd how a strange new portal opened where dissection-related topics, people and items kept popping up in my life.) The cover of the *Gray's* was slightly torn but it was otherwise perfect—I looked up the edition online and it was selling for $50 on eBay.

The classic medical text came out in 1858 and remains in print today after multiple revisions. In my edition, all the credit went to the anatomist, pathologist and surgeon Henry Gray but many of the original 1858 illustrations were done by the apothecary-surgeon, microscopist and gifted artist Henry Vandyke Carter. Professor Susan Standring, the current editor-in-chief of *Gray's Anatomy* said in a 2021 talk that in her opinion, 'Carter's name should have been as big as Gray's'.

'Anatomy is the gateway to medicine. It is the queen of the basic sciences and is the *sine qua non* into the field of human biology,' declared Dr John A. Crocco in the introduction, adding that to 'study medicine without anatomy was folly'.

Excited, I began turning the pages but was quickly left stumped. Like after about two pages. The anatomical language was absolutely impenetrable.

There were flashes of layperson drama, like how to treat an internal carotid artery if one got shot or stabbed or 'a stab from within the mouth, as when a person receives a thrust from the end of a parasol or falls down with a tobacco-pipe in his mouth'. There were also quite a few visceral moments too, like tips on how to dissect the foot:

> The foot should be placed on a high block with the sole uppermost, and firmly secured in that position. Carry an incision round the heel and along the inner and outer borders of the foot to the great and little toes.

But the text felt impossible to pass through or enter. Take the tongue:

> The tongue is the organ of the special sense of taste. It is situated in the floor of the mouth, in the interval between the two lateral portions of the body of the lower jaw. [So far so good!] Its base or root is directed backward, and connected with the os hyoides by the Hyo-glossi and Genio-hyo-glossi muscles and the hyo-glossal membrane; with the epiglottis by three folds (*glosso-epiglottic*) of mucous membranes ...

I flicked the page. Aha! Here was a drawing of a tongue and its little lumps—the dainty-sounding *papillae.* I poked my tongue out and began examining them in the mirror. But underneath, according to Vandyke Carter's drawings, was another world. There were different types of lumps, which can only be seen under a microscope. The *fungiform* had tiny arteries and veins which entwined and formed a little tree, while the *filiform* looked part-jellyfish with tentacle-like legs.

I took Vandyke Carter's work into the garden and began looking at the leaves, plants, trees, bark, dirt, spiderwebs, and branches of the jacaranda tree, and could see that their shapes and curves were exactly the same as the underworld of my tongue. Or my tongue was the garden.

It was the same for the rest of my body. My bladder was a silkworm cocoon. The curves and folds of the upper surface of the brain looked like the seemingly erratic lines left behind by snails. The French anatomist Jean Cruveilhier saw anatomy as 'the most beautiful hymn which man can chant in honour of his Creator'. As an atheist, I agreed with the sentiment and raised my cup of tea to him.

But I wasn't sure how to proceed if only the pictures made sense. I wasn't sure I had the patience to learn the language of Anatomy and Surgery laced through the pages of *Gray's.* Also, who were the drawings based on? In some instances, like in the sketch of surgical anatomy of the arteries of the neck, the handsome man on the page had an almost patrician quality to him. He looked like someone who could be lounging on a couch with a glass of sherry. Neither the introduction nor the rest of the book mentioned anything about him or the dead people behind all the lovely bones, organs, skulls, eye parts and papillae. How weird. How could they be left out? It was like they weren't even there. But they were.

Chapter 4

I was standing at the Dangar Island wharf with my son, waiting to catch the ferry to Brooklyn, and then the train back to Sydney. Dangar is a smudge of an island on the Hawkesbury River in Sydney, a lovely nook where I've hung out over the years as my best friend Jodi lives there. The ferry curved in to the wharf and I turned impatiently to see where George was. I was relieved to see him walking towards me—of course with new book in his hand, which he'd found at a chuck-out on the wharf.

(He is always carrying, reading, ordering or finding books.)

'Here you go,' he said. *Notes of an Anatomist* by F. González-Crussi. I began flicking through the book and suddenly the psychopomps were back.

To be honest, I'd pressed pause on anatomy and dissection. After the excitement of speaking to Goran, it all felt a bit too hard, and impenetrable to me in too many ways. Even though Goran had been championing humanity in anatomy, I suspected he was perhaps an anomaly, and the overall cold objectivity and technicalities of the science were making me unsure about sitting or standing, or where to go, what to hold on to. *Gray's Anatomy* sat on my desk and stood like a guard at the gate.

But here was González-Crussi. Here was a small crack I could wedge my hand into. At last, here was a scientist tearing open his heart about his work. While more pathologist than pure anatomist, he was revelatory. I couldn't believe the way he discussed what it was like to look back at human remains that he had inspected. He called it a 'defilement':

> The dead possess an identity, granted by the living through the agency of intact form; so long as form remains, a cadaver remains

> 'the same one' for associates and relatives, for friend and foe. But without spine or limbs or eyes (which virtually are never removed during an autopsy study), the form is altered and diminished; without ribs, the dead person is a frail mannikin; without jaw, the human face is a grotesque mask.

This was so jarring and gorily exciting. I momentarily flinched, thinking about my grandparents. I'd had a sense of this grotesqueness looking at the old group photographs medical students used to take with the person they had dissected. But what was probably more astounding was his writings about the soul. As he put it:

> The ancients fancied that the soul did not abandon the body on a sudden but even after death it lingered on for forty-two days, departing gradually and as if by stages. Da Vinci reflected on this theme and thought that it was quite fitting that the soul should dally, for the body is so wondrous a habitation that the soul could not find it easy to part with it, and finding it so painful to quit its mortal domicile, it hesitates.

With these words, I saw the hard line of 'science' briefly disintegrate. Yes, it was superstitious and ghosty of me but this idea of the soul hanging around the dead body pulsed with vim.

Not only did Leonardo da Vinci ponder the *senso commune*, aka the soul dallying, but he spent *thirty years* trying to find it inside the body. In his notebooks from 1485 to 1487, he documents vivisecting a frog near its upper spinal cord. 'Frog instantly dies when its spinal medulla is perforated . . . Here therefore, it appears, lies the foundation of movement and life.' Why did Da Vinci dissect there? He had been inspired by the ancient historian Livy who remarked that when elephants became enraged, they would be killed by sticking a spike where the neck joins the spine.

He later mapped the location of the soul in exquisite sketches he did of skulls and an ox brain. You can see where he thinks the *senso commune* is in a sketch known as K/P 42r, which dates from 1489. Using black chalk, pen and ink, he draws a skull and marks two lines—where they meet is X marks the soul. I love how da Vinci was hunting and pinpointing life in death.

Over 500 years later, I spent the next few weeks asking friends if they thought they had a soul. Most said they did, which I wasn't expecting. And where was it? In the spirit of Leonardo, I asked my friend Brigid to draw where her soul was, and she sketched a stick figure with an arrow pointing at the middle, sort of where her heart was. I looked at the picture but felt like mine was in my head.

I'm an atheist but I still had this weird feeling about dissection. I'm dead in the room. For some reason, my soul, lingering after death, is mute and unable to stop me being cut up. I am so vulnerable in this state, my secret, interior world laid bare. But my biggest worry? That I'll need a jumper.

My grandparents were not religious. They signed the paperwork, not worrying that their souls would be lurking around, or that they might be cold. Theologically, they were also clearly not grappling with all the slightly contradictory different ideas about the afterlife:

- That by being cut up, they might not be able to rise body and soul from the tomb on Judgement Day.
- That at the moment of their death, the soul would take flight, and the body was just a shell so cut away.

So with no faith or fear holding them back, something pushed them to take the next step. Perhaps there was more to anatomy than impossible language about the body? Perhaps there was more to what happened to them.

***

A few weeks later, I was back at HQ. Dad was watching a TV show about air crash investigations and I was in Mum's all-purpose room, asking her about my grandparents again, looking at photos, pondering why they donated their bodies, when she casually mentioned Ruby's journal.

'What journal?'

I was nearly fifty and had never heard that Ruby had a diary. Or had I? Facts fall into holes.

Mum went to her astoundingly tidy all-purpose cupboard, Kondo'ed since the 1970s, well before Marie Kondo became a verb. She pulled out a red notebook, and the journal became the beginning of Mum and Dad sporadically and casually mentioning what I felt were massive chunks of information. It seemed like a drip feed but it wasn't intentional—just things would come to mind. *Oh Ruby was quite a good painter. Here are some pictures of her paintings. Oh my bridesmaid worked in an anatomy school.*

I lay the notebook on the spare bed, expecting it would be a normal diary—a ledger of days, feelings, encounters, yearnings, usually chronological. This happened in March. This happened in May. Instead, Ruby's notebook unfolded as one long story, written in what looked like one intense sitting.

Her elegant cursive slanted right on the faintly lined paper for seventeen pages. Some letters—n, s, h, e, i, b—stretched down to the next line with a flourish, and the words were pressed deeply on to the pages. It felt like she wanted the world to know what happened to her. Or perhaps she wanted to just get it down?

Ruby started her red book like this:

This story began a long time ago.

Chapter 5

It began in the deserts of Western Australia in a town called Boulder. Once a howling wilderness, a place where men camped out in hessian tenements and humpies as they looked for gold, by the time Ruby's father Maurice Twomey arrived in 1900, it was blossoming. There were brick houses, well-lit streets, a bookstore and lively music evenings, and weekends were spent swimming at the local pool and punting at the popular horse races. The town toiled along 'the Golden Mile', one of the richest bodies of gold in the world.

Maurice, his mother Sarah and brothers Edward, John and Thomas were starting the new century in a new town. Tumult had defined the past few years. Their expansive dairy farm carpeted with rye grass and overlooking the river in Maffra, Victoria was finally off their hands. Their boarding house went to auction too. Two sisters were dead—little Betsy years ago in a harrowing accident when her clothes caught fire when she was only six; Sarah Jane, a dressmaker, taken by typhoid at twenty-three. Elizabeth and Katie had become nuns and were living in a convent in Abbotsford, Melbourne.

A depression in Victoria meant it was time to leave the east to find work in the west. But it was also time to escape the spectre of Maurice Snr, a violent, mentally ill man, whose addiction to alcohol was slowly rotting his life. His true fate rested inside the bosom of the immediate family, and he became a ghost.

So the family replaced milk with gold, and a twisted father with red dust.

Maurice meet Eleanor.

Eleanor meet Maurice.

At twenty-five, Eleanor carried her own angst. The death of her mother in childbirth snatched her youth as she spent the next decade bringing up her five younger siblings until her father remarried: a blueprint life in the late 1800s.

Eleanor kept house for her brothers in Boulder. She cleaned. She flicked through the paper, the 'Women's World' column outlining how to cook white haricot bean soup and brain cakes. When she met Maurice—tall, good-looking, massive shoulders, a clarity to his eyes—she studied the ring the bank manager in town had given her and soon broke off the engagement. Maurice and Eleanor left town, and their marriage was solemnised in the district of Melbourne in Rev W.J. Palamountain's copperplate handwriting.

It was the 104th marriage in the book. I zoomed in on the photo of their wedding day. Maurice's thick, bristly moustache covered his face and one of his enormous hands clutched at something—perhaps gloves? Eleanor stood in her white, high-collared Edwardian wedding gown, clutching white flowers. They held the moment, although Mum and I can't work out why they went as far as Melbourne to get married.

Back in Boulder, they lived at 17 Hopkins Street, surrounded by Maurice's family—Uncle Edward was at number 19, and Granny Sarah and Uncle John were at number 21. Sometimes Aboriginal people came into town, and Eleanor, fearful, used to sit by the window with a gun. But soon, the world changed in other ways. Ruby writes:

> In the light of what has happened over the years, it must have began before I was born. Because immediately prior to my being conceived, my mother had brain fever as a result of her home being burnt to the ground, and both she and my father, and elder sister escaping in their night clothes. I arrived in due course, and all my life, I had been obsessed with a great love for my mother, putting her before everything, to the extent of altering the whole course of my life.

***

All these years, when I thought about Ruby and Julie donating their bodies, the steps went like this:

A. They donated their bodies.
B. The dissection was part of a medical student's degree.
C. There were some stories about students being disrespectful in the anatomy lab.
D. End of story.

I had not known that body donation was actually a very recent and unusual development in anatomy's long, tortured, dramatic and gory history.

The science—and the darkness—was apparently there from the start when Herophilus and Erasistratus allegedly dissected Alexandrian criminals, possibly while they were still alive.

After these two, the lights apparently went out on human dissection for centuries, reignited again in 14th-century Europe where anatomists were allowed to dissect criminals. In 1540 portly Henry VIII gave a royal charter to the United Company of Barber Surgeons to use the bodies of four hanged criminals per year. In some instances, fights and riots erupted when family and friends tried to stop the dead going to the anatomists. Medical officials took to bribing hangmen and giving money to the condemned men to get bodies. In 1752 dissection was added as a top-up to hanging for the crime of murder. But with demand outstripping supply, where else to get corpses? Anatomists, medical men and students took to digging them up from graveyards. Even anatomy's biggest star, Andreas Vesalius, was known to have hung around graveyards looking for bones, and wrote tales of digging up the dead:

> The handsome mistress of a certain monk of Sant'Antonio ... died suddenly, as though from strangulation of the uterus or some quickly devastating ailment, and was snatched from her tomb by the Paduan students and carried off for public dissection. By their remarkable industry they flayed the whole skin from the cadaver lest it be

recognized by the monk who, with the relatives of his mistress, had complained to the municipal judge that the body had been stolen from its tomb.

Grave robbing became so problematic in 19th-century England, guards stood on duty in watch houses in cemeteries and newspapers at the time ran advertisements for double- and triple-layered coffins.

The extreme quest for bodies led William Burke and William Hare to kill sixteen people in Edinburgh and sell their corpses to the anatomist Robert Knox in 1828. Burke was later hanged and dissected. Strangely, it wasn't actually illegal to dig up the dead as corpses were not regarded as property—it was just considered really offensive. The crime was taking items from the grave like a shroud. In 1831 John Bishop and two other men stood trial for killing fourteen-year-old Carlo Ferrari, whom they had tried to sell to two London anatomy schools. Bishop later confessed to supplying between 500 and 1000 bodies over a twelve-year period and that he mostly 'resurrected' them from graveyards. Like Burke, he too was hanged and dissected for his crimes.

Just how awful it became has been exquisitely documented by the queen of British dissection history Ruth Richardson in her devastating *Death, Dissection and the Destitute*, a book which examines the introduction of the Anatomy Act in 1832 and how the law made dissection a punishment for being poor. Basically, parliament allowed the bodies of people who lay unclaimed in hospitals, prisons and poorhouses to be sent for dissection. Richardson tells countless appalling stories, and explores how bodies become commodified largely because the likes of anatomists, artists, physicians and surgeons made their living from them. 'Corpses were bought and sold, they were touted, priced, haggled over, negotiated for, discussed in terms of supply and demand, delivered, imported, exported and transported,' she writes. 'Human bodies were dismembered and sold in pieces, or measured and sold by the inch.' Corpses of the poor had become a profitable London business.

In the US, the vulnerable were also targeted for dissection. Slave owners either donated or sold African Americans to medical schools—in some instances their bodies shipped in barrels of whiskey. From the 1830s, state laws allowing medical schools to use unclaimed bodies from almshouses were also passed. The American anthropologist Kenneth C. Nystrom sees dissection in this period as a 'manifestation of structural violence' against the poor.

When the British invaded and began their occupation of Australia in 1788, they brought their dissection laws with them. As was the case in the motherland, if a convict committed murder in the colonies, they knew their fate: hanging and dissection. But whereas back in Britain, there weren't enough executed criminal bodies, it seems the anatomists in New South Wales had too many. In 1833 the *Sydney Monitor* ran a story which evokes an image of anatomists lounging around on old velvet couches without a body-procurement care in the world. 'While our Judges dwell with a becoming solemnity on the awful crime of murder, in passing the sentence of hanging and dissection, the public know very well that the latter part of the sentence to be a solemn farce,' it read, adding that Dr Bowman, the Inspector of Hospitals, and his two or three assistants, 'have had the dissection of so many bodies in their day, that they are tired of the art, their skill in anatomy being complete ... and of course incapable of further improvement.'

After their death sentence, condemned men and women ended up at the General 'Rum' Hospital—basically where the Mint is in modern-day Sydney—and were unfortunately often not given a proper burial after their dissection. In 1826 *The Australian* reported that 'here where the unfortunate criminal is most generally far removed from kindred ... he becomes indifferent as to the disposal of his body after death, and is most generally consigned to the earth unlamented and unhonored'.

In some instances, the dissected may have even become dog food. In 1835 a convict cook named George Brown ran away from his master—the Scottish surgeon George Frederick Moncrieff, who was in charge of dissecting at the hospital and lived on the grounds with his dogs and horses. In an appalling testimony, Brown told authorities that he ran away because there were 'so many dead bodies in a state of putrefaction lying in the dissecting room, and Doctor Moncrieff was always telling him to go and cut as much flesh as he could off the bones of the bodies and feed the dogs with it'. George couldn't bear to do it so had run—he was later given 100 lashes after the doctor denied the charges.

In the late 19th and early 20th centuries, the bones and skeletons of Indigenous Australians were collected, and sent to museums and universities for study around the world.

Across Australia, as the colonies settled into their occupation of stolen land, they slowly implemented anatomy laws. By 1876 Victoria had a law specifying that if you died in an old person's home, an asylum, a prison or other public place and nobody claimed your body, you could be sent to the university for dissection. New South Wales and the other states slowly followed suit. Over time, it was often the bodies of people who died unclaimed in asylums who were sent for dissection, a situation that likely persisted across Australia in some instances until the 1980s, and sadly continues for many other unclaimed people across the world.

And then you had the Nazis. Aside from the regime's machine-like murder of Jews, prisoners of war, homosexuals and political prisoners, between 1933 and 1945, up to 35,000 bodies were sent to thirty-one anatomy schools in Germany and its occupied territories. Half of these were Nazi victims. As the anatomist Sabine Hildebrandt has pointed out, all departments worked with the bodies of people executed by the regime, 'which were often those of young and healthy individuals'. In some instances, anatomists collaborated with the executioners. Hermann Stieve at the University of Berlin was interested in the female reproductive system and collaborated with the Gestapo to collect data about women on death row. When a woman was to be executed, she was told the date of her death and Stieve studied how this stress impacted her menstrual cycle. Once executed, her pelvic organs were dissected and studied. While it was legal at the time, anatomists now see it as a highly unethical turn.

So how was it that people like my grandparents agreed to enter this world with its dark history and associations with the poor, the vulnerable and criminality? How was it that they were one of the early adopters, in Brisbane of all places?

Mum had mentioned that they wanted to do it for 'the science' but I would soon discover that body donors were not at all a straightforward bunch of people.

Chapter 6

The 18th-century Swedish biologist Carolus Linnaeus started putting nature into categories such as animals, stones and plants, then later got serious with animals, dividing them into species, phylum, kingdom etc—the system we all studied at school. In the spirit of Linnaeus and objectivity, I decided to be really organised about the donors—I wanted to try and categorise, bring order to this group. I was thinking I could put them in a tribe, like the Amyrgians or Emishi but they weren't always bound by blood, dress, food or words—their only connection was that they were the dissected. Perhaps a movement? I wasn't sure, as movements hold meetings in halls and fervently want to change the government or social thinking, and I hadn't found any organising—just yet. I could frame donors in a more sociological way but the medical establishment tended to refer to them as specimens or cadavers, so perhaps they were more biological? I could have framed them in terms of traditional customs—I was noticing it was something Anglo-Saxon people tended to do more than people from other ethnic backgrounds. I didn't know. I could see why classification had haunted the world since the time of Aristotle.

How do we divide up and categorise reality? As the cognitive scientist Pablo Andrés Contreras Kallens and his colleagues said of categorisation: 'A dog can be an animal, a pet, a friend, a police officer, or something soft.' So I asked a basic question—who were the donors? I started a list called 'Willingly Dissected People' as in the early days the term 'body donor' wasn't used much. My list was to lengthen over time into a Buzzfeed-style Top 11, then 17, but I had no criteria as it was not easy finding candidates—either then or now. But as I trundled along, a pattern emerged.

***

The earliest Willingly Dissected person written about in English I found was John Knill, a man with a penchant for plotting elaborate plans for his death. In 1777 Knill sat for a portrait, which gave no indication of the eccentricity that would tinkle from his biography. It's a classic, formal work—thin-faced, thin-lipped with dark, thoughtful eyes in a dark blue suit. Frill-shirted and ruffled, in his long, slender hand he clutches what looks like a book or perhaps even a parcel, a possible reference to his life in Customs. Within five years, he'd made a splash on the landscape when he commissioned a large three-sided pyramid made of granite to be built on Worvas Hill overlooking St Ives, a seaside town resting on the fingertip of south-west England. A stone coffin was built inside the pyramid, which was to be his grave. He'd been mayor of the town and was winding up his job as Collector of Customs.

The unusual structure came to be known as Knill's Steeple and although *Gentleman's Magazine* claimed it was called Knill's Folly, 'a near relative of John Knill' wrote to the same publication correcting that claim and many others, including the allegation that the mausoleum looked Egyptian. While Knill built the odd structure for his burial, to help the ships coming into port and to give work to local men who were suffering through hard times, the eclectic scholar and Anglican priest S.Baring-Gould claimed in his 1909 book *Cornish Characters and Strange Events* that 'it was strongly believed that he was in league with smugglers and wreckers'.

Not long after building his elaborate grave, Knill moved to London, where he apparently resisted invitations to dinner and was noted for having a silly sense of humour. A person who builds a stone sarcophagus and large stone temple for themselves probably thinks a lot about the afterlife so when it came to his unusually long, thirteen-page will, written in secretary hand—an elaborate European-style of handwriting—he not only gave 100 pounds here, there and everywhere, he also put 25 pounds towards a ceremony he'd first put on in 1801 and wanted to keep going.

He willed that every five years on 25 July, ten young girls, one fiddler, two widows, various dignitaries and townsfolk were to walk up to his pyramid and sing and dance around. (This tradition continues to this day!) But aside from organising a dance party at his death pyramid, John Knill also willed his body to science.

Mum can read secretary hand so spent hours transcribing the section of his will where he left specific instructions that his body be sent to the 'Anatomical Dissector Wilson Esq. Who is Surgeon Keeper of the late Dr William Hunter's Museum in Windmill St or to his Successor'. He offered ten guineas 'provided that he shall dissect'. He also asked that a surgeon named George Davidson Esq of Southampton Buildings Chancery Lane 'attend the said dissection by the aforesaid Anatomist & assist'. He was also to get 10 guineas. Finally, Knill then requested that after he was dissected, his Bones (with a capital 'B') would be placed in a Wainscot wood coffin for the dimensions of a man of his size—which was 5' 6 1/2". It was only quite late in my research that I found out that even though he had willed his body to the surgeons, when he died, his medical attendant considered dissection unnecessary. Or perhaps the attendant considered it an appalling thing to do? Knill was thus never dissected, and was instead buried in the unostentatious vaults of St Andrew's Church in Holborn and not his lovely pyramid.

***

The next entrant on my list of Willingly Dissected People is the British philosopher Jeremy Bentham, a man I vaguely and initially recalled from a political theory class in my first year of arts at university before I dropped out to go scuba diving and get a job as a shitkicker in a publishing house. Aside from espousing utilitarianism, I didn't know that Bentham also had a favourite walking stick he called Dapple and a cat named Reverend Dr John Langborn, and that he invented the panopticon, a large rotunda in which all the prisoners were watched by a single security guard in a central watchtower. He rarely went out. He also left behind a massive body of philosophical work on topics ranging from animal rights to law reform. In 2006 researchers Philip Lucas and Anne Sheeran published a paper positing that Bentham had an 'autistic condition', which may account for his genius, social oddness and 'strikingly unusual cast of mind'. I'm wary of diagnosing people from the past but his different mind may have contributed to his fervent plan to get dissected.

I liked this idea that my grandparents were in fact neo-Benthamites, in a group who wanted to donate their bodies to the greater good. I would eventually learn that altruism was the main reason why people donate their bodies. Bentham too donated his body for the glory of science but what distinguishes him is that he wanted it to happen publicly.

Even as a toddler, little Jeremy demonstrated a precocious intellect, reading Latin and history books. He arrived at Oxford at just twelve and by fourteen, watched a dissection, writing to his father:

> Dr. Smith also begins his Course of Anatomy to day; and as he will have the Man that is to be hanged here to dissect, I imagine a good many will attend him.– As the time will soon come for me to go out of Mourning I must beg you to be so kind as to send me my Silver Shoe buckles and knee buckles and buttons if you can find them.

Dissection must have struck him as intriguing, coupled with his dislike for the church, stemming from when he'd first arrived at Oxford and had to sign the Thirty-Nine Articles of the Church of England, most of which he disagreed with. Thus, when he came of age at twenty-one in 1769, Bentham wrote a will leaving his body to his friend Dr George Fordyce to dissect, declaring he was doing it 'with the desire that mankind may reap some small benefit in and by my decease'.

At the time, it was an abnormal final wish to have. His body would have shared the anatomy rooms with criminals charged with murder and sentenced to hang—anatomised and dissected as 'a further

Terror and peculiar Mark of Infamy'. Bentham, an atheist, held no such terror of his body being dismembered and was fine with infamy.

You could almost call him a dissection activist. Bentham founded and funded the radical newspaper *Westminster Review* and in 1824, published 'Use of the Dead for the Living' by his friend Dr Thomas Southwood Smith. It's a rousing, eclectic and informative paper, filled with passionate descriptions of all sorts of interesting and gory medical cases saved through anatomical knowledge. It could also ultimately be entitled 'Why anatomy is bloody important and we need more bloody bodies'. Take amputation, a practice surgeons rarely undertook as people usually bled to death. The surgeon would cut through the flesh with a red-hot knife in an attempt to stop the bleeding, which usually returned anyway. 'Plunging the stump into boiling oil, into boiling turpentine, into boiling pitch, for all these means were used, was attended with no happier result, and after unspeakable suffering, almost every patient perished.' But as Smith points out, people were now surviving the operation due to anatomists' work.

Another curious section took the reader into the dead-house, where dissecting is described as 'a severe and laborious study', 'highly repulsive', and 'dangerous'. 'A winter never passes without proving fatal to several students who die from injuries received in dissection.' The tome, however, is ultimately a reasoned argument that the bodies needed for study should come from the poor who 'die unclaimed and without friends, and whose appropriation to this public service could, therefore, afford pain to no one'. Southwood Smith understood that while the attachment to the corpse was as a result of the 'noblest and sweetest sympathies of our nature … the promotion of the happiness of the living is a duty from which we can never be exonerated'.

Bentham later helped write Britain's 1832 Anatomy Act—which basically echoed what Southwood Smith had been calling for—and he died on 6 June 1832, just as the Bill was being passed. He left behind rings bearing his effigy to twenty-four people, the miniature portrait having been painted with strands of his hair, which was a fashion of the day. He also left behind quite a few plans for his corpse. First, he wanted his friend Southwood Smith to publicly dissect him, and give a lecture in front of scientific and literary men.

Ask and you shall receive. Three days after Bentham's death, invitations to his dissection at Webb Street School of Anatomy and Medicine were sent out—for this historic event, guests were given a plus two. Southwood Smith gave a very long speech over the corpse of his dear friend, although the physician Dr William Monk reported that he delivered his lecture 'with a clear unfaltering voice but with a face as white as that of the dead philosopher before him'.

As he spoke, a thunderstorm broke out, flashes of lightning filling the room, adding a sense of occasion or portent. The painter Henry Pickersgill sketched *Mortal Remains*—the first known portrait of a soon-to-be Willingly Dissected person. Bentham is lying on the dissecting table, bare-chested and draped in a white sheet in a manner reminiscent of a toga. The subtext to me appears to be that as all great men in Rome wore togas, so too should this great philosopher. His balding white hair hangs scraggily, his mouth slightly downturned, and his quite dainty feet peep out from under the sheet. He looks skinnier than his usual portraits but peaceful as he lies on a slab covered with plain fabric.

Or as Southwood Smith put it during the oration: 'Can you look on the sweetness, the dignity of its expression and ever forget it? Can you dread the aspect of death assuming such a shape?' I couldn't find an actual account of the dissection taking place at that moment—perhaps it was considered too unpleasant to document? Nonetheless, in terms of a hyped event focused on dissection—not a massive canon to choose from—the energy in the room that day must've been akin to Muhammad Ali and George Foreman's 'Rumble in the Jungle' in Kinshasa in 1974.

But there was more in the will. Bentham did not want to be buried but wanted to be turned into what he called an 'auto icon', and it seems he and his friends had been experimenting with how to do it. Their inspiration had been the Mokomokai, the preserved New Zealand Māori heads, and they'd had a go at drying out human heads in his oven.

John Bowring, who was Bentham's executor to his will, a British politician and later Governor to Hong Kong, recalled a conversation in which Bentham said he was getting a human head from the anatomist Dr Grainger. Bentham also wrote about his experiments, 'which promise complete success, by the slow exhaustion of the moisture from the human head. Specimens exist in the College of Physicians. In colour only is there any considerable change; and colour may be easily supplied.'

Southwood Smith followed through on Bentham's wishes—the body was dissected and skeletonised, and dressed in his fave black clothes although the head didn't work out so well so they had to get a wax one. You can visit him today, propped up in a chair with glass eyeballs, at the University College London.

Bentham's whole post-death palaver was extraordinarily radical for the age, motivated by his loathing of the church and his desire to show the beauty and knowledge to be gleaned from the human body. When the Anatomy Act was passed in 1832, the option to encourage body donation was on the table but the parliament instead opted to go after the poor and the mentally unwell.

While he was ahead of his time in spruiking the wonder of the dissected human body, Bentham's different cast of mind made it hard for him to see the fear the idea of meddling with the body after death invoked in others. As his friend the philosopher John Stuart Mill said of him: 'the faculty by which one mind understands a mind different from itself, and throws itself into the feelings of that other mind, was denied him by his deficiency of Imagination'.

***

Years pass.

In most Western countries, it is still only the mentally ill and the poor who end up getting dissected. But something is happening—it's not just wealthy Brits jumping on the dissecting table. In 1876 a group of atheistic French anthropologists founded the exquisitely named Society of Mutual Autopsy, a club which vowed to prove there was no soul by dissecting each other's brains upon death.

It ran up until just before the Second World War and carried out many autopsies on their members' brains. As the historian Jennifer Hecht put it: 'For people who rejected religion so strenuously that they saw burial as an abhorrent, cultish ritual but could not bear utterly disappearing, the society provided great comfort.'

Aside from this wild, politically driven club, donors from other strata of society also began appearing. They were often in the US or the UK, and when they announced their intention, it was so unusual it made the Australian newspapers.

In 1853 when she was twenty-three, Miss Elizabeth R. Branson was staying in a Cincinnati hotel when she was one of a number of guests poisoned. She would spend the rest of her life unwell. 'From that time, she dated her illness, and for twenty-six years had abscesses, fistulas, and cancers,' says the story in Queensland's *Warwick Examiner*. She went on to study medicine. While the newspaper doesn't mention this, she would have attended and taken part in dissections—women had been admitted to dissecting rooms in the US as early as 1847, even though there were ongoing worries that cutting through fascia would turn women into hardened creatures.

In the nine months before Branson's death, she contacted the New York Medical College and Hospital for women and asked if she could be a patient there for free, 'offering as inducement to permit her body, after her death, to be dissected for the benefit of science'. The hospital was obviously not interested in the trade-off, so her friends got together and footed her bill. Resting on the ward, the forty-nine-year-old dying from her cocktail of diseases, decided to give her body up for dissection anyway.

'She requested that her skeleton be hung up in the college. She talked with composure of the will that she had made, and spoke of the benefit to the college that would follow the dissection of her body. Her friends met in the dissecting rooms on Wednesday, and the body was dissected.' Whoever wrote the story in 1879 found it 'peculiar'.

Fifty years on, to donate one's body was still unconventional and newsworthy. In 1931 Arthur Polkinghorne, a well-known Brisbane journalist, bequeathed his body to science for cancer research after suffering from 'the dread disease'. Described as a humanitarian, he had particular interests, playing 'a leading part in publicity against sterilisation of Alsatian dogs in Queensland, and against vandals who destroyed the beautiful trees along the streets'.

Other stories start to appear but they are fists from the page: people killing themselves and leaving a note asking to be dissected or prisoners in jail agreeing to the procedure. That suicides and prisoners were offering their bodies to science makes sense: dissection would have been firmly in the consciousness of this poorer, more vulnerable class of people. Throughout Australia—and many other parts of the world—it was law that if you died in an asylum and your body was not claimed, you would be sent to the anatomists. Technically, this outdated law is still on the books.

In 1910 in a Melbourne city court, Frederick James appeared with 'a suggestive bandage round his head and a dazed look in his eye', charged with attempting suicide. The court heard he'd left a note before trying to shoot himself in the head: 'Dear Sir,– Will you be good enough to hand my body over to St. Vincent's Hospital for dissecting purposes. There is no person in Australia having any claim to be next of kin, so I kindly see that it is handed over.'

In 1938 the glamorously named Seraphin Desire Casile, remorseful on being sent to a prison in Etampes in France, offered himself up for cancer research. 'I am 44,' he wrote. 'I am free to do what I like with my body. The most celebrated doctors have always been seeking a cure for cancer. They have not found it because they need some one on whom to experiment. If my offer is accepted I shall have rendered at least a service to society. My family will forgive me.'

The most dramatic story on the Willingly Dissected list is that of a young man who poisoned himself at the entrance of Melbourne's Royal

Botanic Gardens in October 1923. It was a time when the city was rolling into spring but instead of enjoying the warmth, a miserable but distinctive young man lay dead, albeit with a lot to say.

The headline in the paper doesn't do much for the body donation cause:

DISGUSTED WITH MANKIND
Suicide's Strange Letter
REBEL AND ATHEIST
Body Bequeathed to Science

When the police inspected his body, they found a series of clues as to why he killed himself. There was a letter in his pocket and a photo of a 'prepossessing' woman, 'My only pal' written on the back of the photo in pencil. They found a handkerchief laced with poison and the novel *Out of the Wreck I Rise* by the British writer and suffragette Beatrice Harraden.

They opened the letter, which had the heading: 'What Cato, Zeus, Cowper and Marcus Aurelius approve of cannot be wrong.' The young man wrote: 'I pass out of life as an uncompromising rebel and atheist. I die bitterly opposed to the accepted social conditions of today. The more I see of man, the more I appreciate flowers and animals. I look at the attainments of man, and thus die, disgusted.'

He left no name or address, and declared that he wanted to die unknown, and had no friends for the police to contact anyway. He also wrote of a desire that his body be given to the students practising anatomy at the Melbourne General Hospital. 'I fear not dissection as I have lived a clean, pure life. After they have dissected me in the most minute form, cremate my mangled parts. Do not bury, as I hate all that is called civilisation. In life I was insignificant. In death science may lengthen by having the disposal of my body. And now, farewell all base bred mongrels of mankind.'

Another sheet of paper was found, with the heading: 'My Last Hour'. He discussed having a good meal, and shaving with a steady hand.

He marvelled at his own calm. 'A little child plays on the lawn. How beautiful he romps about and how unconscious he is of the real world in this ephemeral atmosphere. I feel like an artist inspired to death by beauty. Almost a story for a newspaper.'

Definitely a story for a book 100 years later.

But you see this slow pattern elsewhere in the world—more people okay about donating. In the late 1890s in Vienna, a rumour spread that the Institute of Zootomy would pay the poor if they left their bodies for dissection. Working-class people responded and between 1898 and 1908 wrote letters advertising their uniqueness, including having 'peculiarly shaped upper body', 'various inner and outer injuries of the head', and 'two different feet, one normal and one 2/3 thinner'.

Anna Astl-Leonhard, however, was more motivated by science than money, and believed she had a male brain in a female body. Her letter—where she declared she was 'never hysterical but, as all spiritual human beings often are, very nervous'—was quite the pitch, and I imagine she would have been a fun person to get drunk with. Not long after in 1930, a Thai professor of literature donated his body, inspired to do it so he could teach after death—his skeleton is apparently at the anatomical museum of Siriraj Hospital in Bangkok.

Oh, and there is a poet! Her name was Laura Evelyn Dixon and as *The Sun* in Sydney reported in 1953, for seven years she had carried her will bequeathing her body to the University of Sydney in her handbag.

A 'poetess' and former nurse from Harbord on Sydney's northern beaches, she wrote verse under a few names, and her work had been broadcast on local radio. 'Mrs. Dixon requested that her bones be placed in a bone bank. If possible, the corneas of her eyes should be used to restore the sight of a blind person,' said the story. 'Mr. Dixon said he doubted whether his wife's request about her eyes could be fulfilled. "Our local doctor told me the corneas would be useless unless removed within 25 minutes of death."'

Looking at the Willingly Dissected—John Knill, Jeremy Bentham, Elizabeth Branson in New York, the young man with his extraordinary suicide notes—and patterns and shapes like a Rorschach test begin to reveal titbits about these old 18th-, 19th- and 20th-century donors: they weren't your usual type of person. Back then, it was a very unconventional and radical thing to do.

Chapter 7

Economic elites head to Davos, sportspeople have a go at the Olympics. Anatomists converge on the International Federation of Associations of Anatomists in different parts of the world every five years. Goran had mentioned the London conference and I was planning on going. However, I needed to train first. I wanted to be ready. I had to take a crash course and go off on tangents—I was starting to see that there was A LOT on the history of dissection. Like A LOT from so many different fields.

***

While Aristotle laid the foundations by dissecting animals in the 4th century BC, the title 'The Father of Anatomy' goes to the Greek physician Herophilus. He began dissecting humans around 280 to 260 BC and made extraordinary discoveries, including naming the duodenum, giving the first accurate description of the liver, showing that the uterus was hollow and much, much more. He studied and dissected alongside Erasistratus, who was close to working out how blood circulated. The pair apparently vivisected criminals hauled from jail.

The next man to promote dissection was the prolific Galen of Pergamum. Born in 129 AD, he began his career treating gladiators and went on to write 130 treatises on medicine alone. While he never cut up a human, he publicly dissected all sorts of animals, including monkeys, and building on the work of Herophilus and Erasistratus, made all sorts of claims, some of them wrong. He later came to be personal physician to the psychotic emperor Commodus, who Joaquin Phoenix played so well in *Gladiator*.

We've all seen those historical costume dramas where a very ill person, pale and sweaty, lies in bed, delirious. Soon, a doctor arrives and you think, 'oh no, don't do it', but they do—they start placing leeches on the sick person, or they slash their wrist a few times, their blood pouring into a bowl. 'Stop! You're killing them!' Herophilus and Galen lived at a time where bloodletting was *it* and had just kicked off as a medical treatment, borne from Hippocrates' idea that there were four humours—blood, phlegm, black bile, yellow bile—and being ill meant these were imbalanced in some way, and you'd feel much better if you bled a little.

A millennia on, it persisted. Middle Ages and Renaissance physicians and barber-surgeons may have also checked their Zodiac Man, an elaborate naked male figure with twelve zodiac signs superimposed on his body. If you had a sore head—which was ruled by Aries—it could then be decided when was the right time to do bloodletting or take herbs. No! Not the bloodletting! Widespread bleeding didn't stop until the 19th century.

The sick in early Europe sought help from all sorts of characters: monks, wise women, physicians, healers, apothecaries, surgeons and barber-surgeons. The physicians knew Latin, Greek and the ancient texts, the surgeons did the cutting and the apothecaries dispensed the potions. In addition, for centuries, only the anatomical works of the likes of Aristotle and Galen were considered acceptable. People probably dissected on the quiet but it officially lay dormant until 1315, when the Italian Mondino de Luzzi, dubbed 'the restorer of anatomy', revived human dissection by more than likely cutting open a female executed criminal at the University of Bologna. He published *Anathomia*, a step-by-step guide to dissection, which is considered the first 'modern' anatomy text and introduced the idea that dissection should be in the medical curriculum. His book contains a lot of errors as the doctrine of the day ruled that he had to follow what the ancients said.

I feel for these early anatomists, sitting around the dinner table with their wives and kids, quietly bitching over their sausages and ale that they were over what Galen said about the body because when you looked at one, it didn't quite make sense, and speaking of corpses, how am I going to find one to study? Even though the ancients rarely dissected humans and their knowledge was gleaned from animals, the general explanation for the differences was that the human body had changed over the centuries. There were all sorts of regulations about the criminal bodies they could dissect too—take these from the University of Bologna in 1405:

- permission from the rector
- only twenty people allowed at a male dissection
- thirty people allowed at a female dissection as they were unusual
- a student was only allowed to see one female and two male demonstrations

But everything changed with Andreas Vesalius. Whenever he comes to mind, I see a rock star prancing across a stage in a glittering doublet and codpiece, as aside from being a brilliant anatomist and radical thinker he was a showman. In 1543 the twenty-eight-year-old slammed the more than 650-page *De Humani Corporis Fabrica Libri Septem* (*On the Fabric of the Human Body in Seven Books*) on the table and yelled 'Take that! Galen got it wrong!'* A large format book with precise illustrations and detailed descriptions of the human body, it changed the science forever. Incredibly, it came out the same year that Polish astronomer Nicolaus Copernicus published *On the Revolutions of the Heavenly Spheres*, which claimed the sun was the centre of the universe and not earth.

The cover of Vesalius' book alone suggests confidence—it's a picture of himself looking out at the reader, surrounded by a throng of people in an anatomy theatre and a naked woman who has been cut open, which at the time would have been absolutely shocking.

As the historian Katherine Park puts it: 'Vesalius aimed to increase his reputation (not to mention recoup his large investment in artists' fees), and he would have expected this dramatic and novel image to help sell

---

* Galen got it wrong because he dissected animals.

his book.' Vesalius broke other traditions too—he got his hands dirty and did the dissecting himself. Traditionally, doctors sat at a lectern reading instructions from Galen as an assistant did the cutting.

While seen by some as dense and badly written, *Fabrica* featured more than 420 extraordinary illustrations and to this day is considered one of the most beautiful scientific books ever printed. The shorter and very practical *Epitome*, which had large anatomical figures that could be cut out

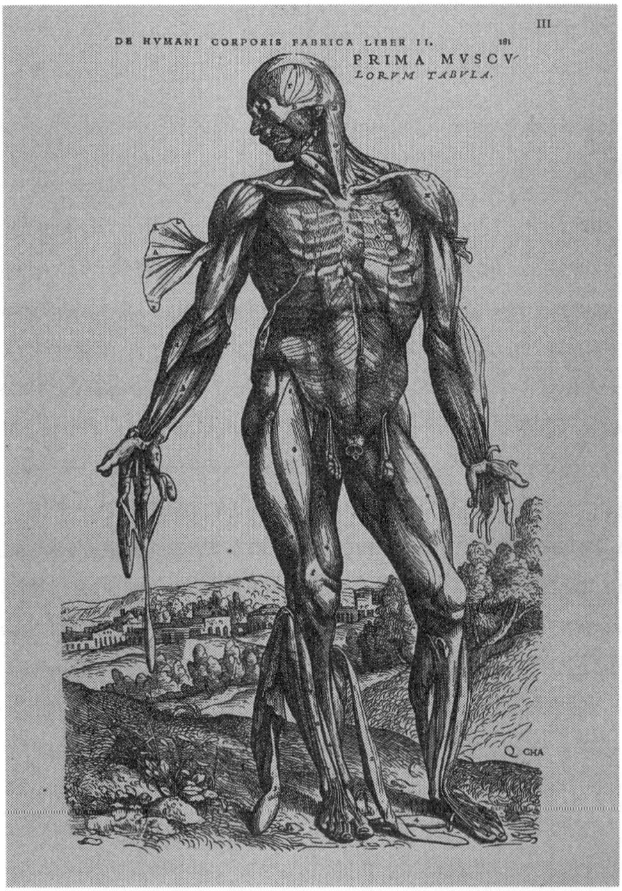

The fifth of fourteen muscle-men in Vesalius' *De Humani Corporis Fabrica Libri Septem* published in 1543. The background is believed to be hills near Padua, Italy. *Wellcome Collection.*

and posted to the walls of a dissection room, accompanied it. A fusspot about quality, Vesalius paid extra to have the book printed on the best paper with wide margins. It was thus relatively expensive, costing the equivalent of thirty-four meals with meat at the time. While a copy sold at Sotheby's in 1998 for USD$1.6 million, you can pick one up in 2022 for around USD$300,000.

By the 16th century, many gross (as in 'whole' rather than 'disgusting') anatomical structures were known but some were yet to be described. It was also a period when anatomists didn't quite know how the parts

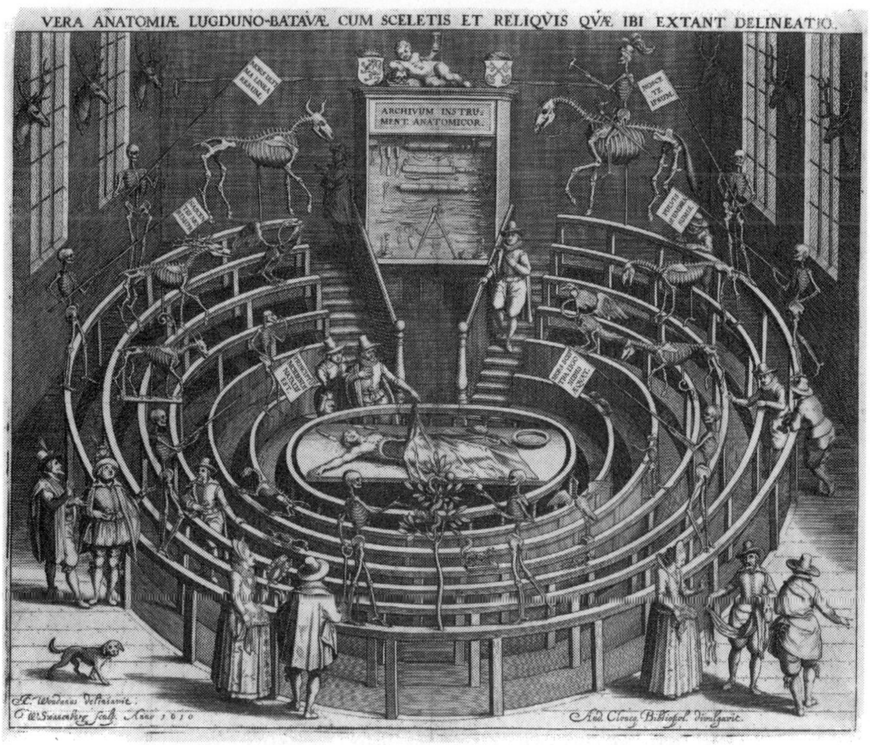

This 1610 engraving by Willem Swanenburgh and drawing by Jan Cornelisz depicts the end of a dissection at the Leiden anatomical theatre. The crowds have left but the corpse remains centre stage. Note the moralising banners and the skeletal figure of Death riding on a skeletal horse. *Wikipedia Commons.*

worked. How did the blood get around the body? To allow students and dignitaries to watch dissection better, specially-designed anatomical theatres began popping up across Europe in Montpellier, Basel, London, Padua, Pisa and Leiden. Some of these beautiful wooden ampitheatres still survive.

Whereas contemporary dissection halls have OH&S rules pinned to their walls, these theatres had human skeletons holding banners breezily declaring *memento mori* like 'death is the last boundary of things' and 'we are dust and shadows'.

Sometimes dissection even turned into a party. In the 1540s Bologna's annual winter dissection and carnival overlapped. University management had to do something about dwindling student numbers so decided to put on a show to demonstrate their new anatomical theatre—some spectators even wore carnival-style masks to watch the dissections.

From the late 19th century onwards, microscopes and X-rays meant anatomists and scientists could travel deeper into our cells and tissues. The 20th century brought forth more new ways of looking inside which we now take for granted: endoscopes, magnetic resonance imaging (MRI), computer tomography (CT) and ultrasounds.

For a science that had been built up over 2300 years, it was time to do some housework, and it was 19th-century anatomists who got out the broom. The first clean-up was anatomical nomenclature, a chaotic language built up over a millennia in anatomy textbooks written all over the world: Latin, Greek, Arabic and Hebrew. Meticulously and erratically created, who could pronounce it?

The cleaning began when a group of European authors of influential anatomical textbooks pondered how to fix the problem. In 1880 the Viennese anatomist and linguist Josef Hyrtl did a review but could see it was too difficult. 'It did not occur to me,' he wrote, 'to wish to reform the anatomical language. That would take an ad hoc elected committee of linguistically educated anatomists.' So in 1887 the German-language anatomical society launched an official naming project at a time when classification and standardisation was exploding around the world in medicine and other areas such as time measurements, weights and coins. The Leipzig anatomist Wilhelm His led the charge. The Swiss anatomist Albert von Kölliker directed the committee for the project. (Years later he had a lizard named after him.) They came up with a couple of rules:

- Each body part could have just one name.
- It would be in Latin and as short as possible.

You could produce a historical drama about what happened over the next eight years but eventually, the English, Italian, Belgian and American anatomists whittled down 50,000 names to 5000 and in 1895 launched the *Basle Nomina Anatomica* (BNA). For the next 100 years, anatomists would meet in cities over the world to argue about revisions and various editions—the JNA in Jena, the PNA in Paris. Since 1998 it has been known as *Terminologia Anatomica* (TA). It's not all Western-centric either. In 1984 a standardised language for acupuncture was published, after it was generally agreed there were 361 classical acupuncture points.

The current TA has 7800 anatomical terms in Latin and English. Some of the language is inspired. The seahorse-shaped hippocampus—a little part of the brain—comes from the Greek *hippokampos*, which refers to a sea monster. Sea monsters in my head. The sesamoid bones in the feet are a combination of the Greek words *sesame* (sesame) and *eidos* (resemblance). Sesame bones in my feet. Some of it sounds so pretty, the language of a faraway kingdom with elves living in villages called *glabella* (the area of the skin between the eyebrows and above the nose), *dactylion* (the very tip of the middle finger), and *malleus* (a bone in the inner ear).

But for some, the TA has an ugly side, particularly the use of eponyms, which are the body parts named after a specific person, such as the circle of Willis, the fossa of Sylvius and the follicle of Graaf. Even though eponyms have been out of the TA since 1998, they persist. In 2020 Dr Kirsten Small (@birthsmalltalk), a Queensland specialist obstetrician and gynaecologist, tweeted a stern comment at the perception that it was just too hard to use different names. She wrote: 'I teach anatomy and have found there is always an alternative to the dead man's name for body parts. Fallopian tube = uterine tube. Pouch of Douglas = rectovaginal pouch. We have a personal choice to decolonise our language. Make use of it.'

In response to the tweet, doctors Robert Buttner, Jessica Lee and Mike Cadogan evaluated the idea that there is always an alternative and in reviewing 700 eponymous anatomical terms, found only one was named for a woman—Raissa Nitabuch's fibrinoid, the internal fibrinoid layer of the maturing placenta. While the trio said it unlikely that there is always an alternative, they had a stab by publishing an online de-eponymification database.

In 2019 Allison Draper, an American medical student, saw red when she looked up the nerve which gives sensation to the outer female genitalia and saw 'pudendal' meant 'to be ashamed'. She checked the TA and saw the Latin for 'vulva' was ***pudendum***, 'the part to be ashamed of'. Incensed, she started a campaign to get rid of it and while ***pudendum*** was taken out of the TA, it was considered a step too far to cancel the pudendal artery, canal and nerve as it was used for both sexes.

Perhaps at TA's next revision they can substitute the name of the discoverer with the name of the dissected. After all, it is technically their tube, pouch and follicle that were found. There must be one instance where their name is buried in the historical record. Isn't there?

***

Philosophers have Rodin's *The Thinker* as their pin-up. Image processors once used 'Lenna' or 'Lena'—a photograph of the Swedish model Lena Forsén taken from a *Playboy* centrefold—as a standard test image. Anatomists have their 'anatomical position', which sounds like an interesting sex move but is actually a person facing straight, their arms down their sides, palms forward. Legs are straight and feet are parallel to each other. Next time you go to your doctor, check—there might be one on the wall.

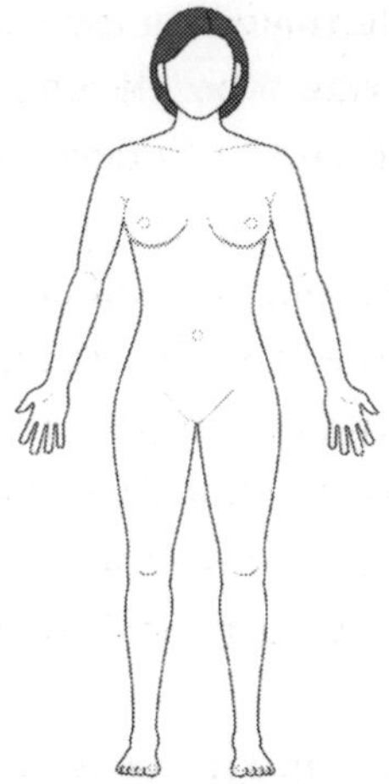

This is the standing anatomical position. If you lie down face up in this position, you are supine. Face down is prone. *(Access for free at https://humanbiomedia.org/)*

To get to this position—and trying to find out how it all started—wasn't straightforward. I initially thought it dated back to the Zodiac Man from the early medical charts but couldn't find any proof, so the official line is this: it was 16th-century anatomist and rock star Andreas who adopted it, and it was decided to stick with this 'orthograde' (i.e. standing up) pose for the 1895 BNA. Decades later, in the 1930s, a group of German anatomists doing a mini-revision of the BNA decided the better position was 'pronograde', which is more like how a monkey would stroll along, the long axis of the body parallel to the ground. They thought it suited the common anatomy shared by humans and other vertebrates. Hey! We've all got spines! We're in the same club!

In 1945 a group of Stanford anatomists agreed, declaring in an essay in *The Anatomical Record* that the standing-up position was a 'rather artificial concept'. They continued: 'The cadaver is never dissected when in that position; the physician and the surgeon deal mostly with patients who are supine [aka lying down]; and, if either of them were confronted in his office by a man who approached him with his palms directed forward, he would probably leave hurriedly by the nearest exit.'

Attempts to quash this 'artificial concept' stance—one which clearly spooked Stanford anatomists—fizzled out. In 1956 when the *Paris Nomina Anatomica* was published, the anatomical position graced its pages. The decision to go with the standing position triggered a long period of breakups—the mammalian and avian anatomists broke away from the human ones, and would go on to form the World Association of Veterinary Anatomists (WAVA). In 1968 they published their *Nomina Anatomica Veterinaria.* Twenty years later, the mammal and the avian vet anatomists also broke up. Perhaps one day we will be reunited with our vertebrate friends? When I read about all of this my first reaction was: 'How in any way is this objective?'

The TA also contains another realm of adjectives to describe where parts are in relation to each other. Our eyes are 'superior' to our mouth. Our feet are 'inferior' to our knees. I know what the anatomists mean when they say 'dorsal'. I was fixated by *Jaws* as a child, and clutched the couch every time that dorsal fin gently rose out of the water.

The TA describes moving differently too—when an anatomist hits the dance floor, they pull off flexion, extension, abduction, dorsiflexion. I may see myself as a fun-loving person who enjoys pina coladas but to the anatomists I am respiratory, cardiac, nervous, muscoskeletal, digestive, lymphatic, integumentary and the list goes on. (I'd never heard the word 'integumentary' in my life, which is pretty bad as the main organ of it is the skin, and I look at it every day.) They've also colonised me in other ways, turning me into a nation with eight regions—Head, Neck, Back, Upper Extremities and so on. We are also hypothetical planes: midsagittal, median, coronal, transverse.

Stop!

It never stops!

As you can see, it is the rare club that can even begin to speak fluent Anatomy. It goes on, on, on, on ... to the nth degree and I now understand why medicine is such a hard university degree. It's full-on rote learning. Mnemonics help. Take the twelve cranial nerves, which allow you to see, hear, smell, and move your head and neck, and basically exist.

I. Olfactory
II. Ophthalmic
III. Oculomotor
IV. Trochlear
V. Trigeminal
VI. Abducens
VII. Facial
VIII. Vestibulocochlear
IX. Glossopharyngeal
X. Vagus
XI. Accessory
XII. Hypoglossal

To remember them, students and doctors use the first letters of the nerves to build twelve-word sentences. Some are fairly straight: 'On On On They Travelled And Found Voldemort Guarding Very Ancient Horcruxes'. Others seem penned by someone with a camp sense of humour—'On Occasion, Oliver Tries To Anally Finger Various Guys. Vaginas Are History!'

Chapter 8

Professions have their stereotypes—shonky real estate agents, bead-wearing psychotherapists, holidays galore for school teachers but anatomists? I close my eyes. Do I see lab coats? Tinges of the odd because they dismember people? I text random friends asking what they think an anatomist is like. One says: 'Quirky. Bow tie. Looney Tunes socks. Pen in top left pocket of short-sleeved, collared (but lightweight) button-up shirt. Never knowingly met one mind you!' Another suggests a skinny tall pale guy in a lab coat who is intelligent, clinical, detached, introverted, and a bit like a mortician.

If the starter gun for anatomy went off with Herophilus and Erasistratus studying dead humans in ancient Alexandria, I would come to find that anatomists have gone through bouts of both being respectable and detestable in their 2300-year history. For a spell they had status: anatomists worked for emperors, popes and grand duchesses. They cut up the dead alongside philosophers, artists, magistrates, writers, sculptors, poets, the educated and students. They could earn a decent wage in Renaissance Europe. Some rich men wanted to be like them, and had their own dissecting rooms, like the one that appears in the Marquis de Sade's 1813 Gothic novel *La Marquise de Gange.*

But I get the sense anatomists don't have the same social or professional ranking as they once did. It's not a sledge. Who has status these days? I can't quite tell any more—some people hate prime ministers and value American celebrities selling undies. I think a big part of the problem is that whereas chemists can go around studying chemicals, and mathematicians pick up a pencil and work on equations, the anatomist studies through cutting—the *tomy* in anatomy—dead bodies, and for centuries, this has immediately placed them in an edgy position, even if they can lighten the mood with their playful mnemonics. As F. González-Crussi said in his *Notes of an Anatomist*, these cutters are 'viewed with distrust'.

Corpses have long exerted all sorts of powers, superstitions, thoughts, rituals and fears over the living. As the historian Thomas W. Laqueur sums it up: 'It is really the greatest possible history of the imagination.' He describes the work of the dead as a form of magic, and he's right—they cast spells over us and make us do strange things. Even when they are gone, mute and unmoving, they fire us up. We feel sad looking at a tomb without lettering. We flock to visit the graves of people we don't know—kids get stoned in front of Jim Morrison's or used to kiss Oscar Wilde's stone before a glass barrier was put up to preserve it. Some dead people exude a potency so strong they must remain secret—the world still doesn't know what happened to Osama bin Laden's body.

Corpses also create unease. You can see it as far back as 500 BC in the laws inscribed on old stones and marbles on the island of Cos, which ruled that the dead body was a source of pollution, and everyone and everything that came in contact with it was also polluted: family members, the house, the water supply and the fireplace. Relatives of the dead were polluted for months afterwards and banned from all shrines, and each time they visited the grave, they again became polluted and needed to perform purification rituals. Again and again.

Corpses at one point had superpowers. King Charles II of England drank a potion containing forty-two drops of extract of human skull when he lay on his deathbed in 1685. Dr Christian Friedrich Garmann's 1709 text *Concerning the Miracles of the Dead* documents the wonders of the corpse, including that their sweat can treat haemorrhoids and tumours, and that a dead arm can heal an arm, a dead leg a leg etc. In a weird way, was he predicting organ donation? Christians flocked to see and touch saints' bodies, skulls, hair and dried-up toes while monarchs and aristocrats collected these bits and traded them.

But this fear of the corpse persists. In 2021 when Gregory & Carr Funerals wanted to open a parlour for viewings in Woollahra, one of Sydney's poshest areas, the community revolted. A spokesman for worried residents said diners at a neighbouring restaurant would have to contemplate people viewing the dead as they ate and that children at the nearby primary school would have to encounter coffins wheeled out of mortuary cars. As Harriet Price, a local councillor, put it: 'A cloud of grief and bereavement is not compatible with fine dining and shopping for bespoke retail offerings.'

This cloud has also long hovered around all sorts of death workers. In 18th-century Florence, a porter named Giancinto Guidetti collected bodies from one of the hospitals and took them to the museum La Specola, where they were used as casts for their anatomical wax models. The poor man complained in a letter that '… in times of rain or snow' he could not take a break anywhere since he carried with him 'the basket of dead bodies', a task which made him detestable to the point where he was treated badly at the coffee houses he used to go to.

Even today, funeral directors—those midwives to the most profound of human rituals—are paid surprisingly poor wages. Job seeker websites advertise the position around $60,000 a year. And what about people who go that step further and dismember bodies? An anatomical prosector can earn between $70,000 and $80,000 a year. There are reams of myths where dismemberment brings about renewal but in our cultural imagination, it is the work of psychopaths. Whenever I think of chopping up the dead, I see the sweaty manic men in masks with saws and axes I watched in horror films as a kid in Manila. In reality, for a while, drug lords in Colombia dismembered their victims to send messages to the community.

At this stage, I'd only met Goran on the phone and wasn't sure how to meet other anatomists or get a sense of them and their work. So I turned to the new Oracle at Delphi for answers: YouTube. After struggling through reading *Gray's Anatomy*, I wish I'd found dissection TV a lot earlier—it was akin to a divine disclosure.

I thought public dissection was something that only our allegedly unwashed ancestors could watch but in 2022, it was everywhere online.

If I had to generalise, I'd say they were wholly educational, of varying quality and each anatomist definitely had their own schtick. They were also 1000 per cent confronting—skulls were sawed open, flesh was sliced and spines were cracked with hammers. As a couple of them rightly suggested: VIEWER DISCRETION ADVISED.

The anatomist was often a narrator speaking Anatomy, explaining the body in Latin and Greek terms as hands, scalpels, scissors and forceps methodically picked away at the dead person. The camera was often so close I felt I could press my face into the dead flesh, which was usually reminiscent of turkey or chicken meat. Depending on the lighting, dead human flesh was grey, pale pink, dark red, vibrant pus-yellow and creamy.

I felt a bit sick every time I started watching one and couldn't concentrate on what the anatomist was saying.

We are so meaty.

I am meat.

Fuck we look like dark turkey meat.

I was also unsure about how to see the dead person on the table or their part that was being dissected. I was falling, tumbling from the sky seeing blue, green, blue, green; the person was a subject, object, subject, object, loved, meat, loved, meat. It was an uneasy place—disgusting and compelling.

But once the nausea and psychic blowout settled, my face shifted from rictus to curiosity, and I would fall in with my chosen anatomist. The Great Gloved hand—and at times UnGloved—would unpick, fossick, scrape, saw and clean away a back, arm or face. As they followed the path of the sciatic nerve, I shapeshifted into Theseus following the ball of thread Ariadne gave him to escape the Minotaur's labyrinth. We were heading somewhere with this picking. I came to see why with a jammed medical program, professional prosectors and dissectors stepped in: it takes time and true craft to precisely cut through fat and fascia to get to the good bits.

You could see the skill in Romed Hörmann and Hannes Stofferin's amusing, elegant and weirdly mesmerising short film *How to Dissect*

Muscles and Fascia made in 2021 for the Anatomy Innsbruck YouTube channel. It features a donor's ribcage area being dissected. Hannes was droll: 'If you want to be the king or queen of anatomical dissection, you have to do it the right way. The sharp side of the blade points *away* from the structure you want to dissect. That's the only way if you're going to succeed and impress everybody in the wetlab.' At the end he thanked their body donors and signed off: 'We wish you happy dissecting!'

In the deep sub-sub-culture of online dissection, I also quite liked the liveliness and matter-of-fact manner of Dr Sanjoy Sanyal from All Saints University in St. Vincent and the Grenadines. Sanjoy got straight to work, and it was raw—no fuss about lighting or rose-colouring the reality. In his *Exonerated Eyeball 1–Conjunctival Dissection with Clinical Aspects* an unblinking eyeball surrounded by crumpled flesh lay on a paper napkin, staring at the camera. Sanjoy, speaking Anatomy, slowly picked apart the thin layers and tissues. It was not easy viewing; it felt like the eye was watching me. Sanjoy dissects everything: spinal cords, a penis, hands—and I loved that he had a written disclaimer at the start some of the videos declaring that the bodies were willed.

There were other genres where the anatomist was the frontman—a bit like David Attenborough with his animals or Nigella Lawson with her cooking. The anatomist Dr Satheesha Nayak from Manipal University in India, in a collared shirt and trousers, was relaxed, professional and sanguine as his colleagues used a hardware-store handsaw to open up the skull of a corpse lying on a steel table. A large tree out the window added a gentle, natural touch.

The hue and vibe of the vintage dissection films reminded me of the days when I could smoke cigarettes at my desk at work. In a 1974 video, Dr Donald Huelke—an anatomist who went on to become a leading researcher into car crash injuries in the US—dissected a man's face without gloves. (One anatomist told me when gloves started appearing in labs it was a bit odd at first—like when people first wore masks during the pandemic.) In the Texas Tech University Health Sciences *Caring for the Cadaver* Lab Video series, a man with a 1980s haircut wore a lab coat paired with shorts and pool slides as he casually rolled over a very stiff dead man.

But the biggest dissection influencers would have to be Jonathan Bennion and Justin Cottle from the Institute of Human Anatomy, a private human cadaver lab in Salt Lake City, Utah. With their black t-shirts and layperson content like 'What's it like working with dead bodies?', 'What happens if you swallow gum?' and 'How much poop is stored in your colon?', the pair have racked up millions of views and fans on YouTube, Facebook and Instagram by dissecting dead bodies for the camera.

Their gift store stocked branded merchandise—black hoodies, leggings, mugs, socks and iPhone cases. Jonathan, a trained anatomy teaching assistant with a degree in health promotion and education, and Justin, a former US marine, massage therapist and marketer, were naturally charismatic, and had the vibe of chilled rock climbers. Hey guys and gals—check this out. As Justin said: 'Let's do this!'

In one video, the pair explained how they collected the bodies from a body donor program in their pick-up truck. They showed a body in a bag in the back. Jonathan and Justin are respectful and professional in the dissecting room but I doubt these videos could be made in any other Western nation outside of a university context, largely because America is the Wild West when it comes to dead bodies—it's not that hard to buy them or get parts. People donate their bodies to companies in exchange for a free cremation. The bodies or parts are then sold locally and internationally to medical researchers and educators. Heavy hitters in the anatomy world have critiqued the phenomena and dubbed this emerging trend 'Bodies R Us'.

I later asked an Australian anatomist what he thought about the Institute and he said they 'aren't that bad'. While Australian regulations forbid him from making dissection films, if he could, he'd create ones which were more aesthetically pleasing.

Chapter 9

Thus, somewhat prepped and totally jetlagged, I float into ExCeL, a bland and barn-like conference centre in the Docklands area of East London, to attend the International Federation of Associations of Anatomists (IFAA) 2019 conference. Checking in, I also feel staggered at the $450 day pass as I put a lanyard around my neck. An anatomist later tells me it was prohibitively expensive for many people in the scene and there are better conferences out there anyway.

It's the final day of three days of talks and I've already missed the presentations on dark humour in the lab and anatomical aspects of transgender surgery. I'm particularly bummed not to have heard a talk from Professor Susan Standring, the current editor of *Gray's Anatomy*.

I've obsessively studied the form guide for weeks and head straight to a series of discussions on body donations in Asia, keen to hear Professor Guo-Fang Tseng from Tzu Chi University in Hualien, an isolated, sleepy and luscious-green city on the east coast of Taiwan. The university's medical school has a curious backstory. In 1966 an idealistic nun named Master Cheng Yen left her family's movie theatre business and founded the Buddhist-inspired Tzu Chi Foundation—Tzu Chi meaning 'compassion relief' in Chinese. Her foundation later opened a hospital to look after the poor and a medical school that would train doctors who would stay on to work in what was an underprivileged area. But to get the students, administrators knew they had to do things differently. Thus, Hualien is not only known for its dramatic gorge and handsome marble, but in some circles, for its approach to dissection.

It's early Sunday morning and I'm confused to see that the large generic room is almost empty—there are about nine of us waiting in various poses on plastic chairs. I expected it to be more packed, as from all the reading I've done so far, I imagined the professor as a sort of Elon Musk of anatomy, a disruptor at the forefront of one of the most radical shifts to have taken place for the dissected in the discipline's history.

But no, there are eight of us. The other guy is checking the sound.

I take a seat in the back row, subconsciously thinking it's a comedy set; that by being in the back row I won't get heckled or asked questions. I'm also tapping my foot and looking around the room. Am I doing something wrong by being here? It's not a case of imposter syndrome—there are no competency issues as I have absolutely no idea about anatomy—it's more a sense that I'm going to get in trouble for intruding in this secret society.

Guo-Fang, bespectacled and in a dark suit, takes to the podium, a large PowerPoint presentation flaring behind him. He starts out by saying that many universities use willed bodies but the students know nothing about the person. 'It's a practice I would describe as emotionally detached,' he says, adding that the use of phrases like 'donated bodies' or 'unclaimed bodies' have a 'scary meaning'. He says the best term he has encountered is 'gifts that teach'.

'But still, we look at the thing on the dissection table as a gift, not as somebody.'

Guo-Fang says there are newspaper articles about medical schools shaking off their dark past. 'Are we?' he asks. 'How do we treat the bodies in the anatomy lab? Do we treat them as a specimen or do we treat them as a person?'

Taiwanese tradition decrees that one is supposed to protect ancestors' bodies from any damage. As a way to gently counter this cultural belief, the school developed the notion of the 'silent mentor', where donors offer their body as a teaching tool. Faculty and students also hang out with the surviving family to get a better sense of their 'great body teacher'. A few months before the dissection lab starts, the students will visit the donor's family in their homes.

'In the process, they learn the life of the donor, they get acquainted with the surviving family; and for the surviving family, they know exactly who they are talking to. By knowing they learn the life of the donor,' he says. Even surgeons doing surgical training on bodies are required to do home visits. The professor says they might be arrogant in the hospital but in the homes of the donors' families, they are humbled.

The students and family members also share elaborate blessing ceremonies. 'They go through some of the rituals so that the surviving families can be more comfortable about the donation and be at peace.' Students also organise an annual memorial concert and he was expecting 700 families that year.

He tells the story of a woman whose fifty-two-year-old husband died suddenly and who had willed his body to the university. Her husband's family were strongly opposed and thought that the wife was doing it for revenge. But she persisted and her husband's body went to the medical school. At a ceremony, she declared to the students: 'I would rather have you make twenty practice cuts on my husband than see you make any mistakes on patients.'

When I mention to people that I'm researching dissection, the first response 100 per cent of the time is about how the students will treat the bodies. Do they respect them? Guo-Fang's talk finishes and someone asks a question about jokes in the dissection room. 'I think it's fine—as long as it's not a criticism aimed at the donor,' he says. 'Jokes lighten up the learning environment. If we are very strict and very tight in the dissection room, I don't think that's a good atmosphere.'

There are some nights when I get into bed and feel gentle with myself, and smile, knowing sleep will soon take me. This moment is often brief, a pulse of contained pleasure. This is what hearing about the medical school at Hualien is like—it's so pleasant, there is no uneasiness. It is deliberately kind and loving towards the dissected, albeit a process which seems intense and time consuming. As much as I wish it were the case, I'm not sure Ruby and Julie were as revered as the donors in Hualien.

***

Perhaps my friend who envisaged anatomists wearing silly socks wasn't far off—I'd seen on Twitter that I could potentially score a pair covered with little organs at the American Association of Anatomists stall. It feels like serendipity as I'd emailed Goran the day before, letting him know that I'd be at the conference, and he replied saying he would be at the American stall at 11.30.

I have a bit of time to spare so start checking out the other stalls. I spot a large operating-size table with 'Anatomage' written on the side. A friendly Italian sales woman touches the screen and literally flicks through a body, explaining one can access thousands of CT, MRI and prosected images of four real dead people. She explains that it's version 7. This virtual dissection table sells for $78,000, which seems a lot cheaper than having to run a body donor program. I later ask an anatomist why they don't all have these tables. They remarked if you need ten of them, the costs add up, particularly as there are annual licensing fees to upgrade the software. It can thus be cheaper to use real bodies. (This was in 2021 so perhaps prices have changed since then.)

Nearby is a stall for von Hagens Plastination, where preserved kidneys and other organs are on display on a small table. It's a humble outing for Gunther von Hagens, the German anatomist who in 1977 invented plastination, a revolutionary preservation process, and went on to create his *Body Worlds* exhibition.

He and his wife, the German anatomist Dr Angelina Whalley, put on their first exhibition in 1995 at the National Science Museum in Tokyo, Japan, and over the decades, millions and millions of people have gone to their shows around the world. From their point of view, they have democratised who gets to see the dead. Gunther has given a lot of interviews but I found the most compelling discussion of *Body Worlds* was a 2008 interview Angelina gave when their show was on in Salt Lake City.

'We touched somehow a taboo in exhibiting human remains in public,' she says, and then explains while anatomy once flourished in Europe in the 17th and 18th centuries, and it was 'absolutely accepted to do public autopsies', over time it 'was finally hidden in the ivory towers of the universities—so lay people never ever had the chance to see what a real human body looks like. And now we revive this old tradition.'

'I think the understanding of the body interior and what anatomy is about ... is unfortunately, very much determined by the Hollywood industry and the horror movies around it. So in people's mind, anatomy is something very ugly and dirty and smelly, and better hidden in the basement,' she says. 'And even if people come sometimes with trepidation and say, "Well, I can hardly see a droplet of blood when I go see my doctor," they are positively surprised once they enter the exhibition that everything is so beautifully done, and that the specimens look so aesthetically appealing, and they're often extremely overwhelmed and feel that they had gained indeed, quite a different perspective of their own body, of their own inner self.'

I found it interesting to hear in her interview that they initially displayed the plastinated bodies straight, like anatomical models. But at the first show in Japan, the visitors said they looked interesting but also 'a little frightening because they look so dead'.

'And that was the moment we felt immediately reminded by the old Renaissance artists and anatomists,' she says. 'For them, it was absolutely natural to see the body in nature. And if you look at these beautiful drawings they left behind, you see, they are all in very natural, lifelike poses, and sometimes even put in nice landscapes. And we thought, "Yes, this is what we have to strive for," we have to make them appealing for laypeople, because laypeople have never been confronted—perhaps—with a dead body, and they need to look at something that is appealing, and also is relevant to their life.'

Not everyone loves their work. At a London show in 2002, a man poured red paint on the floor in protest and put a blanket over a flayed mother with a baby in her womb. One exhibit was later attacked with a hammer. In Berlin, Pastor Ernst Pulsfort held a requiem mass for the displayed corpses. 'As a Christian, I say a dead person is not only material. The human being has a spiritual dimension that is torn away here,' he declared.

Von Hagens' work splits the anatomy world. Is he an artist? Is he a showman, part of a long tradition of embalmers pushing the boundaries of what we can do with a corpse? Some are simply unimpressed. In 2018 the ethics committee of the IFAA published a paper raising 'serious' ethical concerns about von Hagens' use of plastinated human remains in commercial exhibits, as well as questioning whether it was appropriate to inspire morbid curiosity in the public.

Even though he is controversial, he's still in the serious anatomists' club—evidenced by the little stall here at the conference. It seems he's well aware of his critics, as the stall offers a one-page hand-out which addresses their objections. One side spruiks their educational materials and on the other, the headline 'Body donation—an ethical question'. In it, von Hagens outlines how all the bodies and body parts come from people who donated with willed legal consent 'for the education of future generations' and notes that many donors register after going to a *Body Worlds* show. It's definitely a shift as a few years earlier, in a Channel 4 interview aired on British television, he'd been quite comfortable talking about using unclaimed bodies.

***

I hope for some sort of anatomy osmosis experience and settling-down period but I keep feeling surreal and a little shocked, particularly looking at the LEEC Anatomical Sciences stall where there is a large metal rotational anatomy table with a dummy in a bright blue full-body leotard and curly wig lying on the bottom shelf. I called her 'Sheryl'.

On the wall beside the dummy is a poster that reads:

Rotating Anatomical Tables
Cadaver Embalming Tanks
Mobile Anatomy Tables

Prosection Cabinets
Power Assisted Cadaver Trolleys

I'm finding the list macabre, particularly the cadaver embalming tank. I pick up a Dodge price list, which is sitting on a metal tray above Sheryl in her blue leotard. Dodge is the world's largest supplier of all things embalming-related so the twenty-page price list is likely the ultimate cadaver-care shopping list—arterial chemicals, arterial dye, embalming powders, metal screw skull clamps (a pack of twenty costs around $50) and the Dodge Embalming Machine.

There's fashion too: boots, scrubs, and six different types of gloves. Later, I look up the company, which was founded in the US in 1893. In 1906, their founder Asa Johnson Dodge wrote a vivacious text called *The Essentials of Anatomy, Sanitary Science and Embalming*, which he says in the preface is basically all the questions embalming students could be asked in their exams. The book is written in a very simple style with thousands of questions and answers, which I found super informative and could've quoted for pages:

> Q: How soon after a death should a body be embalmed?
>
> A: Many would say as soon as may be after the fact that the death has taken place has been established, but my own opinion is that the work is more satisfactory if the body is placed on an incline and the blood allowed to gravitate to the dependent parts for several hours after embalming.
>
> Q: How many muscles in the human body?
>
> A: About 500

I spot Goran near the American stall. We've not met in the flesh before but I recognise him from his university headshot and go over to say hello. He's tallish, maybe in his fifties or sixties but I can't tell as there's a boyishness about him. He's politely in a rush so doesn't have time to talk but points out that Andreas Winkelmann is nearby.

The Andreas Winkelmann?

I look over and see a noticeably tall and slender man, talking to somebody, and mull over whether I should go and bug him. If I'm right, it's the same Andreas Winkelmann who published one of the most unusual documents in the history of cartography: the world's first body donor map, the one Goran had written about. Andreas, alongside Juri Habicht and Claudia Kiessling, started out wanting to know how medical schools across the world were getting their bodies.

Of 165 countries with medical schools, information was gathered for seventy-one. Of the sixty-eight countries that use cadavers for teaching, 32 per cent exclusively used donated bodies. Most other countries relied on unclaimed ones. Some countries imported cadavers from the US or India.

I go and introduce myself to Andreas.

'Why did you decide to do the map?' I ask him.

He explains he was driven to do it as he's been interested in ethical questions in anatomy for 'quite some time'. He also currently chairs an ethics committee within the IFAA, which in 2012 published recommendations that body donation should be the standard for obtaining bodies.

'If an anatomist wants to work on a body, they should do it with the informed consent of the deceased person,' he says simply. 'That's the recommendation but I was interested in what is the situation around the world. I knew that in many countries this is not standard. They are still using unclaimed bodies.

'You have countries where you only have donated bodies but you also have many countries where you just have unclaimed bodies and no donation at all—like the Arab countries and some in Africa, or East Europe.'

With data missing, Andreas says he was meeting anatomists at the conference from places including Israel and Myanmar who were going to give him more information. 'Many people do not publish on this,' he says.

He says the issue of where bodies come from is getting more important in the global anatomy community. There are more panels on body donation at conferences, and recently there was a special issue on ethics in *Anatomical Sciences Education*, a major journal. But still, not everybody cares.

'I wouldn't say that all anatomists are interested in asking this question and we will still have many anatomists who just don't care—I think? I've got no evidence for that but it feels like there's a growing interest in it,' he says.

I point out that near us are stalls selling computerised teaching models and plastinated body parts and ask if we really need dead bodies any more.

'Well, this is an ongoing debate,' he says. 'I'm quite impressed that still most anatomists in the world will say that cadavers are the basis and the most important. There are not that many that say you can replace them with 3D imaging and with your visual means.

'And even with these images you have ethical issues because as you may know The Visible Human?' I nod. 'That was one of the first projects digitising the entire body, and it was based on the body of an executed criminal, an executed murderer. And that's kind of floating around now on the internet. This is difficult from an ethical point of view. So, there are other ethical questions attached to digital images of cadavers on the internet.'

The National Library of Medicine's Visible Human Project he refers to is a dataset of a man's and a woman's cadaver, sliced into thin pieces, photographed and reconstructed. The man was 'published' in 1994 and the woman in 1995, and they have since been used to teach, in art projects, in industry and diagnostically.

The man was Joseph Jernigan, a Texan, convicted of stabbing and shooting an old man in his home during a robbery, and sentenced to death. He was killed by lethal injection in 1993, aged thirty-nine. *The Los Angeles Times* reported that as he had exercised and pumped iron for years in prison, he 'contributed a well-developed body that—though it lacked the appendix and one testicle—was a near-perfect teaching specimen'.

I looked into *why* Jernigan chose to give his body to science and there were all sorts of reasons. One report said he gave his consent to the prison chaplain. His sister said it was to save on burial costs. His attorney said, 'It was a gift.' A former cellmate said he did it so his family could sell his life story for a true-crime book. I pause when I read these—it's reminding me of Ruby and Julie's reasons, although they would not have suspected their granddaughter would write a book all these years on. And I probably won't make that much money.

It isn't clear if Jernigan consented to being frozen in a block of ice, scanned, cross-sectioned, photographed and transformed into 15 gigabytes of data accessed by the likes of scientists, artists and goths in perpetuity. People put their faith in God, body donors put their faith in anatomists, and I wonder if Jernigan really knew what was going to happen? Perhaps he was okay with his body, etched with his dragon tattoos, floating through the years. From some angles, he looks really tense, though, as if he's resisting someone about to hit him.

Even if Jernigan consented, some doctors have argued that the death penalty means any medical engagement before, during and after an execution is unethical, no matter what. The University of Colorado saw otherwise—they had been offered the prisoners on death row in Texas who had willed their bodies to science and after some discussion, saw no legal or ethical issue with it. They tried to use the body of one man who died by lethal injection but it deteriorated within 24 hours. A panel of anatomists and radiologists later had a choice between three cadavers and chose Jernigan, using a different method of preservation.

I tell Andreas I've just been to the talk about the medical school in Taiwan, and ask where this push to honour the dead is coming from—the public or anatomists themselves? Andreas was pragmatic in his reply: it is coming from anatomists who are facing a shortage of bodies, as many places do not have donation programs for cultural reasons. 'The anatomists recognise that they need relationships with the community to have donations,' he says.

I wander back into the merch area and see that Joseph Jernigan has floated to London: his life-size scanned image is emblazoned on a banner for a company called VH Dissector, which produces a computer platform for anatomy students with step-by-step dissection instructions based on his dataset. The company is managed by two people who worked on the Visible Human Project all those years ago.

***

I find a room where there are rows and rows and rows of boards with posters of anatomical research pinned to them. The odd anatomist stands in front of their little 'shop' but mostly the room is empty as people are sitting in on talks. I wander through. 'Anatomical design of a tissue engineered in vitro model of the human flexor digitorum profundus enthuses.' 'Academic body donation programs in the US: a systematic review of disclosure statements in documents of gift.' 'Body donation in Novi Sad.'

I pass poster after poster—poetry from students about body donors, technical information on breasts and skulls, anatomists as teachers, anatomists on Twitter—and feel like I'm getting in there. In my white nightgown, following the psychopomps, I feel like I'm patting away more and more cobwebs, getting closer to the outskirts of anatomy. But I also sense that people like Guo-Fang and Andreas represent one faction in one culture in the anatomical world, and there are a lot of others, including those dealing with alternative anatomical universes.

***

At this stage, I didn't like the idea of being dissected and still couldn't work out why Ruby and Julie had signed up for it. If I fantasise about my afterlife, it's usually me relaxing at Maya Maya Reef Club in Batangas in the Philippines, a seaside resort I used to hang out at when I was a child and then a teenager. I haven't been there for years so it might be a bit rundown these days but it was nirvana when I was younger. (My mum told me recently that she thinks the bartenders put alcohol in the kids' Shirley Temples, and that's why they were all so happy.)

In my afterlife, I wake up, and walk out of one of the nipa huts—traditional Filipino homes made of leaves and bamboo—and dive into the swimming pool. Next, I'm lying on a banana chair, the palm trees gently bobbing in the perfect tropical weather, and all my friends are magically there. The sun shifts in the sky and it's lunchtime, and after enjoying some BBQ chicken and rice, I hear the whirr of the blender and know that someone is making pina coladas. I don't think dissection will interrupt my afterlife fantasies but my problem with it is that even though I'm dead, I'd want someone to put a blanket on me.

I don't mind the idea of being cremated but in the various studies that have been done into body donors, they would rather be dissected as a form of body disposal, although it's a bit weird as whatever is left will be cremated in the end. We all have different fantasies and reasonings about what we want done with our bodies. It's for this reason, I find it sad that people who didn't sign up to it—especially the poor and fringe dwellers—are the ones who are likely to be dissected.

There is obviously a category of people who are absolutely fine with the idea of being dissected, including my grandparents, my partner George, some of my friends and quite a few random people I've discussed the topic with.

Some also don't see any ethical issues with using unclaimed bodies either—so what, they are dead, why let them go to waste? George is particularly passionate on the topic, arguing that we don't really own our bodies anyway. 'You could get called up for conscription to fight a war. You might be needed to work for the harvest.' He also says he's sick of the liberal, individualistic attitude towards life—he sees dissection as something you do for the community. I argue back that it's often the poor who are unclaimed. George says you could have an opt-out scheme.

I tell him that when the Anatomy Act was passed in Britain in 1832, there was an opt-out scheme where if the poor had said in their lifetime 'I don't want to be dissected' they weren't, but it was rarely adhered to. So in some parishes, the priests were getting the poor to sign a ledger which was proof they didn't want to be dissected. 'The priests were impugning shame to body donation!' declares George. 'It's okay to die of dysentery in trenches but not to be dissected in a table in a medical school!' I agreed that there was a great shame to dissection but it wasn't the priests who had instilled it. The argument continued ...

As I wandered among the posters, I wondered if perhaps there should be an annual dissection lottery so some of the rich are thrown into the mix, especially as they are the ones who often have the money to buy the best medicine. I have my moments thinking I should just do it for science, that I should answer the anatomists', doctors' and surgeons' call for the dead. They need a dead me.

I spend the next few hours wandering, talking to various anatomists about their work. Dr Bryan Bergsteedt, an anatomist at the Stellenbosch University in South Africa, studied 340 limb specimens with his colleague Linda Greyling.

The sciatic nerve starts in your lower back, courses through the bum region, and travels down the leg to the heel of your foot. It's the largest nerve we have.

Bryan and Linda dissected limbs from different backgrounds: 232 were white, seventy-eight were mixed race and thirty were Black. They found the majority of the people had a sciatic nerve and a piriformis that related to each other in a 'normal' way while around 13 per cent had variations. Donors and the unclaimed were used in the research. Some universities in South Africa have huge donor programs while others struggle. Bryan explains that some of the time his university has unclaimed bodies and the families find out that their loved ones are there. 'But because of the fact that funeral arrangements and costs ... are so high, the person prefers that the body stays at the university,' he explains. 'We will then give them a ceremony at the end and cremate those bodies and then bury them.'

He says they strive towards body donation but it's just not always possible, especially as they have such a large number of students—in the undergraduate medical program, they have 400 students in third year.

I ask him if he they have ethical discussions on the topic.

'Definitely,' he says.

Part of the issue is that there is a lot of migration from other African countries to South Africa, where men work in the mines, often not in the best of conditions, and send money back to their families. If they die, they don't have family to identify their bodies at the hospitals or at the university, which is where they end up. It can become quite complex establishing where the person is from.

Forensic scientists are now involved with identifying people and putting their details into databases. Bryan's anatomy department takes photos of the body and includes identifying markers like piercings and tattoos. This way, if an identification is somehow made, family members can be contacted to say that their person is at the university or if they are already using the body, the family can at some point find them.

Bryan stresses that he is always very respectful of the bodies he works on. 'It can be very humane,' he says. 'I went into a dissection to look at 340 limbs and some people might lose that touch but I think it's so important to remember what you are doing and what these people are ultimately giving back.'

I keep cruising the posters and stop to speak to the amiable Dr John Ahenkorah, who is the head of anatomy at the University of Ghana medical school.

I ask him what the scene was like in Ghana and what sort of research was he doing? He tells me his specialty is the placenta and I ask him if it's hard to get hold of them for research. He says, 'Well in the UK it is a different story. When I came here to do my PhD, that's when they passed the Human Tissue Act. Actually, it's not easy to really have access to the placenta, unlike back home in Ghana—it's very easy.'

'What are your body donation programs like?' I ask.

'Well, this story is different because people don't usually donate. It's coming up now—a few body donations where people come and sign up. Where we get our bodies from are from the police—unclaimed bodies.'

John explains that the police put an advertisement in the newspaper saying they were doing a mass burial and that people must claim the bodies. The dead aren't necessarily criminals either—they might be an unknown person found in the street. The bodies that aren't claimed end up at the medical school and John estimates they get between twenty and twenty-five each year.

My next stop is Dr Htin Linn from the University of Medicine in Yangon, Myanmar who says they only use donated bodies, and a large percentage of them are monks and nuns, who also actively encourage people in the community to donate. He says from January to July in 2019, nearly 2000 people came into the university offering their bodies for medical research.

Htin says while they have enough bodies, they can only really accept old people who died from heart conditions and can't take cancer patients because it can be difficult embalming them. He says they are testing new methods of preserving people that use low amounts of formalin.

I wonder why. 'It is more expensive?'

'It is more expensive and another thing is most of these techniques—no formalin or low formalin need cold chambers, freezers to keep the bodies.'

'And you don't have any of that?'

'Yeah. We are trying to get one.'

I'm trying to stay focused on body donors but absolutely cannot resist the poster entitled: 'The "good", the "bad" and the "ugly"; anatomical accuracy in pre-Vesalian British mortuary sculpture by Christina Welch and Wendy Birch'. There are two women in front of the poster but as they are busy talking to someone, I lean in to read the blurb:

> Introduction: This poster shows images of three carved cadavers each presenting a different anatomical aspect of a British cadaver sculpture from the late medieval / Early Modern period. Cadaver sculptures are a marginalized research area per se.

There is a photograph of a sculpture of Bishop Richard Fox at Winchester cathedral, who died in 1528. His life-size, naked and emaciated face and body—made of grey stone—isn't looking too good. His cheeks are sunken. His mouth is ajar, as if he is gasping for breath. The poster blurb claims that the sculptors of this macabre artwork had access to recently dead and emaciated bodies, as the upper arms show signs of rigor mortis. What sort of complex religious thinking was going on at the time that would lead a wealthy cleric to be portrayed on his grave naked and anorexic?

The two women have finished their conversation and are ready to talk.

'How did you end up here today?' I ask them.

Christina explains she's been working on the cadaver sculptures for eight years, and that she's a religious studies scholar. She runs a masters program in death studies at the University of Winchester and one of her keynote speakers was the anatomical sculptor Eleanor Crook, who told her to speak to Wendy, who does 'proper anatomy'.

Wendy introduces herself and declares: 'I'm a forensic anatomist. I work at University College London, I teach medical students anatomy by dissection, and I found a new passion.'

A few years earlier, Christina showed Wendy photos of Bishop Fox, and straight off the anatomist could see that whoever sculpted the work had first-hand experience of bodies with rigor mortis, and that other sculptures suggested some knowledge of evisceration and disembowelling.

But in others, they weren't so sure what inspired the art. Wendy points at Sir Roger Rockley of Worsbrough's quite cute-looking cadaver circa 1524 and remarks: 'These intestines are completely round the wrong way. However, you get a similar sort of effect if you are disembowelling someone.' She's right about the intestines—they are vertical in the body.

Christina adds: 'The sculptor may very well have gone to see a hanging, drawing and quartering, and hence the strange intestines.'

Wendy is also a forensic osteologist and says she used to look out for 'skulls and things' in churches but is now also on the lookout for soft tissue on the skeletons.

Another picture on the poster is of an unknown individual—perhaps a priest—laid bare in the church of St John the Baptist in Cambridgeshire. His backbone peeps out from inside the ribcage. You can see vertebrae discs distinctive in the pale wood.

'I had the wood radiocarbon dated to around about 1400,' explains Christina. 'By the time that had dried out and been sculpted, it probably comes from around about 1410–1415. It's probably the earliest in England. But this is unique. I've not found a single one anywhere else in the world. He's just really amazing and eviscerated.'

A sculpture showing signs of rich anatomical knowledge before Vesalius in the UK seems like major historical news.

'Have you sent ripples through the anatomy world'? I ask.

'No,' says Christina. 'I write and put stuff in humanities books, because I'm a Religious Studies scholar. But now, we're bringing it into anatomy!'

'This is its introduction to the world of anatomy,' says Wendy.

'What's the story with the different feet? Can you just talk me through them?' I point to the poster, which features eleven different carved feet.

'The anatomy of the feet is completely wrong,' says Wendy sadly.

Part of the reason is that the particular scooping tool the artists used—according to artist Eleanor Crook—would've made it quite difficult to make it anatomically correct.

Christina then really throws me when she remarks that she's also looking into the theology behind the sculptures and part of it is related to thinking around the bowel. 'The theology of the bowel?!!!' I scribble in my notebook under 'Eleanor Crook'.

My jet lag is starting to really kick in so I say goodbye and find coffee. I move to another room to watch an impressive 3D anatomical software presentation, and start to see why people argue that the anatomists can get by without bodies. I doze, and fall into a cycle of nodding off to sleep and then jolting myself awake.

I drift to the train, and hazily daydream about the treasure box of anatomy content now on my lap—the gold coins of body donation, the ravishing ethical dilemma silks and strange theology of bowel amulets, all illuminating my face in a pale yellow light.

I really study my lanyard for some reason, and notice the crest for the anatomical society features a lion with its paw on a skull, a dissected man and a female nude. I later read that the lion represents the veterinarians and the female nude is for the artists. The motto *ex conformatione usus* means 'from structure comes function'. (A motto applicable to writers too.)

So while I have this treasure, I know I'm missing the most precious item—an insight into the anatomy labs where Ruby and Julie went all those years ago.

Chapter 10

The anatomist Dr Walter Wood taught anatomy to University of Queensland medical students from 1973 to 2001, not long after Ruby's body left and while Julie's was there. In 2016 Walter gave an interview to ABC radio, which was billed as his discussing 'first-hand how body donors advance the cause of medical science'.

I was anticipation personified listening to it, a cat poised and frozen, waiting to pounce. What was he going to say? Much of the interview was about Walter's work in Papua New Guinea but eventually presenter Richard Fidler asked him about his time with the body donor program.

'What was the procedure?' he asked.

'The donor, when they pass away, the body is removed very quickly to the university precincts, usually within a day or two of death and it is immediately embalmed,' said Walter. 'It takes about three or four months or more for the embalming fluids to completely spread through the whole body, destroy all the bacteria and fix the tissues.'

'How does the embalming fluid spread through the body without a heartbeat or a pulse?' asked Fidler.

'What has to happen is that a little incision is made in the groin into the big artery that's just in that region called the femoral artery, and they put a catheter into the artery and they connect the catheter to a pump and a cylinder full of embalming fluid,' he said. 'Or it may be just gravity, they lift the bottle up to a certain height, and gravity will force it through the blood vessels so it spreads around the blood vessels. There is blood in them but it's basically clotted, but the fluid works its way past and gets right out to the fingers and the toes and the head.'

He explained that the body was then placed in a cold storage room, and kept at around four degrees centigrade, which stops the body from deteriorating. 'The only thing they have to look out for is if a mould may develop sometimes on some of the bodies.' Mould?! 'But they're stored in a storage room until the following academic year, when they would be brought out and placed on a table in the dissection room and over the next twelve months—the body is usually fully dissected.'

Fidler asked: 'Every part of the body?'

'It depends on the actual body itself. Some bodies may have parts that are not usable. For instance, a dentist is more interested in the head and neck. The physiotherapists are very interested in the limbs and the back. Surgeons are very interested in the abdomen and the thorax.' He went on to discuss what happens when they are finished with the bodies, as well as donor ceremonies.

I suddenly had this startling new sense of the size of the cave and universe I was walking and swimming into by the end of the interview. Embalming? Mould? I slumped a little. I really don't like mould. Glancing down, seeing my nightie was still quite clean, I knew it was going to have to get a lot dirtier. Did I want this?

***

In March 1967 Ruby had to quit a job she had been doing since she was fourteen. She was just sixty-three. Julie had that morning dropped her off at the grand-looking Norman Park Primary School, which opened in 1900, the year education for children aged six to twelve was made compulsory in Queensland. She stood in the street, and looked up at the school, the charming old brick facade framed by trees, and walked up the formal entrance stairs.

At the top, she looked back over the city, taking in the expansive view over Brisbane. She headed inside for what she knew would be the last time, dreading saying goodbye to all the children she had watched grow up, as well as friends she had worked with for years. Her red book says:

> I had worked all those years and God knows it was hard. Big classes up to seventy-five—year in, year out.

But she felt loved as a teacher:

> My life for the past 11 years at Norman Park School has been a record of 'well done'. Before my marriage, the late Mr. Faron in my presentation speech said 'Miss Ruby not only has had the knack of teaching children, but in making their lives at school something to remember always'. And I can say without hesitation, the same is said today. The parents of Norman Park School hold me in great esteem.

She sat at the kitchen table that night, glancing at the phone, wondering if she should call her estranged sisters Dolly and Kate. Even though they weren't talking, she felt it was time to patch things up and let them know about her diagnosis: adenocarcinoma of the uterus. Cancer.

Ruby was to die two years later from this disease, which also killed actress Anne Bancroft, first lady of Argentina Eva Peron and 19th century computer programming pioneer Ada Lovelace. She was killed by a condition which has been possibly recorded since antiquity but has always been difficult to diagnose.

As the British gynaecologist Edward Rigby wrote in 1857:

> an accurate diagnosis of this disease in its early stages would indeed be most desirable, but from the nature of it, and of the organ it involves, a medical man has seldom opportunity of examining it at this period, and even if he has, symptoms are at best of an obscure and doubtful character.

When Ruby fell ill with cancer, treatment options were better than they had been in the past, when cancer of the uterus left untreated was a slow, painful, and terrible death. Women bled violently. They secreted foul-smelling substances. Opiates often didn't control the pain. The suffering was so awful that doctors were moved to try radical treatments, and the dying process was so repulsive that women were often abandoned both by their families and charities.

This is what makes a young widow named Jeanne Françoise Garnier Chabot all the more fascinating. In 1842 she founded *L'Association des Dames du Calvaire* or the Association of the Ladies of Calvary in Lyon, France for the sole purpose of caring for women with advanced uterine cancers. In her fascinating biography of cervical cancer, the medical historian and feminist Ilana Löwy writes that these pious widows 'washed these women, changed their dressings, and attended to their daily needs, persuaded that overcoming their disgust while doing these tasks allowed them to be closer to Christ'.

Luckily, when Ruby was diagnosed—unlike the women before her who had died in such dreadful pain—there were better treatment options but in her case perhaps she left it a bit late. She had noticed spotting, some bleeding, but didn't think it was anything. But when it worsened, she didn't go to the doctor. In the 1960s most doctors were men, and she—like most women back then and some today—would have been embarrassed about discussing female issues as it would have led to an examination.

She eventually saw a doctor, and then a specialist.

In Australia in 1967 to 1970, treatment involved radiotherapy, followed by a total hysterectomy, a lymphadenectomy and bilateral sapling-oophorectomy, which is the removal of tubes and ovaries. The treatment varied depending on whether the upper half or lower half of the uterus was involved, and the degree of the spread.

Ruby had surgery but continued to decline over time, and was eventually admitted to Princess Alexandra Hospital in South Brisbane. She died on 6 December 1969. She was so young, really: only sixty-four. Whereas some donors cannot be accepted because of their cancer, this wasn't the case with Ruby.

It was a warm December day in Brisbane. A man from the funeral company Cannon & Cripps drove to the hospital to collect Ruby but there was a problem once he arrived.

***

Mum mentioned that Ruby was interested in disease so I went back to her diary, looking for signs of illnesses.

Back in Boulder, as Ruby's mother Eleanor stood watching her home burn to the ground, did something tip over in her mind? Ruby wrote that her mother subsequently had a 'brain fever', which is a term that doesn't exist any more but it was certainly a condition described in medical textbooks and 19th-century novels. When Heathcliff returned to Wuthering Heights, Catherine was so stressed out, she developed 'brain fever' and later died. Madame Bovary fell ill with 'une fièvre cérébrale' after she read the break-up letter from Rodolphe, her lover. Fyodor Dostoyevsky gave various characters 'brain fever'.

At the time, the condition was seen as some sort of inflammation of the brain, severe and prolonged. The Scottish doctor Alexander Tweedie described it in 1833 as caused by famine, fatigue, and those events which give 'a severe shock to the nervous system. The various kinds of mental emotion—fear, anxiety, disappointments, long continued watching on a sick bed, intense study, want of sleep may individually be ranked among the predisposing causes of fever.' My great-great-great-grandmother Caroline Clowes was a diarist; in an entry from April 1828, she wrote of friend John Lea that: 'He had not returned from London, but from over exertion was taken with brain fever, & died at his brother's house at Hampstead.' So it was also potentially deadly.

Eleanor's brain-fevered illness followed the family to Yarraman, an obscure, tiny timber town in Queensland enveloped in pine forests. From milk to gold to wood. Elder brother Thomas was going to run the Queensland Pine Company mill and Ruby's father Maurice was promoted to foreman.

Yarraman's wide, main dirt road was scattered with a handful of new buildings made from pine and hardwood cut down from the thick bush right on its doorstep. There was no running water but there were horse races, a pastime that Eleanor would get pleasure from for the rest of her life. It was quiet but for the whine of the sawmill and the intermittent boom of falling logs.

In 1913 a train line finally came to the tiny community of 400 people, its opening day luring smart businessmen in motor cars from nearby Nanango, and bearded and legginged timber selectors and getters from the rugged hills and scrubs. They watched the speeches and the school children singing Australia's national anthem. The ruggedness meant it was common for local men to go for a stroll and get completely lost—in one instance a man went missing for days, only to be discovered just one kilometre from the post office.

Surrounded by heavy bush and the main street lit only by the moon at night, the remoteness of this frontier town made Ruby fearful of her mother Eleanor's death:

> As a child, I can remember crying myself to sleep every night, my fear that my mother would die before help could arrive. She had varicose veins, which later on were operated on. But at the time, we lived in a small country town and I was continually told that if they burst she would bleed to death. My eldest sister also shared this worry, but I did not know of this till many years later.

But it was Maurice who was to nearly die when he was jammed between two timber trucks, and left badly hurt across the back and the stomach. Luckily he was found.

The sisters—there were three of them now—stood out in the small town but Eleanor wasn't that interested in what they did or wore. 'Our mother never took us anywhere that was left to our father. Those little girls the prettiest in the town we were called but allowed to run wild and never properly dressed.' Eleanor rarely went out. The only time she did venture into public life was after eight years of living in Yarraman. She had no choice—the family were leaving for Brisbane and the town held a public send-off for her husband, who had been held in high esteem:

> At that time, my mother would have been in her 40th year and yet people had never seen her. Why? She was young and good looking, and yet a recluse*, and bought no clothes herself. We weren't poor. My father was foreman, later manager of a timber mill, my mother carried on a guesthouse for a few years.

Eleanor's deep lack of interest in dressing her daughters didn't really matter in obscure Yarraman. But it did in Brisbane. At just fourteen, Ruby was a pupil teacher at Dutton Park Primary School but was, mortifyingly, sent home one day. As Ruby wrote: 'The headmistress of the school sent for my mother to tell her to improve my standard of dress.'

There's a buzz to Ruby's early frontier life, shared by millions of white Australians rolling out of the cities into the wilds to get by. But it was also the start of—again not a unique story in an age where there was no penicillin—illnesses nonetheless. Eleanor's terrible varicose veins could have ruptured and led to a serious amount of blood loss, even death. But what about her mental state? Was it brain fever or what we would nowadays call PTSD? Or was she just lazy? Ruby grappled with it:

> All my life my mother has posed—I use that word freely now—as an invalid for it is beyond all conception that any person could reach the age of 81 without considerable medical attention, if such were the case and this she never required.

It reads as if Eleanor lived with some form of depression or hypochondria in an era when so little was known about mental health, nor was there

---

* Dad doesn't think Eleanor was that reclusive. She was running a boarding house.

much therapy. In 1931 the American psychiatrist Smith Ely Jelliffe referred to hypochondria as 'a strange child in the psychopathological family'.

Hypochondria aside, I find illness and disease interesting too. My friend Mel says I love a bit of medical drama in my life—which is true. When I'm sick, I often wish I could watch a cartoon of the story of the infection or ailment.

Is there some genetic memory in all this? I can't gauge if the idea that some form of memory comes down through the generations is good, bad or pseudoscience, but it's curious to contemplate. In trying to feel and grasp the motivation behind Ruby's donation, I share her interest in disease but not the donation part just yet. Or is my interest in disease different, like my mother's? She was a nurse so obviously into medicine. And did Mum in turn inherit it from Dr William Clowes, her great-grandfather nine times back who was a barber-surgeon and influential medical writer in England, publishing *A prooued practise for all young chirurgians, concerning burnings with gunpowder, and woundes made with gunshot, sword, halbard, pike, launce, or such other* in 1591 and *A right frutefull and approoued treatise, for the artificiall cure of that malady called in Latin Struma, and in English, the evill, cured by kinges and queenes of England: Very necessary for all young practizers of chyrurgery* in 1602?

I imagine Ruby standing by the kitchen sink, weary from a long day of teaching, doing the washing-up for her mother, who lies inexplicably in bed. Feeling powerless, she thinks to herself: if only the doctors, if only the experts, if only someone knew what was wrong with her mother. What on earth did she have?

Chapter 11

Gareth Jones, a professor of anatomy at the University of Otago, did the first ever study into body donors in 1992. I ask Gareth—who is now retired—what prompted him to do it in the first place and he says simply: 'Just out of sheer interest. I mean why? Why do people bequeath their bodies? It's not a normal sort of thing to do. I'm inquisitive. I ask questions all the time about everything and this is one of the questions,' he says. 'If you are surrounded by these things—at that time, we had all these filing cabinets full of all the paperwork on all the donors. I would be fascinated to know why people are acting as they do. That's what led me to do it.'

A questionnaire was sent to people on the bequest list whose names started with 'J', some of whom had been signed up since the 1960s. Replies from 108 women and sixty-one men soon drifted in, with the majority of donors saying they wanted to aid medical science and teaching in some way, and to thank the medical profession. Around 10 per cent wanted to avoid funeral costs and six people specifically said they disliked funerals and unnecessary rituals. Some donors also thought that perhaps the students might find their illnesses interesting—things like albinism, multiple brain surgeries, gynaecological abnormalities and artificial joints.

While these responses were collected two decades after Ruby donated, I could see her in the research: altruism, helping science, an interest in disease.

Since Gareth's 1992 study, the identity of donors has itself been anatomised and analysed. Some of it is just straight data. At Peking Union Medical College in China, they tend to be men who are significantly older than the general Beijing population. In Brazil, single, widowed or divorced white women who are religious, middle-class and highly educated tend to sign up. In Thailand, the average age of donors is sixty-nine. Women are more likely to register than men but men are more likely to arrive in the dissecting hall. Overall, they tend to be non-religious. In the US, African Americans are 50 per cent less likely to donate than white people.

But more intriguing are the donor's motivations. From studies in Turkey to Hong Kong to Denmark to Mississippi to Otago, wanting to help science and medicine in some way always tops the list, followed by variations on having no family to put on your funeral, avoiding funeral costs or a dislike of funerals or cremation. Saving relatives money and inconvenience also pops up. But I think my favourite reason would come to be that some people found their bodies interesting and thought doctors might too.

There are of course rich, distinct cultural motivations. The anatomist İlke Ali Gürses studied the tiny pool of body donors in Turkey, and while he found they largely did it to be useful to medical education and research, some had anti-religious reasons: 'I believe in science and nature. So I wanted to leave my body to either one. It would be hypocritical to leave it (my body) to Islam or God.' İlke also found some body donors became angry during interviews when they found out their next of kin could stop their donation—it was clearly a wish that was important to them.

In Hong Kong, where body donation is rare, researchers in 2012 interviewed two body donors—women from poor backgrounds—who also basically said they wanted to contribute to their society but a Ms L also mentioned she didn't want to waste any space in crowded Hong Kong when she died.

On the whole, some form of altruism is a common pattern but those bothersome researchers wanted to unpick this idea a bit more. One of them was the Dutch cultural anthropologist Sophie Bolt, who I would describe as the queen of body donor research in this extremely small space—she has really gone for it in terms of studying this group.

When we eventually meet online, I behave like a fan-girl of sorts, as not only has she looked deeply into this tribe, her curiosity seeps through her academic papers. I also feel like I'm meeting a long-lost friend as we'd been emailing on and off for months, and then she was struck down with Covid-19 for seven weeks. Sophie now works at the not-for-profit Fiom, which is focused on issues surrounding unwanted pregnancies, adoption and donor sperm.

'Sorry! This is the noise of our coffee machine,' she says as soon as we start talking.

'I can't hear it.'

'You cannot hear it? I can hear it,' she says, laughing, and then launches into how she fell into the unusual world of whole-body donation by chance after being offered a spot doing a PhD in the Department of Religion at Radboud University in the city of Nijmegen, near the German border. The university has the rather friendly motto of *In Dei nomine feliciter*, which means 'Happily in the name of God'.

The department was running the Refiguring Death Rites project, which wanted to look into new rituals and religious ideas around death and dying, and they asked her to research alternative body disposal. She initially looked into cryogenics—people who are frozen after death in the hope they can come back to life—but found herself more fascinated by body donation. At the time, only around 650 people in Holland donated each year—a tiny 0.1 per cent of the population were registered as whole-body donors. This small number is enough though and medical schools regularly have to stop accepting them.

In 2008 Sophie started working alongside Peter Gerrits, an anatomist at the University Medical Centre in Groningen, a pretty university town in the north of the country. Surveys were sent out to 996 body donors on their database asking them why they wanted to donate, and if they were open to being interviewed in a more in-depth way about their motivations. Sophie was stunned when they got 759 replies to the survey, and that nearly 500 wanted to be interviewed. Clearly, the donors wanted to talk! Sophie sat down in the homes of seventeen body donors, including four couples, and spoke to three on the phone.

From there, she travelled around Holland visiting eight anatomical institutes, touring their labs and interviewing anatomists, secretaries and prosectors. Sophie also spent time with first-year medical students, watching them, and taking notes about their behaviour as they looked at prosected body parts.

She interviewed the undertaker who drove donor bodies to the crematorium, and hung out with staff who helped cremate them. Sophie climbed on board a boat and watched the donors' ashes scattered in the North Sea, their final resting place. She went to donor funerals and spent time with their families.

The notion of altruism and 'doing good' dominate theories about gift-giving but Sophie was drawn to the work of the French sociologist and anthropologist Marcel Mauss, who pioneered work on gift giving in the 1920s, which he saw as binding people in ways that went beyond the gift itself. He was particularly interested in this idea of *do et dis*: 'I give so that you may give,' which entails some sort of obligation to reciprocate. Basically, he believed that gifts are never free and Sophie saw that his ideas could be useful in understanding the meaning-making that went into body donation.

So by giving, what were the donors getting? It seems all sorts of things. Sophie found that some donors had ongoing arguments in their families and they knew that when they died, their relatives would manage their funerals. 'They didn't want that. By giving their body away, they had some control,' she says. In some instances, they didn't want a specific family member to be at their funeral. It was also a way of expressing their identity. One man named Paul was proud to finally have the opportunity to go to university. His daughter told Sophie he was always telling people at birthday parties, 'When I die, I'm going to university', because it was something he'd always wanted. 'The university had status,' says Sophie.

So while the donors' answers collectively showed an overwhelming desire to be useful after death in some way, Sophie and her fellow researchers got a sense of donors' motivations. She then came up with the radical proposition that instead of donor campaigns just focusing on altruism, they could also include the idea of personal achievement. *Hey! Reach your goal by getting dissected!*

After spending more time with donors, Sophie also started noticing something quite striking: an intensity. 'We have a word for that in Dutch—when someone is strong-minded we call them "pittig", which means spicy. If you eat something and it's spicy we say "Oooh! It's pittig", but we also give it to people as well,' she says. 'The body donors had strong opinions.'

Whereas sons and daughters will follow their parents into law or farming, Sophie also discovered another unique family tradition: whole-body donation. It was also a thing with couples. 'When the husband dies, he asks his wife "Oh, I will die and if you die, we can end up together in the dissection lab, like in a romantic way?!"' Sophie's voice is initially filled with amazement but then turned to concern as she thought about one of the donors she spoke to. With too many body donations in the Netherlands, one woman she spoke to is concerned she won't be needed by the university and will be unable to fulfil her husband's dying wish. 'She was really worried. "I promised him. It's so important that I go as well but then maybe I won't be accepted. It would be horrible."'

'I told the anatomists—you should really think about the person left behind ... you should really let her know that she will be accepted.' She asks me if my grandparents were in a Romeo and Juliet scenario—if they had a pact to go to the dissection hall. I don't think so, but can't be sure.

Chapter 12

Dad lies on the couch watching *Hogan's Heroes*, the 1960s sitcom about a group of Americans in a Nazi prison camp during the Second World War. He's fine with me researching his parents—I think he quite enjoys it—but he is not at all effusive in his revelations about them. I'm sort of getting a grip on what happened but still can't work out why. How did they hear about it? Did someone mention it to Ruby at lunch one day? While Mum says they did it for altruistic reasons, I ask him why he thinks his parents donated.

'To save money,' he says casually, still watching the show.

Oh.

I wasn't expecting that answer but it is an issue that has popped up in the donor research.

For decades, as an enticement to get people to donate, universities covered the costs of a body donor's cremation or burial, effectively saving a family a fair chunk of money. These days, a simple cremation in Sydney can cost up to $4000. Getting dissected is certainly a way to save money but really?

A worry about money certainly permeates Ruby's red book throughout her life, beginning when she was a teenager:

> Later I have learned that not only my father was a racing man but she [Eleanor] as well followed the horses. These little things I point out as they have to my mind a definite bearing on all our lives. We sold our home in the country and moved to Brisbane. Soon, all the money was gone on races and the only thing left a block of land taken in payment of a debt.

> I always wanted a nice home, and was always spending any spare money to make things more livable, but did not have a great deal at my command. Every Saturday, saw my parents at the races, then I began to pester my father to build on the land he owned before that went too, and after many negotiations, we were able to start a home of our own, let me say that it was eventually furnished room by room by me as my mother was not a homemaker. I thought in those days that my father squandered all the money on races and I deemed myself responsible over and over to give her a nice home.

Stresses about money hovered in the lives of most people a century ago and in 1928, a particular agony struck Ruby and her family. It was the summer holidays. Ruby's younger brother Maurice lay in his tent on a camping trip on the Gold Coast with family friends when he complained of feeling sick. A day or two passed. He vomited, pain laced his body. Perhaps the friends initially thought it was just a stomach bug but by the time they drove back to Brisbane, the thirteen-year-old's appendix had burst, releasing deadly bacteria into his abdomen.

The blood drained from all their faces as they waited in the halls of Rochford Private Hospital on Gregory Terrace, one of a number of private hospitals scattered throughout the city and the suburbs. While penicillin—the drug that could have saved him—was invented that year, it was not widely available until 1946. Surgery was risky.

> I became engaged to be married and was to go live in Richmond. Then tragedy struck and my only brother met an untimely death. At that time, I was teaching in Charleville and I obtained department leave for a year to be in Brisbane and during this time, I gave my mother my paycheck to do with as she wanted, as a big expense had been incurred with my brother's death.

An ache seeps into me as I read through Maurice's 1928 death certificate. So young.

> Occupation: Schoolboy
> Age: 13 years
> Duration of illness: 1 week
> Cause of death: Gangrenous Appendicitis, Septia Absorption, Heart Failure
> If deceased was married (where, at what age, to whom) = a blank box
> The names and ages of children = a blank box

The specialist bills at the Rochford Private Hospital on Gregory Terrace threw the family, as did the funeral costs, the equivalent of nearly a month's wage for an average worker back then:

> Then followed the depression. The man I eventually married was among the unemployed, which delayed our marriage for some years.

These days, the free cremation on offer is undoubtedly an inducement for some people. One anatomist told me that the university gets calls from people saying, 'oh my mother died and she really wanted to donate' and he can sense they are looking for a free cremation. Other anatomists have said the fact that only poorer people tend to donate is an issue that needs to be addressed more broadly in the profession.

As I slowly sift through the canon of studies into body donors and why they do it, only a small percentage say they are doing it to save money. I suspect that on some of these surveys people tick altruism to appear more noble—or as pollsters call it 'the social desirability bias'. Perhaps the respondents to a 2022 British study were daring to be a bit more frank with nearly a third saying there were savings to be made in donation.

Ruby, Julie, my dad and his brother Maurie lived with Eleanor for quite a few years. Ruby writes in her red book of being obliged to look after her mother—practically an invalid and still suffering from her mysterious illness—and even paid her mortgage in the belief that one day the house would be theirs.

Julie won 1000 pounds in the Golden Casket, Queensland's lottery and wanted to move out but Ruby frustratingly stayed. I too at this point am screaming *Move out! Move out!*

The lottery money went towards a new car and a final mortgage payment, and it was then Ruby discovered that the house wasn't hers at all. While Eleanor had said it would be, the reality was different—her will said it would go to Ruby and her two sisters. 'You have just been paying rent here,' Eleanor said. Others in the family also saw it that way. Ruby was devastated and the family moved out. Despite the troubles with her mother, she loved Julie:

> Much might be said against my husband but his jealousy was his only fault. Otherwise, a kinder man could not exist. I blamed the depression for that it did something to decent men's souls but we have loved each other dearly all our lives and had it not been for my mother's indifference we could say we had a happily married life.

Chapter 13

The dead man lies on a table, surrounded by Dr E.S. Meyers and six dental students in white coats. Some smile, some don't. A board reading 'Dentistry 1927', a human skull and neatly arranged dissection tools rest against him. He looks like the bog man, mummified in peat or an unwrapped Egyptian pharaoh, his darkness in contrast to the white lab coats of the students. The photograph may seem cruel to us now but back then, it was the norm for students to pose with the person they were dissecting.

As far as the genre goes, this one emits an unusual warmth—there are no cigarettes in the dead man's mouth or playing cards in his hand. These portraits often show the dead in a silly pose, which many attribute to a coping mechanism—gallows humour. But in this portrait, the man is not mocked in any way.

The dead man in the photograph was the first person to be dissected at the University of Queensland and he was more than likely from Goodna, which at the time was Queensland's oldest and largest mental asylum, and a major source of legal bodies for dissection. It still exists today but under a different name. It is estimated that between 1865 and the mid-1980s, over 50,000 patients lived there.

Who is the man on the table? He may have been the man who escaped in January 1927 and told police that he wandered around, and survived on grass and water. Perhaps he overheard attendants at the asylum discussing their plans to strike that year over demands for increased wages, extra uniforms and better working conditions. Whoever he was, in 1927 Queensland Cabinet had approved that he and fellow inmates at Goodna, as well as patients from the Diamantina Hospital, could be sent to one of the six tables at the anatomy school.

During the war years, bodies also came from Dunwich Benevolent Asylum.

The photo comes from the collection of a Mrs Bagnall, which means it's more than likely that her husband, Ernie Bagnall, took the shot. Ernie started out as an errand boy at the Anatomy Department at the University of Sydney in 1923 and was poached to be 'Technical Assistant' at the new Anatomy School in Brisbane. In applying for the job, Ernie wrote he had 'good general knowledge of the requirements such as the preservation and preparation of bodies for the Dissecting Room with colour injection, the mounting of specimens, maceration of bones, lantern-slide making and histological technique'.

So much of dissection—in fact its whole history—is about the 'great' anatomists, surgeons and scientists, many of their names living on inside our bodies despite the campaign to stop this happening. There is also a lot of focus on the medical students—anatomical papers are about the best ways to teach them, how they coped during Covid-19, how they feel about the bodies or learning from computers. You don't hear much about the technicians—people like Ernie who made the place tick over.

I volunteered for a project in London years ago where I visited old people who were lonely. As I'd volunteered in a hospice in Sydney, they assigned me people who were dying and I began visiting a sweet woman in her seventies, slowly fading from lung cancer. I saw her at her home and then in hospital in Hackney, where she would eventually die. The youngest of three sisters, two of them already dead, she didn't really have anybody else in her life and I was eventually to find out why. As we drank tea, she shared aspects of her existence, including the one job she'd had all her life—one I'd never really heard of before.

For decades, she cleaned hospital operating theatres—all the silver trays, knives, tubes and sheets, all the blood and fleshy bits left over from surgery. It was a time when they didn't chuck everything out so literally everything had to be washed, sterilised and ready for operations the next day. She always worked the late shift—often cleaning until midnight—which meant she never really made friends nor had time for romance.

I once asked her why they kept her on that shift for so long; why she didn't ask for better hours.

She remarked that she never thought to ask, that it wasn't her place. I empathised with her—all those years cleaning up blood, fat and guts at night, alone, not going out, not having the confidence to ask for something better. But her ghost will forever be in that operating theatre. She made surgery happen. She helped it tick over. She's also voiceless.

The cliche is that there are two sides to a story but it should be rewritten to say there are nine, fifteen or twenty-two sides. I knew I needed characters like her and Ernie as I began hunting around for people from the past.

Chapter 14

At fifteen, Lorraine Sampson's parents moved to a cattle farm in Central Queensland and she spent the last two years of high school living in a girls' hostel in Brisbane. She didn't want to go back to the farm, a place so hot in summer she wasn't sure if she'd ever survive it. In that era, girls focused on their glory box, and collected items for their trousseau. They got married, they embroidered. If you weren't at the altar by twenty-two, *tut-tut she's too old and unlikely to find a husband.* Lorraine didn't care about any of that: she didn't want to settle down. She wanted to be a doctor and in 1957, she arrived at the University of Queensland. 'There was a lot of status in going to medical school. There was a lot of status in doctors and in science,' she recalls.

Those first few days she quickly realised she had a powerful incentive to study: a lot of people were destined to fail—40 per cent in the first year, 50 per cent in the second year and 30 per cent in third. 'There was no specific mark for entry but staying in the course was like winning an Olympic medal.' The situation was particularly brutal for women—their wages were so low that without wealthy parents or a scholarship, they could not earn enough to study and live for a year. It was less of a problem for the men, as they could earn enough money to repeat if they failed a subject. Sexism was hard-wired into the system. 'It was full-on straightaway and extremely difficult,' she says. 'It was very hard work.'

I'm speaking to Lorraine on a hot summer's day just before Christmas, at her apartment in Darling Point overlooking busy New South Head Road, the air-con buzzing in the background. Lorraine studied at the University of Queensland twelve years before Ruby's body arrived but I feel a wary excitement as to what she is about to say, her words the first thread into the dissecting hall.

Lorraine managed to survive as she had a Commonwealth scholarship and the support of an aunt who was a war widow without children, and who gave her 100 pounds to buy textbooks and use as a small living allowance. Throughout her degree, Lorraine lived with women in various apartments, and always made her own clothes as she couldn't afford to buy new ones. They didn't go out much either and even if one had a pretty dress, where to wear it?

Lorraine also found Brisbane boring, and backwards. 'There was censorship of books, there was censorship of plays,' she recalls.

Once Lorraine finished her medical degree, she moved to Sydney. I really feel the sigh of reassurance and relaxation in her voice when she says it was a relief to leave Brisbane behind. 'You could read whatever books you liked. Roman Catholics could be friends with Protestants,' she says. I suddenly have an image of her as a cultivated and frustrated young woman, lamenting on the lawn at the University of Queensland to her friends that she couldn't read D.H. Lawrence's *Lady Chatterley's Lover* or Balzac.

She began anatomy at the end of first year, studying arm and leg bones, and more detailed structures of the arm. It was around this time that she also purchased a box of bones—it was a full skeleton. 'My skeleton had betel nuts on his teeth,' she says, adding that she later sold him on to another student.

In second year, Lorraine arrived at the anatomy lab, which in those days was in one of the large wooden US army huts in downtown Victoria Park left behind from the Second World War. The first day she walked in, as the distinct smell of formalin hit her, she could also see two long parallel lines of bodies laid out on big benches. They were wrapped up in cloths so they didn't dry out.

'They didn't put them in the fridge at night?' I ask.

'No,' she pauses. 'Not at all. And you must remember, Brisbane is hot. But they were all preserved in formalin.'

She was allocated a body according to her surname—she was in the S to T group—and there were twelve students to a group, six on each side.

A lecturer would talk about a particular part, and then the demonstrators would help the students with dissecting. She thinks she also worked bare-handed. 'These days, you couldn't contemplate doing dissection without gloves,' she says.

I'm obviously curious to know how she saw the person on the table. She remembers it was a man. 'I don't know anything about the age of the guy we had. I suppose it really wasn't very relevant. He was just a cadaver that we're working on. It wasn't as though he was a person.' On the table next to her lay a somewhat plump woman. Another group discovered their man had tuberculosis and stopped working on him. One body had a tattoo. I tell her that in a handful of medical schools these days some students come to know the person they are dissecting and their family, and she's not really into that idea. 'I wouldn't have liked to meet the family members of the cadaver. You could disassociate from the person if it's impersonal. It's just learning.'

Lorraine doesn't recall any stress about dissecting, or her fellow students feeling overwhelmed by it. 'It was just very straightforward.' If anything, it sounds like anatomy as a subject was more terrifying. Lorraine spent up to three days a week in the anatomy school and the rest in physiology and chemistry. But anatomy dominated her world—there were so many medical terms to remember, so much to know. She'd heard stories of students resorting to amphetamines to stay up to study.

The door buzzes and it's Dr Terry O'Connor, greying, in a polo shirt, chatty, and an old friend who was at the University of Queensland's medical school as the same time as Lorraine. He's now retired after spending decades variously as a GP, in emergency medicine at a hospital and doing locums in Central West Queensland. The pair soon slip into talking about old friends, old professors, women who dropped out, someone with schizophrenia. At one point, Lorraine recalls that their dissecting days started with a cockroach. I ask if that's hard—don't they crunch? They look at me like I'm being silly.

'No,' says Lorraine.

'No, no, no. Anything is dissectible,' says Terry.

'They had very nice-looking white muscles that moved their legs,' says Lorraine. 'Do you remember that?'

'No,' says Terry.

Terry and Lorraine worked on different tables so I ask Terry if he remembers the person he dissected. He thinks it was a man. 'They didn't have a name nor did we have any history of them. They were just a body. My attitude was that most of these were people who couldn't afford a funeral, and were somehow acquired by the anatomy department. I never went into it either.'

'They were cadavers,' says Lorraine.

I ask them if anyone ever felt sick. 'I tell you what,' says Terry, smiling. 'There's only person I know that fainted in theatre.'

'That was me!' says Lorraine as the pair start laughing.

Terry recalls they would take turns dissecting and that some were better at it than others. 'We sort of tended to let them do it and so I did very little dissection. They dissected while we were looking at the books, and then we'd come and have a look and say, "Oh, yeah, I can see what's going on, I can see what that muscle is,"' he says. 'There were a lot of students, and only one person could dissect at a time.'

We eat a ploughman's lunch, and afterwards, just when I think we're winding up, Terry mentions that he once took a human brain home from university on the bus in a paper bag. I'm a bit surprised, and ask him how it happened. He recalled that he and a friend went back into the anatomy lab one day to study the brain more.

'I could never understand it—could never understand the anatomy of the brain. It's very complicated. And, anyway, this brain was being thrown out,' he says. 'How they threw them out—I don't know. I suppose there was a certain reverence and carefulness of that but anyway, I thought "Oh well, if they are not going to use it any more, I'll take it home and have a look at it." I didn't learn very much from it, but maybe I did?' He can't remember what happened to it then. He thinks he might have taken it back to the uni but he's not sure.

***

Months later, I call Terry to say hello, and discuss this and that, and he mentions that like Lorraine, he too used to own a skeleton—a small man—which he bought from a Brisbane bookstore. 'The skeletons were from India,' he says, adding he used to wonder about his skeleton, what the story was behind it. Back then, it wasn't talked about but these days, he says he would certainly ask more questions. 'Where did this come from? Who was he?' he asks.

We talk about the brain he took home and Terry says he still feels bad about it. I ask him why. 'I suppose it was some religious thing? You thought that everybody has a soul and the brain was somehow intimately associated with the soul. It was something like that?'

But I can see why he had this curiosity about the brain—it really is a very strange organ. During my watching-dissection-videos period, I couldn't believe how seriously mysterious—and soft and squishy—it was. How were all our thoughts stored in it?

The first body to be willed to the University of Queensland was in 1931 but body donor programs didn't really kick in until the 1960s. I mention to Terry that it's likely many of the bodies in the late 1950s were from Goodna mental asylum. 'Oh really? You're kidding. That's incredible, isn't it?' he says. 'It's a bit of a shock.'

***

I think about who else knew my grandparents. My Uncle Maurie hadn't been interested in speaking to me about them—he'd been unwell and I didn't want to bug him. With Covid-19 galloping around the world, I figured I would visit him on Bribie Island with Mum and Dad once we were all free again. I knew that he'd been so upset about Ruby's death he couldn't bring himself to visit her in hospital during her dying days.

Who else?

My Aunt Lindy married Uncle Maurie in 1965 and they'd divorced in the 1970s. I'd seen Lindy at my cousin Kelly's wedding years ago and although we'd not spoken since then, I knew she was interested in the past as she'd written a few local histories, including one on South Stradbroke Island. I emailed her and she promptly wrote back, and I was jolted to read yet another reason as to why Ruby had donated. She wrote: 'I do have some memories of the time when Ruby died. She got the idea of leaving her body to the university, mainly to save the family the bother and cost of a funeral, etc. She would have been horrified with how that all worked out.'

Horrified?! Worked out?

Lindy wrote that when the university was notified of Ruby's death, they had told the family they didn't pick up bodies, and they would have to book an undertaker. She also mentioned that even though Ruby donated her body to avoid a funeral, Julie insisted on holding a memorial service at the local church in Holland Park anyway.

She wrote: 'This blew up even more, when their house at Holland Park was burgled whilst everyone was away at the service! Of course, the only person who would have known exactly what was missing from the house was Ruby!' [In those days, people put their home address in the notice that went in the paper—so all their neighbours would know. This made it very easy for the thieves!] Mum and Dad had never mentioned Ruby having a memorial service nor the house being broken into. Fair enough, it did happen fifty years ago.

In the email, Lindy was also surprised that Julie had left his body to science after all that had happened. 'Unbelievable!' she wrote.

I ring up Lindy to talk more about my grandparents, and what she remembers of that time. She speaks fondly of Ruby. 'You could talk to her about anything,' she recalls. 'She kept the family going.' Julie, however, she remembers as more difficult and that he was always a bit distant. 'He'd had some head injury at some stage of life. He was often grumpy. I think Ruby had a hard time.'

Lindy said she thought it was Ruby's idea to donate. 'She must've persuaded him to do it. Nobody in their right mind would do it,' says Lindy, and I soon find out that she speaks from experience as extraordinarily, she herself used to dissect bodies one night a week at the University of Queensland in 1963 as part of her physical education degree. She found it a particularly unpleasant place.

'I can still remember the smell,' she says.

Lindy studied the muscles and the skeleton, and can recall a few Latin names, although not much else about the experience, probably because it was never her thing. She didn't bother with her final exams and went to the movies instead. She later dropped out.

She married Uncle Maurie in 1965 and I asked her if she ever spoke to Ruby about her experiences there. She says she doubts it.

***

Avoiding funerals—this was certainly a reason that popped up in the body donor research. What was it about funerals that Ruby wasn't into? The atmosphere? They were depressing? Perhaps Ruby hated funerals after the death of her beloved little brother Maurice when he was just thirteen. Sophie Bolt in the Netherlands mentioned that in some instances donors had ongoing arguments with family members or didn't want a specific person at the funeral. By the time Ruby died, she had reconciled with her two sisters. Dad mentioned Ruby had donated her body to save money. This obviously fits in a little with what Lindy was saying.

With no contemporary body donors who were planning their fate in a dissecting room to speak to, I burrowed into the funerary aspect of donation and randomly stumbled into next-level funeral avoidance in India. It would be the Indians who could turn dissection and funerals into an extraordinary social and political movement.

Western dissection has long been seen as a vile practice in India and even when Mahatma Gandhi himself was considering a medical career, he wrote in 1949 that his father said to him: '[W]e Vaishnavas should have nothing to do with dissection of dead bodies.' For those who did dissect, by religious law, they were only allowed to do it on children under the age of two. Dissection was also seen as going directly against cremation, a central part of Hinduism. During a Hindu funeral service, the body is burned on a pyre and at some of them, the dead person's skull is cracked open to release the soul to heaven.

In the 1990s Alok Kumar, now a smiley, grey-haired man in pictures, visited the Anatomy Department of the Government Medical College in Amritsar, and noticed the preserved skeleton of the Ex-Head of the Anatomy Department in a glass box. As Alok says on his website: 'On my inquiry, I learnt that he had donated his body, after his death, for the medical students to study the human anatomy.' Back in Delhi, he discovered there was an acute shortage of bodies with up to fifty students at a time studying one body. 'After discussions with my friends, five or six of us went ahead to register our will to donate our body after death.'

Inspired, Alok set up the charity Dadhichi Deh Dan Samiti or Dadhichi Body Donation Society in 1997. Since 2010, 351 bodies, 826 pairs of eyes and eight organs have been donated. Some of the donors are lauded in newsletters and their photos appear on the organisation's website. Out and about, they wear red scarves as a symbol of their commitment.

The social anthropologist Jacob Copeman was in India in 2003 studying blood donation and became interested in the involvement of right-wing Hindu nationalists in promoting it—to the point that they were running their own blood banks. He soon came across Dadhichi Deh Dan Samiti, a unique body-focused social service group which had links to Hindu nationalists, particularly as its founder Alok was a BJP (Hindu nationalist party) politician.

Jacob studied the 'Samiti' for the next two years, spending time with Alok, studying their donor literature, and going to festivals at which donors executed their wills. He found that Alok's carefully and purposely crafted donation theology was centred around Dadhichi, an austere and saintly sage in Hinduism who sacrificed his bones to the devas, who used them as weapons against the demon king Vritrasura. Thus Dadhichi became the 'first body donor'. The idea of asceticism was also turned upside down—instead of retreating from the world, the Samiti were seen as actively engaging with it through body donation, and cremation was reframed as old-fashioned and wasteful. The Samiti had found a way to give religious sanction to something that traditionally would have been absolutely forbidden.

As Jacob said in an email to me: 'The imagery and inspiration of Dadhichi is a very Hindu way of looking at the practice [of body donation]. This doesn't mean all its members are right-wing Hindus, but there is definitely a strong connection between the group and Hindu nationalism.'

Over the years, Jacob has continued to study body donors and found that it wasn't just the Samiti who have taken on dissection for high-minded reasons.

Take this case in 2010. Jyoti Basu, the former Marxist Chief Minister of West Bengal, died aged ninety-five, and his high-profile body donation and documented dissection is possibly a global first for a politician and public figure. At the time, the press offered a detailed and blow-by-blow account of his journey from hospital deathbed to dissecting hall with regular updates on exactly what happened. As *The Telegraph* reported:

> According to doctors, the dissection of Basu's skull started from his forehead. 'After taking the brain out, we dipped it in formalin solution.' ... The doctors also plan to preserve the other body parts over the next four days ... 'We will dissect his body to bring out his lungs, intestines, kidneys, heart and liver. The condition of the body is still very good for preservation of its organs,' said a doctor.

Much of the media focused on his donation and in an obituary on *Countercurrents*, an alternative Indian news website, Vidya Bhushan

Rawat declared: 'Jyoti Basu has created an example. He has proved that a true Marxist remains true to Marxist philosophy or not succumbing to any religious rituals . . . [he] lived up to his convictions, a true Marxist, an atheist and a firm believer in science.'

The obituary went on to argue that the body donation could be a way of taking away a major source of work for Brahmin priests—conducting funerals:

> The racist brahmanical philosophy has preached us that donating your eyes and body is dangerous ... Jyoti Basu ... has saved us from priestly pontification ... If we have to make the brahmanical priestly class redundant, we must follow what Jyoti Babu did, by donating our bodies and shunning the rituals we are so fond of, in the name of our culture.

Dissection has also became a political act for atheists, their primary motivation being fervently anti-religious, and focused on avoiding all the ritual around funerals. Aside from seeing it as a positive and good thing to do, it also serves a political point about religion. Dr G.Vijayam, who heads the Atheist Centre in Andhra Pradesh, said in an interview that 'in recognition of the fact that there's no life after death', atheists are pledging their organs, eyes and bodies for donation and coming up with ceremonies that 'try to improve the quality of life here on earth'. For other atheists, body donation means not having to pay Brahmin priests for funerals and serves as an attack on the caste system. Some also found the practice of having to smash open a loved one's skull during the Hindu cremation particularly unappealing.

Dislike of death customs also triggered people in Greece to donate their bodies. In 1999 the Greek anthropologist Eleni Papagaroufali spoke to twenty-four organ and body donors, and found the body donors largely did it because they were repelled by Orthodox Christian funeral rituals, which involve the dead being buried, then exhumed and the bones placed in an ossuary. A shortage of space meant in some instances bodies were exhumed too early and were only partly decayed, and donors told Eleni they hated the whole process. Cremation was prohibited at the time but since 2016 has been permitted, despite opposition from the church.

'They consider these practices [of exhumation] unjustifiably expensive and time-consuming, as well as superficial and ostentatious. They call exhumation "barbarous", "aesthetically abusive", "meaningless", and "burdensome",' she wrote in a paper in *Ethos*, the official journal of the Society for Psychological Anthropology.

Instead of familiarising Christians with death, they contend, these practices inspire fear and revulsion. 'It's like watching a Drakula film,' one donor commented in the paper.

In a pattern which seems to pop up all over the world, the body donors Eleni spoke to also became furious at the prospect that their next of kin could stop their donation. Another theme for the Greeks was fear of burial—the worms, the dampness. As Maria, a body donor in her late thirties and an atheist put it:

> I became a body donor because it was very important for me not to be buried ... Instead of paying for my flesh to be rotten and eaten by worms I will give it for something useful ... (laughter). I can't stand darkness and very small closed spaces ... [squeamish look]. I am not exactly claustrophobic but it troubles me very deeply ... (brrr) although I know this doesn't happen because you don't feel what's going on afterwards ... but it was a very good way not to get involved in this procedure and I solved this problem once and for all, that is, I avoided the idea of burial altogether.

***

Mum and Dad hadn't seemed to remember much about Ruby's death or her funeral. But after I told them about speaking to Aunt Lindy and what she said, memories of the slight drama came back to them.

Lindy remembered that the university had told the family they needed to book an undertaker themselves. But as Mum recalled it, the issue was that Ruby's death certificate hadn't been signed, and the doctor who was meant to do it didn't want to go back to the hospital morgue. Instead, Dad had to meet the doctor at his surgery, where he came out and inspected Ruby in the back of the undertakers vehicle.

In a contemporary setting, the body donor sage Sophie Bolt found the period immediately after a donor's death was hard for some Dutch families, as it interrupted the normal goings-on and rituals, particularly as their loved one needed to be at the university within twenty-four hours. Families struggled with 'the fast removal of the body, disturbing thoughts of the donor in the dissecting room, and the absence of a grave or urn'.

As bodies need to be promptly embalmed, some families told Sophie they were taken by surprise at the swiftness and that they didn't have the chance to be 'close to the body of the deceased person, being able to touch the body and give it a kiss on the cheek'.

A coffin usually occupies the central position at a funeral so what did families do without one? Sophie attended twenty-six funerals without corpses in churches, pubs, restaurants and community centres and found the donors were represented by photos, flowers or objects. In one fascinating case, a woman named Anna was symbolised by her actual dining room table. As Sophie wrote:

> They transported the table to the hall of the community center where the funeral ceremony was being held and made sure that it looked exactly as it had been on the evening Anna died, with a bouquet of wild flowers, a box with cookies, her last cigarettes in an ashtray, water in a carafe, two burning tea warmers and her last cup of coffee. In the view of the organisers, these objects reflected who Anna was. One could easily reminisce sitting next to her at the table, with the smell of her coffee and cigarettes, eating the cookies, and feeling the tablecloth and the warmth of the tea lights. It made her presence

> tangible and created a sense of closeness, perhaps even more so than if her corpse had been there in a coffin.

Even the funeral brochure included a photo of the staged table instead of one of Anna.

Chapter 15

With so few threads to follow, I come to clutch at any paperwork I can find. Ruby's cremation document becomes central to my files and I return to it again and again looking for clues. Have I missed something? And it is here on the Brisbane Crematorium Limited's Cremation Permit number A9.799 that I spot 'Cremation charged to (Undertaker): CANNON & CRIPPS PTY LTD'.

Aunt Lindy had slightly different memories from my parents about what happened to Ruby after she died so I decide to see if I can find someone from Cannon & Cripps. Within weeks, the Australian Funeral Directors Association Queensland Branch recommends I speak to Rowan Steer, who worked for the company for eighteen years, and also happened to look after body donations. He's now a general manager and partner at Integrity Funerals, running services on the Gold Coast, Brisbane and the Sunshine Coast. I study his LinkedIn photo—he sports a striped creamy tie and has a distinctive handlebar moustache and grey goatee, known as the Van Dyke on some barber beard charts.

Rowan sounds warm and friendly on the phone. He's also matter-of-fact. There's a cautiousness when he speaks about the nitty gritty of his work, asking if I'm okay with the discussion or prefacing certain topics by saying: 'It's not the nicest thing to talk about but ... ' I assure him I'm okay.

Rowan hadn't planned on working in funerals—it just happened, although he did come from a family comfortable with death. His father was a clergyman and (quite bizarrely for me) his grandfather George Lean was the manager of the University of Queensland's body donor program in the 1960s and could have possibly spoken to Ruby and Julie on the phone about their donation, sent them their paperwork and filed it.

Rowan began working at Cannon & Cripps in 1986, which wasn't too long after one of his colleagues would've collected Julie when he died at home, and probably picked up his remains to be cremated a few years later.

A large and old funeral business, Cannon & Cripps was known for its connection to freemasonry and conducting the first cremation in Queensland in 1934. It had an office in Kelvin Grove, a hilly inner suburb of Brisbane, and it was here that Rowan cleaned toilets, vacuumed, washed cars and looked after flowers at funerals. He watched, he learned. Within a few months his role widened and he began collecting donors' bodies.

'I just fell in love with it, Jackie,' says Rowan of his job. 'It becomes a ... it becomes something of a ministry to people, a care of people. I've just enjoyed it.'

Rowan drove all hours of the day all over Brisbane, picking up bodies from hospitals and homes, and taking them to the university. He could get calls at 2 am or 3 pm on a Friday, and a body had to be collected ASAP to be embalmed.

He says it was best to get the person there within twenty-four hours. Even if someone wanted their body to go to the university, some regulations meant they couldn't. They might have died from an infectious disease like hepatitis. Perhaps they had a form of cancer which meant their body couldn't be used—they had already started to decompose inside. Or they might have had too many operations. Weight could be an issue too. Some contemporary anatomy schools will not accept people who are over a certain weight—they are just too difficult to move, particularly once they have been embalmed, which can add 20 kilograms. People can also be too skinny.

Rowan often drove on the 44-kilometre-long stretch of road from Redcliffe—a working-class suburb on the coast—to the university at St Lucia. He recalls the area had a high number of donors. 'They had a group of doctors within Redcliffe who always encouraged it, and who would sort of advertise it for their families,' he says. Part of the appeal was the free funeral on offer. This group of doctors instantly piques my interest—as my concept of how Ruby and Julie became donors is still hazy. Perhaps a doctor in Holland Park where they lived had mentioned it during consultations?

Cannon & Cripps was paid $12 a transfer—it wasn't a lucrative aspect of their business but perhaps it helped a little. Their name was on all the body donor paperwork to call after hours, and if the university didn't accept a person for various reasons, some families would ask the company to bury their loved one.

Sometimes people who were willed to the university still managed to have funerals. 'There's a big hole in this when somebody dies, and suddenly they've disappeared, and they've gone off to the university. "Where did my grandmother go?"' Rowan recalls.

Rowan remembered that often there was no funeral so for some families, their donor would be embalmed at the university, 'and then we would bring them back and we would put them in a nice coffin that the family chose. And then we would do a funeral in a Catholic church or wherever, and then take the person back to the university.'

Chapter 16

Leo Brown sits settled on the couch, a gold light streaming through the large yellow bottle-glass windowpane behind him. The glass was popular in the 1970s, when he and wife Barbara built their Everton Park home in a quiet suburb in Brisbane's north. His tidy and comfortable lounge room is lightly peppered with religious iconography: candles and figurines of little angels praying. The light feels apt. I'm ready for some revelations on body donation from a man who spent forty-nine years in the anatomy school at the University of Queensland. He started in 1962 and retired in 2011, doing all sorts of jobs, including running the body donor program. He may have sent paperwork to my grandparents. He probably signed the registry when they arrived. I also want to hear the voice of someone behind the scenes of anatomy—the day-to-day administration which made it happen, made it function.

Leo has just come from church. He sports an 'extended goatee' according to my beard chart and is turning seventy-five the next day. He tells me he recently spoke to an old school friend he hadn't heard from in decades and they were arranging to meet up. The conversation had prompted him to sit up writing the names of people he went to school with when he was fifteen—so far, he'd come up with thirty-five. (I tried this and got nineteen.) There are bunches of freshly picked flowers around the room, including a large pale purple and pink rose drooping in a vase behind him. He served in the army reserves for years and has an Australian flag and an article about Remembrance Day stuck to the glass at the front of his home. He must have his sweet and tough moments.

I ask him if he vacuumed.

'A little,' he says.

I'd heard his wife had died and asked him how long it has been.

'Seven years ago.'

'How you going?'

'Oh, yeah. Well, you never forget. Lonely all the time,' he says flatly.

Some would move to a new house to start again but Leo says he likes where he is—he gets along with his neighbour across the road, he's near the shops and his local Catholic church is close.

Leo grew up just an hour away in Rosewood, where he would wake up early before school and milk the cows on the family dairy farm. He left school at fifteen and landed a job in the anatomy department at the University of Queensland. Within the first week, he was shifting bodies around. He's not sure why he was fine working with the dead, but he was. He just accepted it as it was his job. But it was a lot to take on for someone so young.

When he first started, he worked at the old US army huts left over from the war—it's where Lorraine and Terry did their dissecting work. In one hut was a large area with bodies on wooden tables, a room for technicians and a storage space. Terry had a vague recollection of bodies being stored vertically in some way but the memory is shimmery, not fixed. Lorraine can't remember seeing that. I ask Leo about this and he says bodies in the storeroom were indeed stored vertically—there was a clamp with pins that went into the ears.

These bodies were 'in stock' in a sense, curing and waiting for the next year of students to arrive. Leo says there was a small donor program and over time, more letters would arrive from people asking for information about how to give their body to the university. The person would be sent a form, which when returned would be kept on file. Leo recalls that most of the bodies were coming from consenting donors by the mid-1960s.It was a gradual change. They never advertised. Perhaps Leo spoke to Ruby?

I mention to Leo the story of Terry taking the brain home. 'You get all these stories,' he says, maybe a tad annoyed.

The anatomy world doesn't like 'the stories', particularly the old ones about young medical students being silly with body parts. They are certainly a ghost that won't go away—I heard a few. Some mornings I'd argue there is a haunting for a reason, and it's time to talk directly to the ghosts and to the public about dissection. Some afternoons I think it came down to students not coping very well. By late evening, I think this is science, and we should let the anatomists be anatomists, they do what they have to do, which I suspect is just cutting up the dead and studying them with no hoo-ha. But then the ghosts return.

I defend Terry. 'Well, I think the thing is he wanted to learn,' I reply. Another old doctor told me that as a young medical student, he purchased fresh brains from a Sydney hospital and dissected them with friends in a garage. While what they did was ethically dubious, these were young people who wanted to learn. There is a huge difference between fresh and 'formalin-fixed' brains: fresh ones are much gloopier and soft.

'Oh, yes. And that's quite possible,' says Leo. 'But that would have only happened back then . . . if it ever happened since I don't remember. I don't know of anyone being able to take anything home. Back in those days, it was a bit more lax.'

In my notebook, I have written 'petal falls'—in reference to the soft pink purply rose sitting behind him. I'll put that reference here.

Just four months into his job, the anatomy department moved to new, modern clinical-style facilities in St Lucia. It was a step up from the wooden army huts—they now had stainless steel tables and refrigeration for the bodies, which were stored lying down on trays. The fridges made a huge difference; they were the saviour, particularly as the warm temperature and humidity in Queensland meant that some of the dead could go mouldy.

In the thousands of years before fridges and formalin, anatomists were always in the ring against decay. They had to move quickly. In 1497 the Paduan Alexander Benedictus, an anatomist who designed the first anatomical theatre, wrote a book with regulations, which alongside stressing that the dissected must be humble and unknown, and not too lean or fat, advised that severe cold was needed as the bodies would putrefy. In 1540 a young student named Baldasar Heseler watched Andreas Vesalius dissect and in his lecture notes remarked that as the thorax of a dead person was much decayed, a dog had to be killed to explain the muscles. The Scottish-born Sir Thomas Peter Anderson Stuart, the man who founded anatomy at the University of Sydney in 1883, was also up against the elements. He tried to preserve the bodies with arsenic but unfortunately, when it rained, 'The Cottage' where he worked became damp. In one instance, the bodies, covered in mould, had to be buried before they could be studied.

But the University of Queensland now had fridges, and a new space big enough for 100 tables, although there were often only around twenty bodies out at a time. Sometimes the second-year students would work on them, then the third years the next day.

Leo's days were eclectic. He would call out names from the roll to make sure all the students were there. He would show slides during lectures. He placed needles into femoral arteries into the legs of the dead and switched on the machine to pump embalming fluid into them. He leaned into cages and fed the rabbits, rats, mice and monkeys. He would collect mail. He collected donors' bodies from nursing homes. He fixed morning tea for his colleagues. 'There was good staff there. It was quite pleasant,' he says.

As technology shifted over the decades, so did medical teaching. One technician looked after an extremely powerful electron microscope—the first in Queensland and one which meant the anatomists and students could peer deep into the cells. Audiovisual technology improved and Leo began projecting professional anatomical movies on ears and lungs for the students. In 1967 he showed slides at a major pathology conference, including case studies of victims from the Black Tuesday bushfires in Tasmania, which burned down the Cascade brewery and other parts of the south, killing sixty-two people. Leo recalls one image of melted coins found in a man's pocket. ('The things we remember.) He also photographed prosected specimens to make into slides. He recalls around the 1970s photographing the autopsies of dolphins and killer whales that died at Marine Land, the precursor to Sea World on the Gold Coast. He also went out with staff to catch dolphins in the wild, and filmed the animals swimming in the wake of the boat.

The dissecting room was not only busy with medical students—there were dentists, physiotherapists, occupational therapists and physical education groups. For most of them, anatomy was hard. Not only did some find it psychologically difficult, they struggled with the rote learning, all those Latin and Greek names to remember. Leo recalls there was always an ongoing debate about how much anatomy should be in the curriculum—did the students really need to know all of it?

The body donor program took up more time and Leo's phone would ring with potential donors wanting information, a funeral director needing details of a pick-up, or a family member with questions. *Mum has died. Could I still have a funeral?* Leo would tell them yes.

'I recommended that people have a funeral or some sort of gathering shortly after death. And it might be the next day or something like that, and then the body can come to the university after,' he says. 'I used to encourage people to make that as part of the grieving process. And if they couldn't organise something within a couple of days, I'd say look, all right, well, what we can do is we can bring the body to the university, we can embalm the body. And then at a reasonable time, we can hand the body back for the funeral. And you can have a funeral with the body in a coffin, or you can have a funeral without a body in a coffin. I'd offer that to them. They were so happy that we were working with them.'

In some instances, mothers, fathers, sons, daughters of donors would come to see him at the university and want to know more about what happened. (It seems I'm not alone in this!) He would take them to the small anatomy museum to show them the research specimens—arms, legs, various organs—and tell them: 'This is what your family member may have contributed to.' Other times, he could hear the strain in the voice of a family member on the phone, unhappy about the donation. 'You'd have discussions with people and you could feel that they weren't happy, and they weren't comfortable. So it was just a matter of talking them through it.'

After all those years, and as a Catholic, were there days when Leo stared at the rows of bodies under the sheets and contemplated the soul? I tell him that even though I'm not religious, I still feel funny about dissection, that it's wholly superstitious of me, and it's totally about feeling like I'd be cold.

'You don't find a soul,' he chuckles a little—the first time I've heard him laugh. I tell him about a friend who worked in the University of Queensland anatomy lab in the 1980s who was very practical and no-fuss about it all too. He agrees. 'Because you're involved with it on a daily basis, you don't go off on esoteric tangents.'

It's not at all rational but some part of me wants the Loch Ness Monster and all the ghosts I grew up with in Manila to be true. I want Leo to tell me that by working with The Dissected so closely for forty-nine years, they had doused him in cosmic answers or actually there was that one time where he'd bumped into a soul on its twenty-second day out of the body when he was all alone in his office.

But no.

He'd only really felt death when his beloved wife died. 'I dealt with death and dying for fifty years—it doesn't make it easy when it comes close to you.'

I ask when he looks back, what does he remember? 'Is anything striking? What snippets come to mind?' I ask. His answer is unexpected.

'Seeing the surgeon doing implants—heart valve implants in dogs as a forerunner for replacing heart valves,' he says. 'There you go. That was back in the mid-sixties.' I then tell him how being back in Brisbane reminds me of a dead rat in a jar that was under our family friend's house.

There's remembering.

And there's knowing.

Even though hundreds of thousands of medical students and scientists are initiated in the labs, it still seems so hard to know. I ask Leo why it's so hidden.

'Death has always been—it's always been taboo to talk about death and dying, and all that sort of thing. It's the black subject. And I think people still have that attitude,' he says. 'Sometimes people want to come and have a look and see what's happening. But you've got to be very careful about who you allow to come in and see what's going on.'

'Why?'

'Because they might get the wrong impression, and say, oh that has been just chopped up, and the students are not very respectful and all that sort of thing. But it's just normal process.' I think what he is saying is that life goes on with and around the dead—bodies do need to be cut up, students do tell stories and make jokes as they learn—but each of us have a mythical ideal of what 'should' happen in the anatomy lab, that everybody stands around like robots.

It's like this in every nook and cranny of life really. I remember my first morning at a breakfast table in Afghanistan at a UN guest house and the conversation was buzzing with the news that a young Western woman had been kidnapped. My perception—borne from where? Why? How?—was that people should have been sitting there solemnly, worrying. Instead, my new colleagues were making light-hearted jokes about it. I felt drained listening to them, a horror sitting on my shoulders, stroking my chest. *What sort of place was this?* I went back to my room and looked at my half-unpacked suitcase, and wasn't sure if I should continue taking out the rest of my clothes and trinkets.

A few months later, an Afghan colleague lost his brother in a suicide attack, and the only way he could recognise him at the morgue was through his foot. Awkwardly, I had just returned from London and had given him and another workmate a pair of socks with the Big Ben clock tower on them. As they tried the socks on, one made a joke about the brother's foot, and as they chuckled together, I sat mute, stunned.

I later scolded my friend, questioning him about making jokes about such a horrific experience, and he scolded me back. 'There's been a lot of misery here—if we've got the option of laughing or crying, what do you think we should choose?' Soon enough, I slowly joined in on making light of kidnappings and suicide bombs. To a 'newbie', I would've seemed heinous.

Chapter 17

Dr Frank Maloney would be fun over a cup of tea, a beer or possibly even just doing something mundane like walking around the supermarket. I feel like a dog being thrown little bits of roast chicken and cheese—he keeps filling me up with treats. 'Treat' comes from the Latin *trahere*—'draw, pull'—and I'm certainly drawn in by Frank's random medical tales over the phone, and as we discuss his memories of dissection, there is a general *joie de vivre* vibe to him.

From 1962 to 1966, Frank was at the University of Queensland's dental school. He then decided to have a go at a medical degree so was back buried in books and classes from 1971 to 1975, and went on to become an oral and maxillofacial surgeon. I'd never heard of this type of surgeon—it has a patrician glamour feel to it—but they help people with injuries and conditions in their mouth, teeth, jaws and face. Apparently the bread and butter of the specialty is taking out wisdom teeth. He's now retired but 'not handling it well', so at the age of seventy-seven has gone back to university to do an arts degree in history.

As Frank told me about arriving in the anatomy labs in 1972—Ruby's body had left by October 1971—an anxiety began bubbling in me, aware that his story was a blueprint of what could have happened. I was finally looking over a threshold and into the past. The thing is once I was on the other side, it wasn't at all what I expected.

According to the historian Richard Sugg, the idea of cutting up, analysing and methodically dissecting a topic in fact comes from anatomical dissection, first spilling into popular culture around the late 1500s. The word 'section' originally came from dissecting a body and was first recorded in the *Oxford English Dictionary* in 1559. It appeared in the engraver and printer Thomas Geminus' rip off of Vesalius' *Fabrica*, which included the line: 'neither in man only ... but in the anatomy or section of any other beast'. But it soon jumped ship or as Sugg puts it: 'the Latin root "sectio" (a cutting, cutting off, or cutting up) was increasingly propelled into a broader vernacular use by association with dis-section', and from 1577 onwards, books began to have 'sections'.

Books with 'Anatomy' in the title also became all the rage, and between 1576 and 1650, around 120 titles were published which 'anatomised' a topic like *The Anatomie of the English Nunnery at Lisbon* (1622), *The Anatomie of Urines* (1625) and the *Anti-duello: The Anatomie of Duells* (1632). The most well-known from this period is Robert Burton's *Anatomy of Melancholy* (1621).

Eighty-four books had 'lay open' or 'rip' in their titles. Sugg also discusses how the word 'analyses' is connected to anatomy—to analyse was to 'undo' or 'break down'—and that between 1585 and 1642, sixteen 'analyses' were published.

So in the spirit of dissection, I'm sectioning Frank into thirteen parts. And in honour of Joseph Maclise's aortic arch drawing, why not some variation? After all, we are all a little different on the inside, and books can be too.

Here is Frank sectioned. It's the only way to tell his story.

1. Frank signed up to dentistry quite randomly after getting a Commonwealth scholarship. 'My friend David said: "Well, I'm going to do dentistry" and I said, "Dentistry? What the hell? Why would you want to do dentistry?" and he said: "My brother's been one for years and already owns a Holden." I ticked dentistry. It was not a serious hard job getting into university in those days.' (The ability to buy a car was a motivation to study medicine for quite a few of the other doctors of Frank's generation I spoke to.)

2. When Frank was at dental school, he heard the story of a medical student who took a scrotum home and later put it in a girl's purse. 'He was kicked out immediately. They did give us on day one or day two

lectures on the ethics of dead bodies—they are actually belonging to someone. So we had to treat them with respect,' says Frank. (I heard and read a few stories about silly things that happened with body parts in the lab. The general theory is that any 'cadaver antics' such as taking a body part or telling jokes is a way to cope with the stress that goes with dissecting or studying the dead. A 2020 study published in *Medical Science Educator* surveyed 185 students in nine countries and found 72 per cent had experienced dark humour in the anatomy lab.)

3. Professor Max Hickey ran the anatomy department at the University of Queensland for years, and was a well-known atheist, and, as a classicist, was also well-versed in Latin and Greek. He was invited by the Irish club in Brisbane to say grace before the annual St Patrick's Day dinner. And when he got up, he said: 'Gentlemen, stand up, stand please. *Levator labii superioris alaeque nasi*.' While this may have sounded like an earnest prayer, it is in fact the longest name of any muscle in the human body. It means 'lifter of both the upper lip and of the wing of the nose'. At one point, Max hired a Romanian in the anatomy department and although the man didn't speak a word of English, the interview had been partly done in Latin as they both spoke it.

4. Frank attended the London lectures of the famous Australian anatomist and surgeon R.J. Last, who was originally from Adelaide and taught at the Royal College of Surgeons. 'He did the most exquisite drawings in colour on the blackboard and was quite eccentric. He wore a bow tie and he took snuff during the lecture. Every now and then, he stopped, put snuff between a thumb and finger and would go sniff, sniff, and then shake his nose and twitch and carry on.'

Frank lauds his book *Anatomy, Regional and Applied*, which came out in 1954. 'It was a nice, clear, concise book, a good read about nerves and stuff,' he recalls. 'And also the other thing he did, there's about thirty to forty pages in the back where if you refer to Wilson's nerve or Johnson's muscle, there would be a little historical vignette on who that person was, what years they lived, and how they became famous for that particular thing.' (You get a vivid sense of anatomical teaching reading Baldasar Heseler's eyewitness report of Andreas Vesalius' first public anatomy at Bologna in 1540. Aside from enjoying dissection, I would come to find that many anatomists also love teaching.)

5. The dead man who taught Frank was old and had a few tattoos. Frank was never told his name but he did wonder who he was. (RIP the man with the tattoos.)

6. Frank owned his own skeleton at university, and still has the skull at home, which he thinks may be from India. He's unsure what to do about it. 'It's a real person,' he says. 'How do I ethically dispose of it? I can't just go and chuck it in a rubbish bin. It's a person. I think legally I have to hand it in to the police.'

7. In Frank's view, they spent too much time dissecting—all those hours upon hours of doing what he thought was unnecessary stuff. He says to get from the skin to the ribs, and then to look around for muscles and nerves around the ribs, took an enormous amount of time. He didn't feel it led to any surgical skills either as operating on a dead body 'is vastly different to a live one'. When he was at dental school, he dissected a person's head, neck and thorax.

With a head dissection, he says it took a week to pull off the skin to find the facial nerve or facial expression muscles. Even then, when they got to the muscles, they were stuck together. 'It was a very difficult thing to do for people of that age group,' he says.

'I think anatomy needed to change and it has, it should be provided for you—you see much more if it's professionally done, rather than me looking for a nerve and find I've cut it off, and thrown it out somewhere.' He also had to dissect a brain, which he described as 'awful', as the brains were in formalin. 'Your fingers always ended up like your hands had been in dishwater for about three days—that crinkly feeling.'

Dissection was also physically difficult as the person had been embalmed. 'Let's say, when I was a medical student, you were dissecting the guts. You'd cut it open, you try and take out all the gear. And the trouble was, those bodies were hard to dissect because it's not like you're doing an autopsy. I was always amazed when I saw an autopsy at Royal Brisbane, holy shit, look at all that. You can actually see this stuff! I mean, it wasn't all stuck together—all the guts just came out like you would see in a dead animal.

'Anatomy was somewhat difficult from that point of view because it was hard to dissect, and you'd put it all back in again and come back again tomorrow as you're trying to find the artery to the liver or something like that. You had techniques—you had to cut the liver out to get behind it. And all those bits were put back.

'So at the end of the day, you cleaned up all the bits and pieces. You had scraps, skin and stuff—there were plastic bags for disposal. But the body was kept together, and by the end of the year, the leg looked like one of those things you see in the old anatomy drawings with sinews and tendons hanging off. And skin hanging off. So it looks pretty raggedy by the end of the year.'

(I found this discussion not easy to listen to, particularly Frank's detail about the flesh going into the bins. Another person who worked in an anatomy lab in the 1990s also told me this detail and I felt it on my skin. Another fact that struck me was that people's faces swelled from the embalming fluid, and it could be hard in some instances to tell if it were a man or woman.)

As dissection was so arduous, Frank recalled that quite a few people avoided it altogether and went for drinks at the Regatta Hotel or the Royal Exchange. But not knowing your anatomy was a risky option. 'A lot of guys would be signing other students in for anatomy to avoid the hours upon hours of dissection, and they would just learn from books. But at the end of the year, not only would you get multi-choice questions, you'd also have to go around and do a test where they had bits and pieces of bodies outlined with tags on them. What is this? Like the phrenic nerve or the pelvic nerve or some artery in the arm.'

Frank recalls that with Professor Hickey in charge, students had to know their anatomy backwards. There was one story that did the rounds about a student who was trying for the third time to pass second year medicine. Apparently the professor threw him a hand bone and the student replied, 'It's a metacarpal,' and quickly threw it back in the box. Max replied: 'Yes, I know it's a metacarpal but is it right hand or left hand?' The kid said: 'Sir, I'm not going for high distinction.' I later ask Frank for more details about the story and he jokes it is of 'doubtful authenticity'.

8. Frank is fine about donating his body. 'I wouldn't have any hesitation! It doesn't worry me. I mean—I'm a Catholic so you're allowed to be buried these days or cremated. Either way, once the hearse leaves the church, that's the end of you seeing it unless you go and specifically get yourself buried. I must admit I . . . yes! I can't see why I wouldn't.'

9. This story is not connected to anatomy but in 1973, Frank was doing a 'weird' class called 'Social and preventative medicine'. 'We had this gentleman who came in, and in his United Services Club tie, conservative, said: "Gentlemen, ladies, today we will talk about the disease of homosexuality,"' Frank recalls. His friend sitting next to him eventually interrupted and said: 'Sir, sir, it's actually not a sin. It's not a disease.' The conservative told him to 'Sit down young man.' Within five minutes, there was an uproar, and the situation was reported to the Dean.

'So the good thing was that the Dean organised a weekend seminar, two weeks down the track on sexual diseases, and that's the first time that guys or girls came out as openly gay in our class. My wife and I got invited to a gay party … I realised that quite a few of the friends I had there were gay,' says Frank. They also attended an AA meeting and visited Boggo Road jail, where Frank recalls listening to a convicted murderer play his Spanish guitar. (Sounds like quite a well-rounded education.)

10. It was Frank who introduced me to the concept of dirty medical mnemonics. When he asked me if I knew about them and I said no, he remarked: 'Oh! You must put those up!' and then reeled off a list of classic rude ones, which were popular at the time.

'Oh, Oh, Oh To Touch And Feel A Girl's Vagina And Hymen,' are the cranial nerves—Oh = Olfactory nerve (I), Oh = Optic nerve (II), Oh = Oculomotor nerve (III) etc.

11. Frank's mother cleaned train carriages for a living and no matter how difficult their financial situation was, she would always starch his white lab coat for university. 'I'd be up there along Main Road catching the Alexandra Road bus and this girl who later became my wife said she saw me every day and thought, "Who is that lovely boy with the gorgeous lab coat?" And it wasn't until years later, I met her and she just happened to remember it.'

12. He says the dissecting room was often very quiet, almost meditative. 'There wasn't much talking—if you're sitting around a table, you might be discussing something about a nerve or different things, but a lot of people by the end of the three-hour sessions, only about a third would be left. The other guys would have just shot through by then.'

I mention I'd heard students used to go outside for a cigarette. 'Yes! One day we went out to listen to the Cassius Clay fight … there must have been hundreds of us all listening to radios.' He also never once saw an Indigenous body in the dissecting rooms. 'I don't know whether that's because they didn't donate or it was a religious thing. No idea.'

13. Frank recently had a robot operation, which demonstrates just how much surgery has changed over time. 'My surgeon basically made five stab wounds, and put the probes in my tummy and pelvis, and he does the surgery with a Mario and Luigi joystick over on the computer, guiding it all. He didn't even have gloves on! Once he got the tubes in there, he went to the computer and did the surgery that way. And I've actually watched it online—you can actually watch your robot prostatectomy online.

'It's fascinating stuff, no blood, no bleeding, and no invasion, so that in fact would be better learned from a computer. They learned their endoscopic surgery by putting those things into watermelons, and moving around inside. The actual anatomy where you're viewing it 3D on computer is probably more practical these days than cutting open the body.'

Some of Frank's observations about dissection affected me unexpectedly—a bit like food poisoning. I'd seen dissection in videos but hearing him say it, and then me writing it down felt too vivid at times. *This is what happened.*

But his comments about all the time it took to dissect have hung over anatomy for a century, and by the mid-1990s—well in Australia at least—the era of students standing around a body dissecting head to toe and knowing it all by rote fell into a decline which persists today. Systems change but I felt oddly disappointed for Ruby and Julie, as if their donation might have been a waste.

***

Every Friday, Robert Sweeney and Edward 'Ted' Weaver stood with four other student doctors around a table dissecting, the pungent, eye-watering vapour of formaldehyde filling the room. They were both nineteen. It was 1972 and their lives were overwhelmed by second-year medicine at the University of Queensland, which involved studying anatomy. They spent a year dissecting an old woman—interestingly they have different memories of who she was—and go on wildly different paths as they recollect that year. It's Maclise's aortic arches again. It's also an insight into Ruby and Julie's world.

Robert was studying medicine but it sounds like he had a thespian, imaginative side. He recalls that at lunchtime, he and his friends would set up on the lawn outside the anatomy building and recreate the *Monty Python* skits they had seen on ABC TV the night before. Once the frivolity was over, he would head back inside to the serious work of continuing to dissect a donor's arm, for example, which they'd been slowly cutting away for two Friday sessions, gradually identifying muscles, tendons and arteries. 'We would work on one part of the body for an extended period and then move on to the next,' he says. While outside they were laughing over the surrealist antics of John Cleese and Michael Palin, inside he says it was never irreverent. They were well behaved.

He was quite diffident about dissection at the beginning. 'I think, initially using a scalpel on somebody's body was quite—it didn't come easily because we hadn't had anything to do with real-life injuries or using scalpels or things like suturing people at this stage. I think only one person in our group had already worked a bit at hospitals or something.' The only real experience Robert had had with dissection was with a toad and possibly a shark. 'It was quite testing at first. But I think after a while, we relaxed and it just became Fridays.'

They named their donor Evelyn, after the English writer Evelyn Waugh, the loose connection coming from Waugh's 1948 novel *The Loved One*, which is partly about the Los Angeles funeral business. 'We didn't know anything about her and obviously the facial features had changed, so we had no idea what she was like in real life. We used to sort of make up imaginary lives a little bit for her.'

Robert would become a GP in Brisbane, and then move to Christchurch, New Zealand, where he still practises today. He was thoughtful to speak with, and of all the doctors, I imagined he may have been an artist or actor in another life.

His table mate was his good friend Ted, who is now an obstetrician and gynaecologist at the Sunshine Coast University Hospital. Ted has a soothing voice—I can imagine him calming pregnant mothers or hosting a podcast—and he is good with details.

This is what Ted remembers about dissection:

> 'Confronting is an overused word but it was an unusual experience, certainly, to go into this large, quite well-lit room with these parallel tables, with a cadaver in a plastic bag, and the strong smell of formaldehyde. And so the first thing that struck me was the smell, and the room was cold. [The cold!]
>
> 'We're sharing our table with colleagues, whom you know—but then there was this anonymous person in the body bag on the table in front of you. We were given I think reasonably poor instruction about how we'd start off, and then we just had to start. We were supposed to have purchased a dissection kit from one of the surgical suppliers ... and we had lab coats on. I can't even recall if we had gloves on, I don't think we did—I think it was just done,' he laughs a little with sheer disbelief, 'with bare hands.'
>
> 'There were various instructors or tutors who would come around from time to time and see how you were going. Our job was to open the lower limb, and then dissect out the various muscles that made up the quadriceps femoris muscles—the four muscles that make up that and then turn the body over and do the muscles on the posterior aspect of the thigh, the hamstrings, and then the calf muscles and so on.
>
> 'Depending on what we were doing, we would have to position the body in a certain way or we'd have to open different parts of it and certainly in the abdomen, you would open the abdominal wall and then rummage around inside and find all the different organs—the liver and the kidneys and the stomach and the small

> and large bowel and so on, and the most important thing I guess we were learning was all the different relationships of the different bits to one another so that in a surgical procedure, you're able to know.'

He switches to 2021.

> 'These days when we teach students now, we don't do anywhere near as much cadaveric anatomy and students aren't allocated a cadaver—they see a lot of what's called a prosected specimen. So in other words, somebody who's an expert in dissection has already done these sorts of dissections. The students do a lot of radiological anatomy. So they might look at a CT scan or an ultrasound or something and have to relate the anatomy to that. So that it's really about trying to find out what's wrong with a patient.
>
> 'I've often looked back to those anatomy days and think it was quite useful having seen what it looked like in a deceased person, but also comparing it to what it's like when you're actually operating on someone for real—so the living tissue compared to the dead tissue, for instance.'

Robert and Ted were on the same table but both remember the old lady they studied differently. Robert described her as eighty-seven. Ted remembers her as being in her seventies and that she'd had a reasonably hard life. He said: 'She had quite a lot of heart disease. And she had pretty beaten-up hands and feet. She looked like she'd probably worked hard all her life.'

The donor on the table was an enigma to Ted: 'Most of us were nineteen, I suppose, and you didn't really think too much about the deceased person but you did have this respect for them. Or it taught you a bit about that people would do this—that they would actually donate their body to science. Or they might be a vagrant who nobody knew.

'They were just in some ways an unknown person who all of a sudden ended up at the anatomy school. So the way that they acquired the bodies—it was always a bit of a mystery. There was always this undercurrent of who is this person? And where had they come from? And how come we were able to operate on them?' Mysteries abounded—the students didn't really know what happened to the bodies afterwards either. 'At the end of the year, once we'd done our thing with the cadaver, then the cadaver went off and got buried, I guess in a common grave or a family plot, depending on who the person was. But again, we didn't hear anything about any of that sort of stuff so the actual governance behind all the acquisition of the bodies and the disposal of the bodies—as a student, we didn't know anything about it,' he says.

Whenever Ted walked into the pathology museum, he passed a portrait of his grandfather—J.V. Duhig, who founded the pathology department and was its inaugural professor in 1937. 'It was quite unnerving to walk into the pathology museum past your grandfather,' says Ted. 'He used to regale his kids, one of whom was my mother, with all sorts of stories about what they take out of bodies and put in the pathology museum. Queensland has got quite a good collection of pathology pots with these removed organs and different weird and wonderful things.' The lady on the table and all the other donors got them thinking. About a lot.

The medicos I spoke to who'd studied between the 1950s and the 1980s were told nothing about the people they were dissecting—they all had to draw on their imaginations. What else did they have? A 2013 survey of over 1150 medical students at twelve medical schools in the US found that the majority of them wanted to know more about their person and that 70 per cent gave them names, which served as a 'beneficial coping mechanism'.

I spoke to one South African doctor who named the body he dissected 'Whisky'. It was the 1970s in Cape Town and students in the year above advised his group that if they wanted a slim body with minimal fat—there was a perception they were easier to dissect—they should bribe Old Man Don with a bottle of whisky, which is what they did. His group ended up with a very slim dead man in his forties.

Albert Howard Carter III, the comparative literature professor who spent a semester watching first-year medical students dissecting in a US anatomy lab, wrote that all the students named their donors: Nero, Little Old Lady, Fred, Quasi, Fatless Man and Rose. While some anatomists and students are opposed to naming and think it disrespectful, the practice persists. A 2006 study of Cambridge University medical students found that not only were all the donors named but they were also apologised to. 'Today when I was cutting I was saying sorry. When I was making the incision, I was saying, "I'm sorry, I'm sorry",' said one student.

Since the 1990s, a wing of anatomy interested in the pedagogy of teaching has arm wrestled over 'to know or not to know' the name of the donor. While the International Federation of Associated Anatomists calls for anonymity, medical schools like Tzu Chi in Taiwan directly challenge this idea—students know their donors, meet their families and have their pictures on the walls of the dissecting room.

These days, there is a spectrum—some schools know what the person died from but not their name.

The anatomist Professor Claire Smith at the University of Sussex in Brighton tells me her students are allowed to know the name of their donor if they want to. 'I'd much rather they had a connection to that person and called them by their name so when they move them, or they do something, or they refer to them, that they do so respectfully. If they don't want to know their name, then they can give them a nickname, but it has to be a respectful nickname,' she says. 'You've got to keep the connection to them, and I think that helps instil respect, and that's very much important in what we do.'

Gareth Jones, the anatomist who did the first body donor study in 1992, has explored the issue of bodies' anonymity, pointing out that in the past, when unclaimed bodies were used, anatomists in some instances could not know who the person was. But these days, while they generally do, anonymity seems to persist, and the reasons aren't exactly clear.

When I speak to Gareth, I tell him I've wondered if I'm being unethical writing about people who were dissected and whether I should be respecting their privacy. Gareth says that the rise of donors being considered 'the first patient' and discussions around whether students should know what the person died from suggests a move within anatomy to 'personalise the whole process'.

'I think what you have got here with these dead bodies are people who used to be like us, they used to be alive, they used to be thinking people with their interests, and whatever. Now they're dead. But they still have a connection with us who are alive,' he says.

'When you get to medical schools or anatomy departments which have no dissection at all, they lose all this because they don't have a real body, which you can say, "Well, look, this was once a person like us, what does this tell us?" I think that is a big loss there.

'I would say that is one of the big things that has come in anatomy over recent years is that this is the first place where you can begin to teach students and medical students in particular about death,' he says. 'Death is seen now more and more as an integral part of anatomy.'

How extraordinary. I had assumed it was there all along but perhaps not.

***

Whereas corporate dudes connect through cycling and soldiers cement friendships on tours of duty, what was noticeable was how the medical students bonded over dissection. I wasn't expecting Ruby and Julie's donations to have created friendships but they probably did.

As Ted describes it: 'It was a useful bonding experience with your colleagues in that you had these long sessions, dealing with this almost bizarre kind of atmosphere with this strong formaldehyde smell and this deceased person that you were doing various things to.' Robert has strong memories too: 'We all got on very well.' Decades on, dissecting table buddies still go for lunches, have coffees and beers.

I spoke to one surgeon in Brisbane who had just spent the weekend at the property of one of his dissecting friends. 'I remember my first day going in as a formal student. You go and stand by your body, and six of us became very friendly because we spent maybe twenty to twenty-five hours a week picking at the poor old body.'

In the late 19th and early 20th centuries, the intensity of this group experience was celebrated in the curious trend of anatomy students getting photographed standing around a dissecting table with their dead person often in silly poses. In other images, grinning women in their dorm rooms cradle skeletons and skulls. To the 21st-century punter, these images are jarring and macabre but according to Yale's John Harley Warner, a medical historian, and Lawrence Rizzolo, a professor of surgery, it became a common way for medical students to commemorate their friendships in an era when it was acceptable to show feelings in the dissecting room. The pranks and gallows humour in the photos were a recognition of the emotional intensity of human dissection, and that the experience helped shape these young men and women into doctors.

Warner and Rizzolo explore how in the 1850s there was discussion in US medical schools about how dissection could harden and change the students' characters. As one professor told students in 1847: 'anatomy, however indispensable it may be, tends certainly to freeze up the springs of human feeling, and destroy our sympathy for human suffering'. Nonetheless, dissection was seen as a way to shape professional character and bring about some sort of moral transformation. Reading this reminded me a little of how dissection was being presented in 2021.

But this sensitivity and recognition of the intense feelings that went with dissection were to be quashed. According to Warner and Rizzolo, anatomy went through a crisis around the early 1900s, where it was seen as not scientific enough and too practical. Being emotional in the dissection lab became 'disreputable, professionally suspect' and to counter it anatomy hardened. As the pair write: 'the norm of silence about the emotional dimensions of dissection was set in place'.

In 1951 Renée Fox, then a sociology PhD student at Cornell University, spent time with medical students in the anatomy labs and observed that their emotions about dissection were considered something to be overcome. She would later develop what she saw in the dissecting rooms into the now-classic concept of 'detached concern'. As Fox wrote in 1959, the doctor is 'to be sufficiently detached or objective toward the patient to exercise sound medical judgment and maintain his equanimity' while simultaneously being 'sufficiently concerned about the welfare of the patient to give him compassionate care.'

I noticed that all the doctors, surgeons and technicians who were in the dissecting rooms from the late 1950s to the 1990s tended to take an 'objective' approach to working with the dead, who were seen as specimens. Of course there was respect, and moments when the donor or the skeleton they owned prodded them into thinking about who the person might have been, but the thought passed, and they returned to their work. It was a strange swaying between objectivity and subjectivity, objectivity and subjectivity. Or as the medical anthropologist Rachel Prentice puts it simply: 'Cadavers are persons and things.'

At first I thought the doctors hung out in objectivity more. *It's the science person in them,* I thought. While these students were in a 'detached concern' period, I could also see it was connected to self-preservation. I have often had moments of not really wanting to know about what happened to my grandparents, and feeling like throwing my laptop into the sea. I didn't like hearing the details. I didn't want to upset my dad or Uncle Maurie or families of donors with my findings. But the fact it was a truth overrode the drama in my head.

Warner and Rizzolo think the 'detached concern' dissecting period shifted when universities started holding memorial services for their dead—when the donors became a person first.

***

Dissection is not a stable, objective act—it's a moody business. I spoke to a few older doctors, some of whom didn't want their names in a book. One saw dissection as essential, while another didn't find the body useful and preferred learning from anatomy textbooks. Some went into excruciating raw details about the act of dissection, others didn't mention the process at all. Others recalled the strange characters, the blackboard drawings or the school counsellor who told them to get into medicine. One student in the 1990s used to take body parts from the city morgue without consent, which at the time wasn't an issue as it was for scientific research.

So I begin to see it wasn't just 'what happened' to the donors—it was also what the donors inadvertently did to the young students too. One donor prompted a young man to study the ear, nose and throat. One donor inspired respect. Donors made students feel pity, contemplate death and build life-long friendships.

Chapter 18

When it came to *what happened* to Ruby and Julie, I'd only ever vaguely thought about dissection. Embalming never remotely drifted into mind. Contemporary embalming for funerary purposes seems so macabre to me and while it obviously makes sense in anatomy, it was just one of those facts of life that I didn't think I'd ever have to engage with.

But spring, summer, autumn, winter—formalin became a constant in all my dissection discussions, popping up then back down again. The chemical compound was so ever-present that I began to see it as a dark, albeit necessary character. It hovered around, a gloomy fluffy cloud in the anatomy lab. It smelt, it stung, it irritated the skin, and caused cancer in certain dosages. I even looked into buying some just to get a sense of this smell that everyone talked about.

Formalin and formaldehyde were interchanged to the point that I wasn't sure if they were completely different, cousins, twins or identical twins. Embarrassed, in conversation I took to pretending to know it, but reached a point where I had to sit down and do some chemistry.

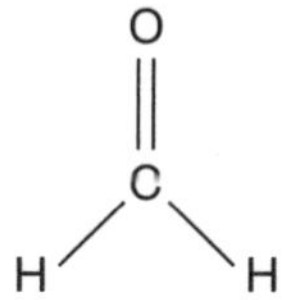

Formaldehyde is made of hydrogen, carbon and oxygen.

Formaldehyde is a colourless naturally occurring gas and formalin is formaldehyde mixed with water. The gas was discovered in 1859 and synthesised in 1868. In 1893 Ferdinand Blum, a young German scientist, when tasked with looking into the antiseptic qualities of this compound, noticed it was an effective agent in killing bacteria and that the skin of his fingers became hardened after coming into contact with the diluted solution. Since that time, anatomists have flocked to the chemical to preserve the dead for study. It had its flaws—it made the bodies rigid and discoloured but it was a good preservative over the long term.

Armed with next to zero knowledge of embalming chemicals, my next step was to find someone who was at the University of Queensland all those years ago. I'd heard about Robbie Boyes from a few people so I emailed him, unsure if I would break through his junk box. A few months passed and just as I was beginning to think he was lost to dissection history, he wrote back and we spoke over Skype.

By the time Robbie, originally from Scotland, arrived to work as a technician at the University of Queensland in 1988—around five years after my grandfather's body had left—the chemical formaldehyde was still being used even though there had long been a push to reduce the amount of it in the embalming fluid as it had been placed on the probably-a-human-carcinogen list.

It wasn't until 2004 that it was classified as a carcinogen although this remains a controversial listing in some quarters. Aside from using formalin, the University of Queensland embalmers were also using phenol, a disinfectant which Robbie describes as 'bloody nasty stuff' as when it got on your skin it burned. There was a constant hunt to try a less toxic embalming mix. 'A lot of us would muck around with different formulas to try and improve it,' he says.

When a donor arrived—at this stage in the early 1990s there were about sixty people a year and Robbie says there was never a shortage—they would be washed down, a ritual signifying the body donor's entrance into the dissecting room. Their heads would then be shaved.

'Interestingly in New Zealand, certainly at the University of Auckland at the time, they didn't remove the hair,' recalls Robbie. 'They were trying to get the person looking as animated as possible. There was a different approach there.' They would be checked for a pacemaker and there would sometimes be a slight delay if people from the cornea bank were coming to take these out.

Robbie would then 'raise' the artery, which involves cutting through the skin and using a stainless steel needle to find the artery and lift it out a little. The needle is about the length of a fork and is basically a very skinny stick. A nick is made in the artery and the cannula is inserted. Usually he would put the cannula in the back iliac artery, which is at the top of the leg. Sometimes, he would also have to raise the carotid artery in the neck as well, and the axillary in the armpit.

I struggled to get a sense of all this so watched an Indian forensic scientist on YouTube do a very straightforward presentation on embalming the cadaver of an elderly man, who he thanked before proceeding. Gunther von Hagens also goes looking for the femoral artery in the opening sequence of his dissection TV series—it's quite deep down.

Robbie says ideally one wanted to embalm the body as slowly as possible. 'Gravity feeding is the best way to do it but you don't always have the luxury of time.' Gravity feeding is where you suspend the fluid and it goes in like an IV drip in a hospital. He says it's the 'absolute best way to do it because you want to try and avoid damaging any structures on the way through as well, as you embalm.' If not, Robbie would pump the fluid through with a commercial embalming pump, the type also used at large funeral homes. 'It's a pressure pump basically.'

He says if the bodies were 'good', embalming would take a couple of hours. The donor would be placed in cold storage for a year or so. 'You certainly wouldn't want to be using them for a few months in an ideal world,' he says.

Having never mulled over embalming fluid but now doing so, I assumed it came in a generic bottle and you just injected it into the dead person—whether for a funeral, for anatomical purposes or to keep Chairman Mao and Vladimir Lenin looking good. But no. Anatomical embalming has long been more art than science—different methods, different 'looks', different textures and countless recipes. Some anatomists have also long kept their recipes and techniques secret. 'There were many recipes for embalming fluid but a lot of them were closely guarded by the universities for whatever reason,' recalls Robbie.

Guarding recipes is a tradition that dated back centuries. The Dutch anatomist Frederik Ruysch, known for his wildly inventive dioramas of fetal skeletons wearing jewels and surrounded by embalmed tissues, used to inject a secret preservative into his specimens, which in recent years has been discovered to contain clotted pig's blood, the mineral Berlin blue and mercury oxide.

But Robbie isn't too secretive about his old 1980s mix. He was using formaldehyde and Plasdopake, a flesh-toned Dodge product from the US that he introduced to the anatomy school. (Dodge, which I first encountered at a stall in London, are to embalming chemicals, instruments and supplies what Nike is to running shoes and sportswear.) He also used a fair amount of glycerin, although he says it had a tendency to encourage mould. I felt a pang hearing this.

Robbie says a perpetual problem with embalming was that the bodies became very hard. He kept baths at the university filled with a mild form of embalming solution but they usually used them to hydrate body parts that were used for routine classes. 'Off and on, the bodies periodically would be put in there to try and rehydrate them,' he says, adding that they also had to keep on top of mould.

Robbie travelled to anatomy conferences around the world, where he encountered the 'secret embalming recipe' phenomenon. 'The most interesting one was I went to a conference at the University of Graz, in Austria. They wouldn't disclose their formula. They were very proud. Their bodies were very dilated, and full of fluid. And when they weren't using them, they kept them submerged in baths of the solution as well, so they would raise them up and down and out of these baths. And what was attractive about it was it created a very soft tissue. So particularly for when the kids started dissection, it was more lifelike—if you like,' he says.

The Graz recipe wasn't secret for too long. The anatomist Walter Thiel, a man who spent his life researching embalming, invented the method, known as Thiel or Soft Fix, and published the 'new' recipe in a German magazine in 1992. I'm not sure why they didn't tell Robbie about it when he visited in 1994 but whatever the reason, the technique was finally published in English a decade later.

Components of the Thiel Solution
Hot tap water
Boric acid
Mono-ethylene glycol
Ammonium nitrate
Potassium nitrate
Chlorocresol-solution with Mono
4-Chlor-3-methylphenol

Thiel-fixed bodies have long been admired for looking so 'real'. Robbie sends me photos of the bodies and they do look surprisingly fleshy. The donors are soft, flexible, not smelly and long-lasting, largely because they have a low concentration of formaldehyde and are saltier. Unfortunately, the Thiel method is also seen as expensive, time-consuming and cumbersome. Once the bodies have been injected with different solutions in different areas, they need to be kept in large metal trays submerged in tanks for six months in a particular solution. In a 2013 interview with the BBC, Friedrich Anderhuber, Dr Thiel's assistant, said they worked on at least 1000 donated bodies to get the technique right.

Aside from hard fix and soft fix, bodies can also be 'fresh-frozen', which is pretty self explanatory. They are frozen and then defrosted, giving the tissue a sort of lifelike feel—although later I would learn that some people object to this term.

***

I read through old 1950s, 1960s and 1970s papers, where anatomists discuss how to preserve museum collections, small mammals and molluscs. I start to see that dissection and body preservation are a bit like Siegfried & Roy, the 1990s duo who entertained the world with their magic tricks and white lions—they are the twin children of anatomy. There is a lot of writing about innovation—try this new apparatus or check out the difference between formaldehyde-water and formaldehyde-methanol. There is nothing on 'The University of Queensland mix 1968 to 1982'.

But then I stumble across 'Human Body Preservation—Old and New Techniques', an article buried in the 2014 edition of the *Journal of Anatomy*. It not only has a detailed list of thirty (!) embalming mixes developed by anatomists in the 19th and 20th centuries—Tutch's 1975 mix was cheap and odourless, Bradbury & Hoshino's 1978 effort wasn't good for fixing brains—but is also a wondrous parade through the history of human embalming, each paragraph worthy of a museum display. The paper outlines how people have been:

- frozen
- dried out in the desert
- covered in the bright red pigment vermilion
- immersed in honey or alcohol
- eviscerated and stuffed with herbs
- injected with wax, mercury and arsenic
- injected with the Leonardo da Vinci mix of turpentine, camphor, oil of lavender, vermilion, wine, rosin, sodium nitrate, and potassium nitrate

It is clear that religious folk and anatomists have been fervent in their quest to find a way to have the dead ready for the afterlife, whether it be metaphysical or on the dissecting able. They've pretty much turned the periodic table and the natural world upside down, inside out and shaken it all about in the quest to find the perfect preservative.

Embalming powder used by Petrus Forestus (1521–1597)
Prepare a powder from:
2½ lbs aloes
1½ lbs myrrh
7 handsfull of ordinary wermut
4 handsfull of rosemary
1½ lbs pumice
4 lbs majoran
2 lot storacis calamata (1/16 lbs, 30 g)
½ lot zeltlinalipta muscate

I feel myself clutching at the edge of a new rabbit hole, legs flailing, trying to stop myself from falling in. But I can't help myself. I let go. I email Dr Erich Brenner, the author of the tome on embalming to find out more about these mixes, and what's going on with Austrian anatomists.

***

When Erich smiles over the internet, the screen comes to life, his big, toothy, friendly grin bursting from under his thick moustache. He's speaking from the alpine city of Innsbruck, where he is an anatomist at the Medical University, which began as a hospital in a nearby town in 1307 and evolved into a medical school over the next few hundred years. He's using a filter to block out his surroundings so I can't make any assumptions about him. But one I can make is that he is into his anatomy department—he's been there since 1990, which is basically his entire adult working life.

'For most people, it's not really interesting what is beyond the skin but I'm interested. I'm eager to see how things work,' he says. 'And what I've really learned for the last thirty years that I've been an anatomist is that ... let's say, when I started medicine, and studied anatomy, I was quite sure there is a general blueprint, a general plan for building up the human. And the more I learn about anatomy, I find out there is no general plan—there's a general concept. Men have to have a heart. It probably would be best to put it on the left side of the chest but there are people who have a spare heart on the right side. And it works. Shit happens.'

Like many anatomists, he fell into the profession by chance. When Erich was in his third year of medical school, he started tutoring in anatomy, an area he liked. It was also a way to earn a few more schillings. One year passed, two years passed, and he decided he wanted to do a PhD. He spoke to different departments but wasn't interested in the topics on offer.

He was complaining about it at a staff meeting when he was asked if he'd ever thought of doing a PhD in anatomy. Weirdly, he hadn't. He was soon studying the *hallux valgus* on the big toe—the dreaded bunion. My partner has one and I ask Erich if he has any tips on surgery or shoes. He says no and that George must consult a surgeon. Bummer.

As Erich describes it—and as Robbie mentioned—anatomists have long tinkered around with their own embalming recipes. Erich's list of different mixes in his paper is reminiscent of those times when something is missing from the bubbling sauce on the stove, and one flings open the herbs and spices cabinet to add more flavour. But in this case the anatomists have got the ethanol, formaldehyde and glycerine in a tub but decide to chuck in some sodium arsenate, salicylic acid and a bit of 6-chlorothymol to fight off the mould.

They try it but hmmm, the person is a bit *too* stiff—so they try adding some potassium pyrophosphate and magnesium chloride. The Anatomy Department at the University of Sydney reported in 2010 using different mixes depending on need, and one combination of pine oil, phenol and particularly di-(2-hydroxyethoxy)-methane completely eradicated mould growth, particularly *penicillium simplicissimum* and *penicillium waksmanii*.

Erich says anatomists would often experiment with mixes after reading an article suggesting that phenoxyethanol, for example, might be good for embalming, so they would try to find an optimal recipe with it to use in their own mortuary. 'Sometimes a recipe spreads to different anatomists because a new head comes and he brings the formulation from his old anatomy department with him. There was no real general scientific approach,' he says.

But the days of art over science may be waning.

As of 2021 the anatomical society for German-speaking countries is trying to unify the recipes and give general advice on embalming. For instance, one suggestion is that when formaldehyde is used, it must not be done with concentrations higher than 3.5 per cent.

Why the shift? With formaldehyde's status shifting from ***probable*** human carcinogen to ***known***, it may be banned for embalming under the European Parliament's Biocidal Products Directive 98/8/EC. Erich also predicts that in the next five to ten years each anatomy school will have to certify their own embalming recipe, which would cost around $475,000 (!) for a test without being sure it will be passed.

With anatomy schools unable to pay this exorbitant cost, Erich says the plan is for German-speaking medical schools to come up with a common recipe to get tested, so as to share the cost of the certification fee. 'No anatomist would be able to afford to certify their own recipe,' he says.

'Is there some debate about whose recipe is best?' I ask, anticipating a brouhaha or competition about what mix to go with. Far from it.

He says they will try to find a common recipe which can be tested across various anatomy schools. 'Because of course, in different settings, maybe there will be different aspects. For instance—moulding. We know that there are some morgues where some anatomists have a higher problem with moulding,' he says.

Nonetheless, Erich is okay with a common recipe. And globally, it's not like every department has its own brew anyway—some opt to buy company-made fluids. I know saving the planet and human health is obviously a positive step but I feel a strange pang of nostalgia for the anatomist who may love their particular mix. Homogeneity sweeps the world and embalming mixes are caught up in it too.

But with surgeons increasingly returning to dissecting halls to practise new styles of operations on donors, the need to have the bodies more 'lifelike' and formaldehyde-free means anatomists will continue to experiment. Perhaps the grumblings in the anatomical scene for more internationally recognised standards will bring more science to the art of embalming.

Day-to-day, Erich's work is literally hands-on. Clinicians will come to see him about a problem with a patient and he will go looking for answers in the bodies of his donors. 'You go to the dissection lab, and do a plain, very careful dissection, and you think, "Oh this could be a solution", and you spread it out to fifteen to twenty dissections,' he says. Erich takes his suggestion back to the clinician and months later, he will get a call saying the patient is better. 'When you see everything went well, you're really glad that you could indirectly help this patient by your anatomical research, by your anatomical knowledge.'

Erich's department gets about 160 body donations each year. He's noticed it's becoming something of a 'family tradition'—grandchildren sign up, following in the footsteps of their grandparents and parents. When he says this I'm reminded of Sophie Bolt's observation of that it was also becoming a custom amongst Dutch families. And my own grandparents both did it.

I confess to Erich that I'm not sure if I could donate my body to science—I still keep thinking about being cold—and he launches into a rousing from-the-mountaintop speech, which could be called 'Brenner's Body Donor Epistle'.

'There are two main reasons you can consider. One—it is actually necessary that you have good treatment for severe illness. Whenever you have a severe illness, you will of course want have the best treatment,' he says. 'Think of this—you had an accident, your knee is almost destroyed. And you have a surgeon who is really trained in anatomy and puts everything perfectly back. And one year after your accident, you don't even think about the accident because you have no restrictions in life. You have optimal quality of life, everything works fine. So the second thought is what kind of surgeon do you want for your next knee accident? Of course, a similar one—one who is also very well trained.

'Your thoughts could go beyond this. You can say "I had an anatomically well-trained surgeon and he did everything properly. I have heard about so many friends, colleagues who didn't have the luck to have a good surgeon,"' he says. 'One thing I could do is donate my body so that more medical students could be well trained in anatomy. Therefore, these things don't happen any more.

'The other idea which actually comes up in the Eastern world is that by donating your body, you become a great teacher.' Erich then says that as I write books I am a teacher. How about I be a teacher not only through books but through my body as well? He says it's about being very altruistic. 'I give the best I have—I give you my body to teach you to treat my children, and my grandchildren in a better way than I was treated.'

I'm momentarily caught up in the spirit.

***

Robbie Boyes would continue to embalm, dissect and prosect donors but he soon found a new interest—plastination, an embalming tool which did not exist when Ruby and Julie went to the anatomy lab. From the 1990s onwards, Robbie would become one of Australia's leading practitioners of this revolutionary technique invented by Gunther von Hagens, in which body fluids are replaced with a polymer and produce a rock-hard specimen, which can last for years. Robbie first trained with von Hagens in Heidelberg in 1992 and set up a plastination lab at Royal Brisbane Hospital, dividing his time between there and the university's anatomy department. He attended international plastination conferences and meetings. He later taught others how to do this extraordinarily time-consuming process, which involves embalming donors, cutting away skin, fatty and connective tissue, placing specimens into a freezing bath of acetone, and then a freezing bath of polymer, and then hardening them with a liquid gas cure. And that's leaving out a lot of details.

He says the ideal person to plastinate was someone who's not too fat, had good arteries and died of old age. 'Having said that, an obese cadaver is not necessarily a bad cadaver if they've been mobile right up until the time of death,' he says, later mentioning a 101-year-old woman who was a perfect donor physically.

'My passion was plastination,' he says and I feel it. 'I was actually very good at it.' Robbie also came to know von Hagens and later sends me a picture of the two smiling at a dinner together. But things weren't as cheery at the university though—it sounds like it was a tumultuous time for him. Due to a variety of reasons, his plastination lab was subsequently closed and he left the university in 2006.

With the end of a Covid-19 lockdown, I finally have the chance to meet Robbie in Melbourne for a coffee—he's tall, lithe and silver-haired, and shows me photos of his equally silver-haired dog Jock, reminding me of that adage about owners looking like their pets. He clearly loves Jock: the two appear together in Robbie's LinkedIn profile pic.

We get back into discussing his plastination days. I'm at times uneasy about the details but his pragmatism soothes it: he has a sort of hard-working, bloody-well-get-on-with-it attitude about it all, which is tinged with moments of tenderness—reminiscing about various surgeons and pathologists in his life as 'absolute gentlemen' and 'lovely'.

Talking to Robbie reminded me we are all in this whole strange life thing together, and he was there to play his particular, unique plastination part. On behalf of the world, I thank Robbie and the other technicians for doing this work, and seemingly enjoying it too. Perhaps if I tried it, it wouldn't seem too bad—at this stage, I imagine it being a horrible thing to do.

Robbie fell into working with the dead by chance when he began at the Dumfries and Galloway Royal Infirmary mortuary in Scotland in the 1980s. He soon found it fascinating but also moving, particularly when he had to show families their dead loved ones, a task he describes as a privilege. He moved to Brisbane and worked at the Royal Brisbane Hospital mortuary, where he did day-to-day work such as eviscerating postmortem cases, skin harvesting for the burns unit and showing family members a dead relative.

He used to spend a lot of time in the postmortem rooms. 'One thing I realised is that with children that die, it's only ever beautiful children,' he says. 'After the postmortem, you are left very much on your own to reconstruct them—that used to upset me a little bit.' During this time his own child died—a stillborn baby who was sent to a different morgue for examination.

I say that after this death, it must've been hard going about his daily work. 'It's not being desensitised but there are a lot worse things than the dissection of someone who has given their body,' he says. 'It's all relative if you like.' He's so perfectly clear and right, and I need to be reminded of this: of course there are far more disgusting and horrific things than cutting up a donated body.

Robbie seems drawn to working in places others would find confronting. Where others volunteer at charity shops or with their local sports club, when I met Robbie he was busy with a few volunteer gigs: taking his beloved Jock to do pet therapy with cancer patients at a hospital, visiting an elderly lady in a housing commission each week, and working as an independent volunteer visitor in Victoria's youth justice centres. His background in volunteer work is varied and extensive—he is obviously someone who likes to help others in his spare time.

I'd spoken to one scientist who said that prosection could be emotionally difficult, and they would sometimes tell their staff to take a day off and go to the beach.

'Are you quite thick-skinned? Did you ever find plastination hard to do?' I ask.

He seems unfazed and I'm surprised when he says he finds it interesting. 'It's only yucky if the bodies weren't properly embalmed and you've gone to a lot of effort and it's not going to work,' he says. He said while a normal specimen only lasted one or two years in a dissecting room, the 'lovely thing' about plastination was that it lasted for years.

Robbie stopped plastinating over a decade ago but remains a cheerleader. 'I always make the point—it's a much nicer way if someone's kind enough to donate their body to science. It's a much more humane, if you like, more civilised way to preserve and respect the hidden identity of that person. I've always felt that with the plastinated specimens that I did—particularly when they came out very nice—I thought: "This is great. If this person could only know what a huge contribution they are going to make."'

He raises a contemporary debate in the anatomy fraternity: to dissect or not to dissect. 'I hope universities are not still fighting to keep cadavers. Really, it should go back, I believe, to the surgeon. Historically, surgeons would teach surgeons. From the day of the barber shop, if you want to go back that far. But they got busy, and they were making lots of money, and they didn't have time to teach these incoming young guys, so they said to the universities, you teach them. That's where it fell over, if you like—I would suggest.'

I'm quite stumped at one point when he says he's okay about the use of unclaimed bodies for dissection—I've not really heard a professional in this area say as such. It doesn't happen in Australia any more but it does in swathes of the world. 'I don't have any problem with that. Otherwise, the taxpayer is going to give them a respectful funeral and that's the end of it. So why not do something more with it?'

I tell him I don't agree. 'I think it's pretty ... I think you've got to consent to this happening.'

'I don't know. I've been there and when you are dead, you are dead, Jackie.'

Chapter 19

I'm sitting in the University of New South Wales medical school foyer waiting to meet up with Goran for a proper face-to-face chat, after meeting so fleetingly in London. I'm a tad nervous as I'm also meeting Professor Nalini Pather, who runs anatomy at the university. I'm not sure what she's going to be like but I can feel a slight angst for some mystical reason, akin to my behaviour at the London conference—looking around, suspecting I am going to be marched out or busted. What was with this paranoia?

I'm yet to find any former anatomists who were at the University of Queensland and I figure meeting contemporary anatomists may give me an insight into the old world, some sort of take on the guild. Of course Goran and Nalini were anatomists from a different age, but would they share some traits, some interests, at least a bauble of similarity with their predecessors?

As a Gen Xer, I have inadvertently absorbed some of the spirit, tropes and tones of 19th-century slum journalism and 20th-century new journalism. As a young writer I read classics like Norman Mailer's *The Executioner's Song* and Joan Didion's work, and saw what worlds they cracked open. I asked George, my partner, what he thought linked him to mathematicians in the past, and he replied: 'An irrational belief that elegance and beauty are indicators of truth.'

***

It was the early 1980s in Belgrade and Goran was a teenager who didn't really know what he wanted to do with his life. Conversations at home nudged him into medicine—how many kids have endured this pressure!—so he tried out nursing for a spell but realised it wasn't for him. He says one of the reasons was that he was too empathetic. He next tried philosophy because as a teenager he'd had an existential crisis. (When he tells me this, I remark that I'm still having one. 'Me too,' he jokes.) He'd always been interested in questions around the meaning of life, and philosophy suited him. 'It taught me how to think, how to explore things, how to reflect.' Although Goran left the former Yugoslavia years ago, he still has a strong Balkan accent.

He collected his philosophy degree but science kept waving in the distance, so he did a masters degree in biological anthropology, a field which explores human origin and our variations, and how we have changed over time. Biological anthropologists like bones: they study old skeletons found buried in mud; they examine our primate relatives. Charles Darwin laid the field's modern foundations. The Leakey family continued the work, unearthing numerous ancient remains, including the 1948 discovery in Kenya of a 25-million-year-old skeleton, a common ancestor to humans and apes. In the 1960s, Jane Goodall discovered that chimpanzees used tools.

There are so many branches to it but one way of thinking about it are those display cabinets in museums with life-size statutes of half-human, half-monkey figures—our ancestors essentially—slowly changing shape over millions of years. Goran was drawn to this realm as it gave him an opportunity to explore questions of who we are and where we came from via the body.

At university, with the fall of the communist government in Belgrade, there was a sense that Yugoslavia was going to open up, and catch up with the rest of the world. It didn't. It degenerated into what he calls a 'nonsensical bloody civil war'.

His studies suffered as he was engaged in political activism against Slobodan Milošević, the dictatorial president of Serbia from 1989. War erupted and Goran ended up moving to South Africa to do his PhD in biological anthropology at the University of Witwatersrand or 'Wits' in Johannesburg. It was here that he got a job as a demonstrator and prosector in the anatomy labs, which stressed him out at first as he'd not had much to do with dead bodies. Over time, however, he got used to it, as he had a good network of colleagues. 'So we did it together, we supported each other,' he recalls.

'There was a bit of apprehension about how I was going to react when I encountered a dead human body. But I think I had the same experiences as many of the medical students. So first time it was stressful but then all the subsequent labs were much less stressful,' he says. 'And then later on you're mainly worried about your anatomy knowledge. Do you know enough? Is your expertise good enough? That's the main stress. But stress from working with dead bodies sort of goes down, and it stays down for the majority of students and me as a staff member.'

Once he'd finished his PhD, there was a job opening teaching in anatomy and biological anthropology. 'Many biological anthropologists are recruited to teach anatomy because as biological anthropologists, we have to know anatomy really well.' He initially resisted anatomy—it's both emotionally and cognitively hard. Students can struggle with dead human bodies. The language is so difficult.

Yet somehow Goran came to love it. Wits university, founded in 1896, was also a mecca for international scientists who had come to examine the thousands of unique specimens stored in the Fossil Primate and Hominid Vault in the Evolutionary Studies Institute, a trove of priceless ancient skulls, teeth and bones of humans, chimpanzees, gorillas and orangutans. It was in this atmosphere that he started meeting like-minded scientists who were interested in some of the ethical issues Goran was starting to confront in the classroom.

He recalls one of his first anthropology lectures where he was teaching human biodiversity, which in the past was referred to as *race*. He noticed immediately the apprehension in some of the African students, 'because in the past, if not them, their mothers and fathers were taught or told all sorts of rubbish about people having better abilities, higher intelligence, racial differences and so on'.

But as he moved through the course, he could feel a sense of relief. 'At the end, invariably, there was big applause to my and my tutor's lecturing, and it was almost liberating that all the knowledge, all the nonsense that was taught about racial differences is just that—nonsense. I felt it a duty to sort of disperse these myths, simply by teaching science, and what we know about racial differences, what we know about anatomy and so on.'

But Goran encountered other issues in the anatomy lab. Why was it that all the anatomy lecturers were European white men, while those lying dead on the dissection tables were usually Africans, who nobody had claimed? The few European bodies that came in had been donated. 'So immediately that stratification that was left over from apartheid was noticeable and was noticeable to students,' he says. It was not really spoken about either. 'It was taken for granted that this is what it is, and this is what you work with.'

With his background in biological anthropology, as he watched the way the classes were taught, he also saw it was schematic, it was always 'average' and what was average was a European white man. There was little exploring of biological variation and diversity—all the textbooks were of male livers and kidneys, for example, and there was absolutely no mention of intersex people, who can have both male and female sex characteristics. It's an issue that persists today—numerous studies have shown how anatomy textbooks largely feature young, white muscular men as 'normal'.

We're talking in his new, generic white office with a glass wall that looks out on to other offices. Behind him are shelves jammed with quite a range of texts: anatomy, anthropology, paleoanthropology, human diversity, primatology, history of anatomy, *Origins* by Richard E. Leakey. I can see his diverse interests reflected in his collection and how they have spilled into his ongoing career.

Goran moved to Australia in 2008, and began managing the skeletal collection and the body donor program at Macquarie University. It was here that he began putting his ideas around humane anatomy into practice, such as teaching students respect for the donors, and looking into the provenance of the large skeletal collection, which he soon found was mostly made up of donations from old doctors who had them left over from their medical school days.

But where were these skeletons from? Goran began networking with anatomists across Australia and they too shared concerns about the provenance of their collections. He and his colleagues studied the skeletons, and he says there was a high likelihood they were from Calcutta in India, brought in either legally or illegally over the years.

An estimated two million skeletons were shipped to medical students around the world from the 1930s up until the ban in 1985. At one point, the trade was so big that the Indian bone dealers had their own union, and had their company brands on small metal plates on the backs of some of the skulls. Goran recalls that they had to rethink their collection. 'When we teach anatomy, we try not to just teach anatomical structural of human bodies, but also professional behaviour, medical ethics, and it's really difficult to do that if you use human remains that potentially came to you in a way that's *maybe* legal, and definitely not ethical.'

Concerned anatomists are now finding ways to supplement these skeletal remains. Goran and his colleagues started scanning bones and 3D printing them, and found they were pretty accurate. Down the track, Goran hopes to use skeletons from donated bodies, and if they have permission, to scan and 3D print them.

Across the hall from him is Nalini, who he met in South Africa, and the colleagues have since collaborated on books, papers and book chapters, which often tackle contemporary issues in the profession. One of their more recent collaborations explored the sex binary. In their paper, the pair argue that the anatomy curricula and textbooks need to introduce intersex and more differences in sexual development, and 'present sex as a continuum rather than two sharply divided sets of characteristics'. They argue this approach is crucial for training doctors but more importantly, stopping the 'problematic practices such as non-consensual "normalising" surgeries'. Alongside Joyce El-Haddad, they also looked into the tricky issue of human fetal tissue and embryos of unknown provenance kept in museum and university collections around the world, and how to ethically deal with them.

I ask Goran what part of the body he likes the most and he says he's drawn to the musculoskeletal system. 'It still amazes me,' he says. 'I like muscles, I like bones, and as a biological anthropologist, bones will be my first love. But what amazes me the most is that humungous variety that each of us exhibits because of our individual backgrounds because of our sex, because of our age, and because of our ancestry.' He uses the example of biceps—the two-headed muscle on top of your arm. Between 15 and 25 per cent have three 'heads'; some even have four. 'So each muscle is structural—it has numerous variations.'

I'm in awe when he says there are still so many different areas that anatomists don't know about—one particularly neglected area is children's anatomy, which is very different to adult anatomy—and that our bodies are constantly changing to the point that the Scottish doctor Gavin Francis called us 'shapeshifters'. As Goran puts it: 'As you look at human anatomy, you have to look at it as a dynamic system, which constantly changes throughout life.'

***

Nalini Pather's office is filled with anatomical bric-a-brac: a small banner which reads I ♥ anatomy, a 3D print of a dissected heart, a whale vertebra and a student's beautiful drawing of her dissection of the gluteal region. It's silly I was so nervous about meeting Nalini as she's open and charismatic, and chuckles a lot in conversation, consistently seeing the amusing aspects of her life in anatomy. But what is more extraordinary is her rising out of poverty and endemic racism in South Africa to become Professor of Anatomy at the University of New South Wales and running the body donor program. (Since we met, she has since been promoted to Associate Dean of Education but is still closely involved with the anatomy school. Goran has moved on too—he is now Professor and Head of Discipline in Anatomy at Flinders University in Adelaide.)

Nalini was originally from the coastal city of Durban in South Africa where as a young Indian girl growing up under the racist apartheid system, her father, Dave, worked as a laboratory chemist as he was unable to study engineering because of his skin colour. Her mother, Radha, was a pattern maker in a factory. 'She was highly creative. She loved doing things with her hands,' says Nalini.

Nalini got the marks for medicine but as she was Indian, there were only a few places she could go. She didn't want to leave her family so changed to a Bachelor of Medical Science degree at University of Durban-Westville, now known as University of Kwa-Zulu Natal, which was predominantly Indian and Black. She had no idea she would end up dissecting. 'I didn't realise that that was what was expected of me.' She felt very afraid that day in 1995 when she first walked into an anatomy lab.

'There was very little appreciation for the fact that we may be terrified walking into that dissecting room. I was actually trying to keep this facade of keeping it all together and all of that, but I was really terrified, especially of sitting in front of this whole body, which was covered in calico, and with the plastic over it.' She would spend the next two years dissecting one young Black man in his early thirties, who she describes as 'really young, perfectly fit'. She clearly remembers him. 'I think the thing that struck me most was—and it struck me more when I came here to Australia than when I was in South Africa—that the bodies that we had in South Africa were very young. Their muscles were well defined, well developed.'

Over the next few weeks, as she grew more comfortable, she and her fellow medical students began talking about who they were dissecting and started asking questions. It was only then that Nalini came to learn that the young man had lain for two years in a morgue and with nobody claiming his body, had ended up on the university dissecting table.

Apartheid was in its final days when Nalini was at high school and heading to university. It was a tumultuous period which saw mass protests against segregation and a lack of equality in education. Nelson Mandela was released from prison in 1990. Democratic elections were held in 1994. Against this background, she became sensitive to the fact that the bodies in the lab were never white or Indian—they were all Black. 'All kinds of questions were raised in my mind. I asked several questions and I think what I came across was a fear of people to actually talk about what was really happening,' she says. 'We accept that this is where the bodies come from, but we actually don't want to talk about it.'

Despite these niggling ethical concerns in the back of her mind, she spent the next two years dissecting the young man. She also learned from the bodies on the other tables around her, and it made her see how much variation there was between people.

I say: 'You mentioned this word "variation". This is kind of quite crucial in anatomy, isn't it? We all think that we're the same ...'

'But we're all quite different, and there's a range of normal. And variation is really important,' she says. 'Variation is really important in clinical anatomy—it is one of the reasons why there could be surgical errors like mistakes made in surgery or why surgical procedures won't work. It's because everyone is slightly different.'

'What would be the differences between you and me? I mean, we're both forty-seven,' I say.

'We are both forty-seven,' she laughs.

'I'm a white woman and you're an Indian woman. I would have thought we were the same.'

'Except for skin colour, we probably are the same, mostly, but there will be lots of variation. So for example, in my hand, there is a muscle that I don't have, it's called *palmaris longus*, and the latest stat is that 17 per cent of people don't have it,' she says, laying her hand palm-up on the table and I follow suit.

'I'm pretty sure if you flex your hand ...' she pauses.

I flex my hand.

'See you've got a really prominent one there,' she says pointing to my wrist area. 'I've got nothing. So you know, that's a really easy one.'

She explains that some organs and muscles are becoming what's known as vestigial, where as a species, because we haven't used them for a long time, they are disappearing.

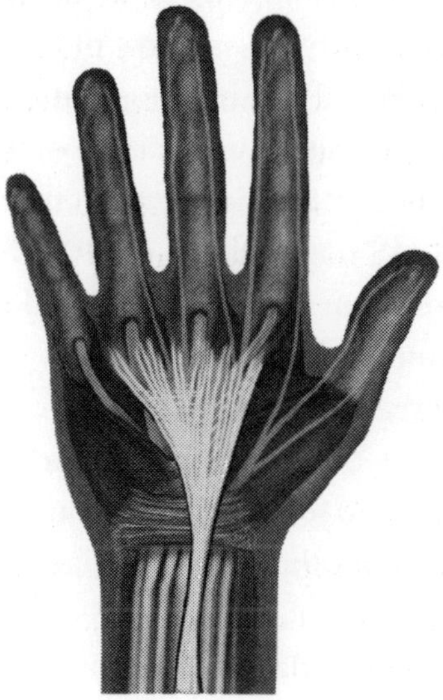

Palmaris longus is the white part that fans over the palm and the tendon that goes down the forearm. It protects the meridian nerve. *Marie Dauenheimer.*

Nalini's dad had a ***palmaris longus*** as do both her sons. 'It's really interesting I don't have it,' she laughs.

'So there's endless variations?'

'There's an endless list of variations. There's a book, it's called a *Compendium of Variations*. And as we find new variations that have a higher probability than just a case report, it's normally put in there.'

She points to two PhD students sitting outside her office and explains that they are studying variations in a different way. One student is looking into the variation of big vessels and ducts that go into the liver and how it varies with age but also how it changes if you have a particular type of surgery. 'So for example, if you had your gallbladder removed ten years ago, how does that anatomy actually change? And what implications does it have for you as you age?' she says. Another student examined a set of eight bones in the wrist. At first they are made of cartilage but over time ossify and become bone.

Based on how quickly it happens or at what point someone is in that bone-forming process, we can say how old they are. Nalini and her student Ehab Matar looked at this in a population of New South Wales children, and found that the rate at which it becomes bone is 'significantly different' from the standard that is used in clinical practice, which is based on a UK and a US population sample. These variations within populations have major clinical implications. (Ehab became a minister in the Lebanese government in 2022!)

I ask Nalini which area of the body she's most interested in. She finds many parts beautiful—the brain, the thorax and the abdomen. 'But the organ I would choose second to the brain would be the heart—dissecting the heart I find amazing but I think partly because it's a funny story—not so funny story actually.'

She goes back to her early days in Durban, when she was dissecting the young man. 'Somewhere in the first quarter of the year we'd dissected the thorax out, and took the heart out and I had the job of dissecting the heart. And I thought it was such a beautiful dissection.' A few weeks later, Nalini arrived at university and there were police everywhere in the department. A family had come to claim the body of their loved one and it was the young man Nalini had been working on.

'Then the story slowly emerged that there was a problem and that body was the one they'd come to get, and so we had to put all of it back. And I remember the professor at the time saying, "Well, you know, there was this heart dissection we'd like to keep it. It was really good," and the family saying that out of everything, the heart was most important to their culture that they have back. And so it had to go back.'

She laughs gently as she tells me, 'And so all of my beautiful dissection was taken away, you know, it had to and I perfectly accept that it had to but I was emotionally tied to this dissection that I had done.' To this day, she remains tied to the heart for that reason.

The end of apartheid saw a large influx of Black students, many unable to speak English, which was the lingua franca at the university. Nalini got a job tutoring these students to help them pass anatomy and realised that she loved teaching, as well as helping people. Her professor could see she was bright, and offered her work on a team researching surgical procedures.

'Coming from a really disadvantaged background and relatively poor family, I was suddenly in a space where I was going to conferences, I was going overseas, I was doing things that were really well respected and I loved it and decided to stay.'

As part of Nalini's masters degree research, she collected specimens from the state morgue. 'And when I went to the morgue, I think the first few times, what really struck me was there were so many bodies and they were all Black—probably because it was the state morgue and it was in the city, a fairly big city. And so I realised then that violence in South Africa was a real thing for a particular group of people who were disadvantaged by the political system, more so than I was.'

She eventually moved to Wits in Johannesburg where she got a job as a lecturer, and did her PhD in an era which she describes as an 'awakening moment' as it was so diverse in so many ways—there were staff from all over the world, and while the bodies were mainly Black, there were also white donors. 'There was quite a lot of variability in lots of ways. But also, I think because the staff was so diverse, I began to understand more about different people's perspectives on studying anatomy, and on handling dead bodies.'

It was in this environment that she met Goran, and Nalini jokes that she's not even sure what he was doing in Johannesburg. 'I actually don't know much about why he came there or when he came,' she laughs.

Anatomists globally are in very different legal situations. Some grapple with having to use unclaimed bodies and even though it might be legal to do so, their efforts to transition to using only donors can be thwarted by management because it's going to cost more.

In Australia, many anatomists are what's known as the anatomy licence-holder at their university, and they are in the difficult position of being both employed by the university but also having to report problems to the public health unit. 'I think we need to have a higher standard than the law expects from us—that we need to be way above board, and we also need to highlight discrepancies that we see. So there needs to be some kind of mechanism where the anatomy licensee has some independence or some autonomy.'

It's important to have independence, as Nalini sees herself as the voice of the dead. 'The anatomist needs to actually rise to the fore and be that ethical advocate for the right thing because the donor has no voice, right? And so who's going to be their voice? It can't be their family because their family actually is not here when the body is here. It has to be the anatomist and so trying to highlight to the larger anatomy community that we are the voice and all of our situations are less than ideal.'

I later realise the seriousness of what she's saying when I learn that prior to Nalini's arrival, the UNSW anatomy department was put on notice in 2007 over allegations that a staff member had inappropriately handled and fondled donated bodies in a surgical training laboratory, and that body parts were piled together in coffins. The University apologised to families. The school went through a series of reviews so they could be compliant.

As we speak, Nalini's office telephone rings a few times. She remarks that she regularly gets calls from donors checking in. 'They ask if everything is okay, just to chat, and to say "I'm still here, and this has happened to me, and I thought you'd want to know that I'm okay, my body is still going to be good,"' she laughs affectionately.

'Our donors are all much, much older than you would find in South Africa. And when we talk to them when they are thinking about donation, I think the tragedy for me is for lots of them, they are alone, and they don't know what's going to happen to them when they die. And so taking care of their body and donating to us is a way of them saying, "Okay, I've taken care of that. So I'm not going to be lying on a bed somewhere and rotting or something," which for me there is an immense sadness in reflecting on that kind of isolation and loneliness that people feel.'

But Nalini has observed that people donate for all sorts of reasons. The donor might have had an affiliation with the university. They may have suffered in life but didn't know what it was, and hope the anatomists will find out the problem and report it back to the family.

Families regularly phone Nalini to find out how the dissection of their person is going or when the body will be cremated so they can get the ashes. 'They will randomly just call and have a conversation,' she says. Families frequently want to watch a dissection; they are not allowed for multiple reasons but mainly because NSW law states that bodies can only be examined for education or research purposes. 'It's not for public display—even though it may be your mother or father or sister or brother, or even child . . . so we don't allow for that. But also, it's not good for them to actually do that.'

She says they put on annual thanksgiving services for families of donors. Students play music and recite poems, and staff do the same. 'We also lay a flower for each person, and their name is read, and we give the family a token of appreciation,' she says. 'When the body is cremated, we give them the ashes back. If they want to know whether something was found, we try to find that information and give them that as well, but we don't allow them to come [to the anatomy lab].'

Nalini makes sure she goes to the labs every day. 'It's the way I stay connected, not just to my staff, which I obviously want to be very connected to. But also it makes me connected to the fact of what is real, and what is the most important thing in our job,' she says, adding that she's also there to teach.

She then pauses, and laughs a little. 'To tell you the truth, I like dissecting. It gets my mind off lots of things. Some people do needlework, and some people do art. I like to dissect.'

Chapter 20

Dr Juliet Gallagher has just finished for the evening at her job as a GP on Queensland's Sunshine Coast in 2021. It's 8 pm on a Tuesday. 'Is it okay if I eat dinner?' she asks. Yes of course. We are speaking over the phone so I don't know what she looks like or if she moves her hands when she talks but I can hear the tink of cutlery on crockery as she eats. Juliet is Robert Sweeney's older sister.

She is also the cousin of Margaret, an anti-war activist I know, and she reminds me a little of my friend—open, easy to talk to, chatting away like we're at a slumber party or hanging out over coffee. (In fact, almost everybody I speak to about dissection is like this.) She seems autonomous and spirited, and I imagine someone who appreciates common sense. A slight anxiety is circling me though. Juliet arrived at the University of Queensland in 1969. Ruby's body also arrived in December 1969 and could have possibly been in the dissecting halls in 1970. Imagine if she tells me she dissected a woman …

***

As a child, Juliet was always interested in animals, nature, frogs and bodies. 'I think I always loved looking at bodies and if there was something dead it didn't worry me. I remember sheep getting killed when I went out to my cousin's out west. So you know, they cut the throat, which is awful, but it didn't revolt me. I just went, "Oh, that's so interesting,"' she recalls. 'I went to the Barrier Reef when I was quite young. My parents took me to Heron Island when I was about eight, which is a pretty good privilege. They were into national parks and walking and streams and things. You weren't told about nature, the way kids are now, where they had nature programs and that sort of thing. It was more just being immersed in it.'

As she grew older: 'I didn't particularly like chemistry and physics. I liked biology, physiology.' Juliet was so young really—like all of them—when she started at the University of Queensland medical school. It was a particular era, a time of formality, of long white coats, when people were referred to as Mr and Miss so-and-so. The girls had to wear dresses, skirts and stockings and pants were not permitted. Ties were compulsory for the boys.

'As a medical student, you were sort of treated like a mini-doctor. You know how in the old days in the movies all the doctors wore white coats? The doctors wore long coats and the medical students wore short ones and that's how you knew whether someone was a doctor or student. Have you seen that TV show *Call the Midwife*? It was a bit like that,' she says, 'with the coats and stethoscopes. It was very formal. But society was very formal then ... it was to show respect.'

Some memories and images of her time in the dissecting hall seem firm. Some facts she isn't so sure about. As she says to me later: 'We were very young, I was seventeen when I started. So when you're talking to me, my memories were not even mature. My brain was still growing.' One thing she remembers distinctly is the way the men dominated the course—she thinks there were only around 30 per cent women.

She pauses and chuckles a little to herself, possibly working out how to best articulate what was going on for women at the time. 'Some women ... there wasn't ... it was pretty ... oh well, ask me more questions and I'll tell you,' she muses and then settles on: 'Anatomy was very much the domain of the surgeons. So if you weren't going to be a surgeon, you weren't given as much to do. You had to let the males do more of the work. That's what I remember—I was a bit cross.'

Juliet began dissecting in her second year.

'The boys would say, "Oh, I'm going to be a surgeon so I want to do this. You watch."' She laughs a little but it's more sardonic. 'I didn't really like it much so I sort of let them do it if that makes sense. How would I know if was going to be a surgeon? I didn't know what I was going to do. I was only eighteen.' One of her fellow students who was slightly older was particularly bossy. 'You know, at that age, a male of twenty is going to boss an eighteen-year-old girl around.'

She did three practicals a week for three hours each, and one was on a Friday, which meant a lot of people wagged it. When she walked into the dissecting hall, the bodies were covered with a white sheet. Technicians in white coats looked after them but she isn't sure if they were taken in and out every day. She isn't sure if they were told the name of their person either. 'What I remember is this person that we did the dissection on was a very old woman, skinny and small, and had grey hair. So she was probably eighty or something.'

I'd been frozen all this time speaking to Juliet but felt my ice crack when she described her person as someone who wasn't Ruby. I began melting and continued to warm at her tales, knowing she could have been in the room when Ruby was there. 'I remember that you *did*,' she says emphatically, 'you treated them with respect but it was a bit hard to always be respectful because you'd be talking to each other and talking about you know, what you do on the weekend, and all that sort of thing. But there was no smoking or anything like that in there. Even though people smoked heaps outside, there was no party or anything. It wasn't rude.'

She thinks there were either ten or twelve students around the table, and usually only two or four people at the most could be dissecting. The others were left to chatter. 'So imagine having an arm. Someone would be doing a wrist, and someone would be doing the fingers. But I think you could only do the muscles in order, you couldn't just attack it, you would have to do it slowly, and you would have to identify every nerve, every artery. And then you got down to the bones. We had skeletons that we actually owned and kept at home. And I think the skeletons you bought from another student weren't anything to do with the donors' bodies. I don't know where the skeletons came from, to tell the truth.'

'So it was obviously a real skeleton?

'Oh yeah, no question. Isn't that terrible? But it was just taken for granted.'

She doesn't specifically remember her first day dissecting but she does remember the *feeling*. 'They probably gave us a talk before we went in there. That's why I remember the whole thing about respect and you had to wear these clothes [lab coats], and you had to do this [behave in a certain way]. Oh, yes, I remember being well—just amazed at how people are dead. They really are dead, you know? They're not people any more, unfortunately—if you've ever seen someone who's died. Their spirit isn't there. It's the weirdest feeling. You just go "Ohhh, their body's here but they're not here."'

I asked, 'Did you ever wonder about who you were working on?'

'Oh yeah I did but we weren't told anything, which is a pity really. We weren't really given ... now maybe they would be. It would have been nice to have her story but I do remember it was a woman and she was old and she was little.'

Whoever this donor was, she gave Juliet superpowers. 'I just know that I know a lot more anatomy than someone who graduates today because, okay, we did nine hours a week, and unless you're completely slack, you must have absorbed quite a bit of it.' She would sit in lectures watching anatomists draw a body part, she would refer to her *Gray's Anatomy* and she had a body to study. She saw how different we all are.

She says when she used to teach young doctors as a GP, she noticed that if someone came in with a numb finger, the students wouldn't immediately think of the anatomy. But she can easily think of what's in the finger, the wrist, the elbow, the knee. 'I've sort of got a 3D image of what's in there still.'

Anatomy was about memorising but biochemistry was *really hard*—it was much more complicated. She worried about biochemistry so much that she didn't learn enough anatomy. 'I found it an overwhelming amount of information. Because I wasn't exactly studious to tell the truth,' she confesses. 'I was a bit of a party girl, unfortunately, but that's probably just my age group—I was eighteen, nineteen. I found it really hard to concentrate on all that stuff and still go out on weekends.' Juliet would fail anatomy and have to repeat again the next year.

Even though she was and is fervently anti-smoking, she'd hang outside the anatomy building while her friends had a cigarette. She'd seen smokers' lungs in the dissecting hall. 'I can still see what happened to them in the person who smoked. They were black.'

It sounds like she didn't get to dissect much—she estimates it was probably a quarter of the time. 'The really "conscie" ones who wanted to be surgeons, they would be just obsessing and you would have to stand back and let them do it. Then you would look over their shoulder and see what they're doing and they'd go, "See that?" and you'd go, "Oh yeah, right oh". That's my memory.' It was always crowded. Curiously, she doesn't remember dissecting the head and neck in third year at all. 'I wouldn't have liked that.'

She does remember her donor's heart and the lungs though. 'Seeing the heart ... you did open up the heart and see the little valves and the little strings. And I'd say that was pretty impressive. Yeah, and knowing that it had beaten for eighty years without stopping that whole time. This thing, this small, little thing—not much bigger than your fist—had been beating all this time.'

It was a peak period for 'detached concern'. 'Everyone acted tough,' she says. Perhaps people were freaking out but they weren't talking about it.

But still, this old lady got her thinking. 'I wondered about her. But I don't remember being told her name or why she gave her body. But would they have known why she gave her body? Who would have asked her? They would have just said, "Oh, this person wanted to donate their body." But I know it was voluntary. It wasn't as if they were taken from criminals or anything—I hope.'

I tell her that in some parts of the world today, many people who are dissected are unclaimed. 'That is so cruel!'

'Would you donate your body?' I ask.

'No,' she laughs a little. 'I wouldn't.'

'Why?'

'I just have a feeling that I wouldn't like people looking at my body,' she says. 'I think you feel a body is part of you—even though you're gone. I'm happy to donate my organs. I put that on my licence but that's different to your whole body, your head and your hair and your face and your legs and feet, your toenails.'

Chapter 21

I loved that Goran said he was drawn to biological anthropology because he could ask philosophical questions about who we are through the body, and that the anatomy lab was a way to explore life and death. My interest in death momentarily felt honourable and meaningful, and not something to be ashamed of.

There are times in sunny and death-free Sydney that I feel like I should be into something with more—I dunno—life? I'm lonely in my interests. I gaze at Jacques Fabien Gautier d'Agoty's *The Flayed Angel*, a disgusting but mesmerising painting of a woman glancing over her shoulder at her entirely dissected back: flayed, creamy ribs and red, pulsing muscles exposed.

I find solace online, like the rest of the world. The Yale Medical Historical Library posts unusual and delightful images—often old anatomical drawings—from their rare book collection. Art historian and photographer Dr Paul Koudounaris' macabre feed features images of old jewel-encrusted skeletons in German churches and countless photos of his cat dressed up in kooky outfits, as well as roadkill. The Thanatos Archive is a collection of eerie yet poignant 19th- and early 20th-century postmortem photographs and ephemera. There are photos of dead people in their coffins, which was a fashionable portrait to have done for a while.

I'm particularly drawn into a site called Morbid Anatomy, a hard-to-define project run by Joanna Ebenstein, an independent scholar, curator, artist, writer, photographer and expert on anatomical art based in Brooklyn, New York City. What started as a blog in 2007 has evolved, and Joanna and various guests hold classes and talks on how to make your own memento mori, the history of embalming and the iconographic tradition of Jesus looking *very* sick on the cross.

Joanna has produced a number of books, including *Anatomica*, a striking pictorial history of anatomical art, featuring etchings and drawings of flayed men dancing in landscapes, little babies snuggled in wombs and delicate maps of human ears. It is in this book that I first came across Maclise's aortic arch variations, which have come to represent a particular truth about life for me. Morbid Anatomy has a library in Brooklyn with hundreds of books and morbid artefacts, and a gift shop. The Instagram account had 402,000 followers at last count.

Joanna has been hard to pin down as she's been busy finishing an illustrated book on the wild 17th-century Dutch anatomist Frederik Ruysch, known for his dioramas featuring skeletonised and embalmed infants in various poses. 'This has been my pet project for years and it took me a long time to find a publisher that was interested,' she tells me when we eventually speak.

She didn't use her real name when she first started the blog in 2007. Working as a freelance designer in children's publishing, she didn't want people to know she did all this 'weird shit'. Although she was shy about her 'weird' musings online, people instantly sent in fan mail. 'They would say, "Oh, my God, I've loved this stuff forever. And I always felt like a total freak,"' she says.

Times have changed. 'I think now it's a lot cooler to look at death than it was when I started. I think Morbid Anatomy cultivates this community and gives it the content that they want that maybe nobody else wants to know,' she laughs, 'but stuff that we find interesting, taken very seriously, I think, but also with a sense of, I hope, accessibility and fun as well.' Curiously, the majority of her audience is women and when we spoke, her taxidermy class was all female.

Like so many 'deathies', Joanna had been interested since she was a child—although she would argue all children are into death but it gets beaten out of them. She kept animals in formalin and her father purchased her a taxidermy kit. She also thinks the fact her grandparents survived the Holocaust—her grandfather essentially lost his whole family in Auschwitz—has fed into her interest in the topic. 'I think for certain Jews who have families that lived in Europe at that time, death is a part of everyday life in our family history,' she says.

I tell her how sometimes it feels like death has vanished in Australia. 'Yeah,' she says. 'We're not supposed to talk about it—polite people don't talk about it.' But she also thinks there's a class connection. 'When you go into—at least the US—neighbourhoods that are disenfranchised you'll see death is not exotic. It's part of everyday life. You see memorials everywhere, you see murals, and you see altars,' she says. 'So I feel for people who are educated and upper or middle class in the Western world, it's not seen as polite. We're not supposed to talk about it. It's seen as morbid.'

I silently turn into a cheerleader, chanting *Give me a D.E.A.T.H! YEAH!*

Something has certainly shifted more broadly in the culture, and she uses the example of a Dutch crockery set depicting human dissection dating from the 1760s. 'This is for drinking tea so I think to me that says that if this was really gross, it's not going to be on a teacup, right?' Joanna says we are the ones who have obviously changed. 'I think a big part of it is we don't believe—I shouldn't say we don't—but many affluent Westerners no longer believe in an immortal soul, or at least it's a questionable thing where for most of human history the body was not all there was. We went on in some way after the death of the body, so there's a different attitude towards the body.'

Death was also part of life. 'I think part of what makes it so grotesque to us now is it's foreign, it's frightening. People died at home all the time, women laid out the bodies. It was maybe not the nicest thing in the world but it was just a part of everyday life. People butchered their own animals, right? So it's like, we're very squeamish about these things. But I think it's a luxury to be able to be squeamish. It's unique to our time and place.'

Months earlier, I'd signed up to one of Joanna's courses—a six-week online course entitled *The Anatomical Venus: Wax, death, God and the ecstatic*, which explored the 18th century life-sized waxworks of anatomised women made by Clemente Susini.

The class was eclectic: artists in Los Angeles, Wales and Nantucket, a funeral home worker in New York, a human remains conservator in Edinburgh. Another member of the class was Marie Dauenheimer, who was the medical editor on Joanna's book *Anatomica*. I looked her up and could see she was a seriously well-established medical illustrator in the US, having created work for the American College of Cardiology, the National Library of Medicine and all sorts of other medical groups and organisations representing different diseases. What were her days like? Did she spend time with the dead?

While some of the lecturers would draw nerves and arteries on the blackboard, as far as I can tell, there were no artists in the dissecting rooms of the University of Queensland when Ruby and Julie were there. Nobody I spoke to ever mentioned seeing an artist drawing the dead. So even though I think donors from there were never rendered in pen or coloured pencil or wax, there is absolutely no way one can tell the story of the dissected without writing about how they live on in so much epic anatomical art, which for centuries was intrinsic to the science.

***

When Marie did her masters degree in medical illustration at Johns Hopkins Medical School in Baltimore in the 1980s, she dissected a donor body by day and then drew the dissection into the evening. She had to draw at night as the next day she and her fellow students would get back into dissecting. 'You need a lot of time to draw these dissections,' she says. 'It was really important to have that opportunity to really do some nice polished drawings before the next day, when you're cutting more stuff.'

Out of a class of 120 mainly medical students, she was one of four illustrators and a handful of biomedical engineers who spent four days a week dissecting for one semester. The man she was studying was in his late forties and while they were dissecting his heart, a visiting cardiologist diagnosed that he had died from a heart attack.

'There was a cadaver a few tables away from us that had a big aortic aneurysm in the abdominal aorta. That was incredible to actually see. You see different kinds of pathologies, you see people who had had different kinds of surgeries. And then you just see the variation. There's a huge amount of human variation, even within the normal anatomy. So that opportunity to see that and maybe even draw from that was really exciting.'

Marie took basic science classes with other medical students but also spent one semester illustrating surgery. Each evening at 8 pm a hand-typed operating schedule would be posted, a 'what's on' in neurosurgery, orthopaedics, ophthalmological, cardiac and the like. Marie would then trudge three blocks to the medical library, go through the stacks and find sophisticated surgical atlases and textbooks to research the operation she was going to watch. She would spend two hours consulting several surgery books and reviewing the relevant anatomy.

'You didn't want to go into that surgery not knowing what they were going to be doing and what anatomical structures you needed to know,' she recalls. 'You really needed to know what you were seeing. Because if you don't really understand what you're seeing, especially in surgery, it can look like kind of a big mess.'

By 6 am the next day, Marie was in theatre, holding her sketchpad, graphite pencils and a few coloured ones—red for arteries, blue for veins and yellow for nerves. Dressed in a gown like the surgeons, she usually stood on a tall stool to watch the surgical field from above. In those days, it was visually interesting—surgeons really cut open the body. 'Back when I was in school in the 1980s, things like gallbladder surgeries and kidney surgeries were done with big open incisions. So you got to really visualise that anatomy,' she says. 'I always joke that as a medical illustrator it was great but for the patient not so much.' These days, if she went into a surgical suite, all she would see is people looking at video monitors. 'They're doing everything through catheters that are being snaked through the body. So there's no surgical field to see.'

As a full-time working illustrator, there was a spell where she was frequently spending time in different dissecting rooms—drawing hand dissections on one particular project or teaching a comparative anatomy class for animation students, who were very interested in the musculoskeletal system. But that was a decade ago or so. As she doesn't spend as much time with the dead any more, I wonder where she gets her inspiration? She's doing a lot of heart art at the moment, so she works from angiograms or she'll watch a video of a procedure. 'I had a lot of time in autopsy and cadaver labs, and saw a lot of really amazing surgeries. I have a lot of reference. I can sort of visualise it.'

Contemporary illustrators are still dissecting—and in some instances more than medical students. Johns Hopkins offers a particular course that the medical illustration students take to give them more time drawing cadavers. 'When you see those kids graduating, those medical illustration students are going to have a stronger foundation in gross anatomy and cadaver dissection than the medical students.'

We're speaking over the internet—Marie has a distinctive Queens, New York accent—and in the background is a home office jammed with books, the pitter patter of her basset hounds Fleur and Ernest, and a real human skeleton, which at times is a little distracting. I eventually ask her about it, and Marie says she has owned it since college and thinks it may be a man from India. Her husband is a forensic anthropologist and one evening after dinner he and a dentist friend studied the skeleton, guessing the man may have been in his forties.

As medicine has become more technical, so has the art. In the ensuing years, Marie has seen her profession move from drawing to Photoshop to working with complex 3D animations and holograms. 'Your audiences are more sophisticated. They are people who grew up playing video games, and are used to three-dimensional environments and pretty sophisticated graphics. When they go to medical school and become doctors, that's how they're going to want that information.'

For twenty-five years, Marie has been taking travellers on art and anatomy tours across Europe, where they visit anatomy museums, theatres, and rare medical book collections. Considering her knowledge, I ask her who is her favourite. She says the German anatomist Bernard Siegfried Albinus, who published *Tabulae Sceleti et Musculorum Corporis Humani* in 1747, which featured the work of the engraver Jan Wandelaar. Marie particularly loves the engraving of a skeleton with a two-and-half-year-old rhinoceros named Clara.

'The pair were really interested in creating this concept of *Homo perfectus* so when you look at a lot of their anatomical illustrations, you can tell that they were done maybe from one particular cadaver,' she says. They worked on the musculoskeletal system for twenty years and had plans to start sketching the gastrointestinal system but Wandelaar died.

Marie points out that with some artists like the Dutch physician and anatomist Govard Bidloo, born in 1649, you can really feel the rawness of the lab.

'You've got the blocks and you've got the flies and you've got ropes and you've got tissue that's just ragged—it looks like it's just coming off the body in this raw manner. And then you juxtapose that with Albinus and Wanderlaar and they want it to look perfect,' she says. 'They want it to look idealised, and you don't see that rawness of what you're seeing in the cadaver lab.'

I ask her how the great old artists would feel about her contemporary work. 'My stuff is ordinary and maybe they would think it's kind of sterile,' she says, laughing with a shrug. Perhaps it's the subject matter—there are no bodies, blocks, flies or ropes. These days, Marie draws medical devices and a lot of 'mechanism of action' imagery, which shows how a new drug will interact on a cellular level.

But still, the donors are a powerful reference for her. 'I think back to taking gross anatomy constantly. A lot of the stuff I do now is cardiovascular. I've got a heart model here,' she turns and points at a heart model, 'and when I think of that experience of learning first-hand on somebody's body, and how things are all put together, how the cardiovascular system—your blood vessels, your nerves and the bones, how everything is linked together, and how unbelievable it is to see it first-hand, to have that tactile experience of taking things apart, to really understand how they're put together—is just really incredible. But I would say there's always been this sense of reverence and also wonder—just excitement—about learning.'

***

Across Etsy, Instagram and other social media, anatomical artists and businesses sell pretty images of skulls, hearts and lungs nestled in gorgeous floral arrangements or painted in colourful watercolours. You can get them on prints, t-shirts and enamel pins.

At the other end of the spectrum, however, you have the likes of Eleanor Crook, one of the few anatomical wax modellers in the world. And when I track Eleanor down and talk to her about how she got into what she does, she reminds me again of how for some us, the deathly-corpsey things we saw as kids steered our lives.

For Eleanor, it was seeing *Carry On Screaming!*, a film she watched as a five-year-old-girl in Birmingham. The black comedy horror was part of the British *Carry On* franchise and featured a mad professor character who kidnapped women and turned them into shop window dummies in a laboratory.

'It's a dreadful film. It's sexist. It's sort of offensive, it's funny but it's also not funny. But even within all that it manages to be very eerie,' she says. The mad professor character relies on being plugged into electricity to stay alive and every so often, he starts to fade. 'It's cheesy, and it was a comedy, but it had a huge effect on me as a child. It raised all those questions about who is alive and who is dead. I used to lie awake at nights thinking about it, and also dreaming of having a laboratory like that one day.'

In some ways, her childhood aspiration has partly come true. From her workshop in a small village in Berkshire, she sculpts anatomical pieces from wax, wood, bronze and lifelike media. She's artist-in-residence at the Gordon Museum of Pathology at King's College, London, one of the largest pathology museums in the world, a space filled with 8000 pathological specimens, some from dissected bodies and some wax. She teaches art students to draw in dissection labs, a place she has spent a lot of time in during her career. As we speak, she shows me a half-completed wooden carving. It's a homage to the British carved cadaver sculptures I encountered at Christina and Wendy's stall at the London anatomy conference, and which led me to her.

Eleanor is both a rarity and doyenne in the small but flourishing medical-anatomical-historical death art scene. I have no other way of describing it. The contemporary medical illustration world is expansive, and at one end is Marie and at the other sits Eleanor, describing her work as 'anatomical expressionism', which is expressive art that has a bit of anatomy knowledge in it. 'I always think of people's art as rather symptomatic of what the culture is doing to their heads at the time. Mine often comes across as a bit violent or a bit uncomfortable.'

As a teenager, Eleanor envisioned a future where she was a professor of classics or archaeology. When she at Oxford, it was all about Greek, Latin, philosophy and a bit of ancient art history on the side. But she got so interested in ancient statues that she started making them out of newspapers and Polyfilla in her small student lodgings. Making it was better than studying it. She left Oxford and went to Central Saint Martins art school but in the early 1990s, conceptual, performance and video art were in and figurative was off the menu. 'Making sculptures was considered extremely reactionary and retrogressive,' recalls Eleanor.

While her art school friends were hanging out at the Tate, Eleanor found herself spending more and more time in anatomical museums such as the Gordon and the Hunterian, the specimens in jars and wax models enthralling her. 'I got more interested in those than I did in the living people I was sculpting.' She drew. She absorbed. She attended an eight-week anatomy art course at the University College Hospital in London. She eventually asked the people at the Gordon if she could bring modelling wax in to make some 3D studies. 'I ended up being the person at the corner of the museum making these little wax figures, really quite honing what I was doing, before I was particularly good at it.' Eleanor became part of the furniture. Eventually, somebody at the Gordon asked her if she wanted to make a model of the bubonic plague.

The wax bubonic plague man she made is a bit bigger than a Barbie doll but not huge, and his poor body is peppered with all the signs of the disease which over time has killed anywhere between 75 and 200 million people: vicious black sores; black, gangrenous fingers and swollen glands. For inspiration, she studied photographs from two outbreaks—one in Brazil in 1909 and another during the Vietnam War in the 1960s.

'So that was your first official commission—a bubonic plague doll?' I ask.

'Official commission doesn't really bring across what my career has been like. My career has been more like a friend says: "Do you think you can make this?" and I go: "Probably,"' she says drolly.

Disease can make the body ghastly: pus-filled blisters, bleeding and ulcerating skin lesions, rashes, masses of warts, emaciation, bubbling cysts, lumps all over the body. Most of us turn away but Eleanor is drawn to these misfortunes found in the museum. 'Some of the older material shows you diseases really running their course in a way that you don't see walking down the street today,' she says. 'I think I describe them as museums of the extremes of human experience.'

When we spoke, she had just crafted a wax model with AIDS, which was inspired by a conversation at the museum. 'We were looking around the museum going, "Oh, all these diseases you don't see any more like glanders. When was the last time you saw a case of glanders?" It's a very dramatic-looking disease.'

'What is glanders?' I ask.

'It's a bacterial infection from horses—it comes up in great big blisters and it looks pretty awful. Grooms used to get it in the olden days. Pre-antibiotics.'

The Victorian anatomical sculptor Joseph Towne made the glanders work. The master modeller of beeswax and spermaceti wax has hundreds of models in the museum, many of them created from dissections and patients who came through the hospital between 1826 and 1879. There is little romance to Towne's work. Eleanor describes it as 'brutally honest'.

'We were looking at [the glanders sculpture] and going well, if that walked into a doctor's office, I bet very few people would know what that was now. The conversation then arose what diseases could we add to this collection that the 19th-century modeller who made our collection—Joseph Towne—would never have seen. And I immediately thought, well, he would never have seen AIDS.

'I was in London when AIDS went through it like a dose of salts [slang for quickly and thoroughly] in the eighties and early nineties, and I knew a couple of people who unfortunately died of it, couldn't be saved before the treatments became as good as they are now. AIDS had a particular set of visual symptoms then which—because the treatment is so successful—you already don't see very often on living people walking the streets.' Eleanor thought it would be interesting to have a three-dimensional document of the disease. 'It was a really painful-looking set of conditions that somebody with terminal AIDS would have back then, which was going to become part of medical history because thank goodness, they could treat it so well.'

The public also don't get to see many medical specimens and anatomical artworks as many of these museums are restricted. My feelings on this issue carousel. It's paternalistic—*oh we must control these dark voyeuristic urges in the public! No, we need to protect the dignity of the dead.* It's exclusive—*oh yes, only doctors know how to best deal with life and death.* This is absolutely not entertainment—*the collections are for learning and healing.*

Eleanor says there is a broad church of opinions about who should be able to access medical museum material. 'I tend to fall towards the idea that the public do have a right to know—it's a part of the human story that the body can do these things to you, that processes can do these things to the body and it seems to me information that anybody who's in charge of a body has a right to know. If it's mediated through photography, or modelmaking—that's fine. But seeing it in the flesh brings it home to you in a very particular way.'

It could also help save lives. Eleanor is friends with a heart surgeon who travels the UK and gives talks about the body. 'He said he is surprised how few people know how close to the surface of the body essential organs actually are. So you get young people getting around stabbing each other, and they don't actually realise that there's something very fragile and irreplaceable within the length of the blade. He often wondered if better knowledge of the inside of the body wouldn't deter some of them.'

***

To look at the massive canon of anatomical art, which really starts to kick in around the 17th century, is to settle into a curious trinity: the dead person, the dissection itself and the way the artist has chosen to depict the scene. The dissected are rendered in all ways: butchered, magnificent, ugly, raw, fleshy, smooth, dead, alive and expressive.

Take Joseph Maclise, the 19th-century Irish anatomist, surgeon and medical artist, whose aortic arches I became unexpectedly fixated on. What is notable in his tome *Surgical Anatomy*, published in 1851, is how utterly gorgeous and somehow alive the dead young men on the page are. Even though anatomical hooks stretch open their armpits or there is a scalpel on the side of the sketch; they could still be pin-ups, their moody faces, Byronic curls, hands, penises, intestines and torsos so gorgeously rendered that medical historian Michael Sappol now posits that Maclise might possibly have been gay. 'Maybe they were a space in which he unveiled himself, sent out flares of homoerotic desire,' writes Sappol.

But while these men are stunning to look at, I also wish someone had picked up their bodies from the hospital or the asylum in which they died

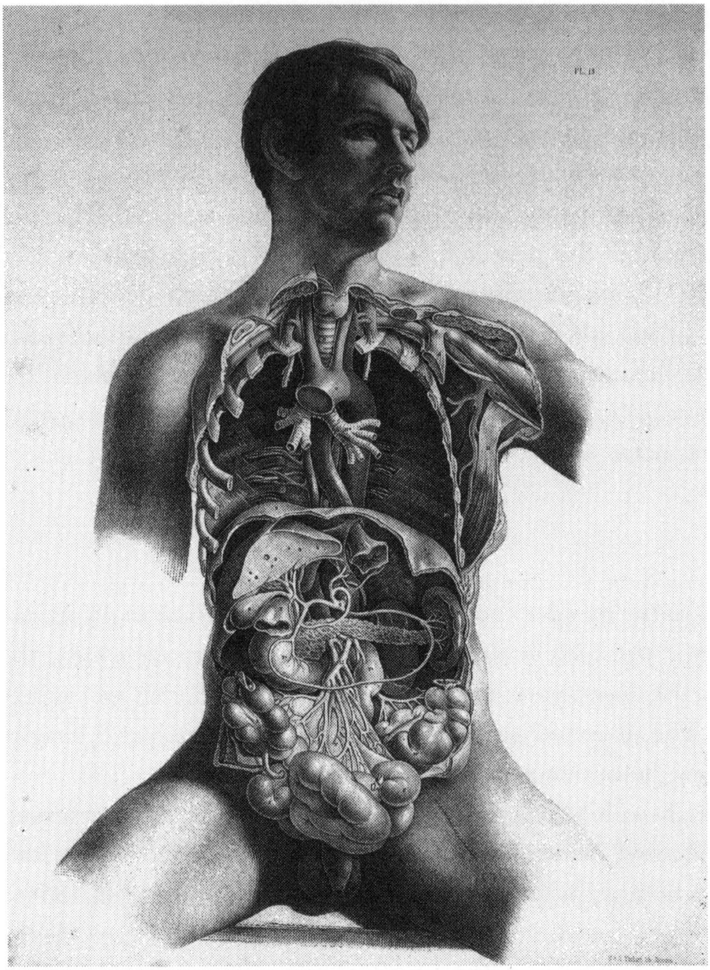

A lithograph by Joseph Maclise of the cadaver of a young man's dissected trunk, showing the arteries and blood-vessels supplying the viscera of the thorax and abdomen. The image is from his 1851 book *Surgical Anatomy. Wellcome Collection.*

and given them a proper burial. How sad that it was only in death that these friendless, poor and sick men were transformed into Apollonian gods on the dissectors' and lithographers' slabs of stone. If only they'd felt that love when they were alive.

The Italian Clemente Susini also breathed life into the dead and did so using wax. His female models are particularly striking, exuding what viewers describe as outright, shocking sensuality. They are life-size, recline in glass cases, wear pearls or a golden tiara, and one can unpack their organs. Made at La Specola, a natural science museum in Florence, they were used to teach anatomy. One model known as Venerina, 'Little Venus', is based on a small, delicate and probably teenage girl who was pregnant. Apparently Susini worked directly with her body and contemporary scientists have studied it, and think she died from a congenital heart disease.

All that is known about Susini's subjects is that they came from the local hospitals—the adults from Santa Maria Novella and the children from Degli Innocenti orphanage. A lot of dead people were needed to create the sculptures—around 100 to 200 body parts each year—and the modelling workshop was often in competition with medical men at the hospital for the dead. Sometimes, La Specola had too many bodies and didn't use them, and sent them off for burial. In one instance in 1794, Susini bitched in the margins of a list of dead bodies he got from the hospital that a man from the cemetery had called one of his staff 'a fucking vagabond' for returning dead bodies without operating on them.

Where Maclise and Susini made dissection sublime, the British anatomist John Bell is at the other extreme—his 17th-century drawings are brutal and ugly, showing no mercy to the dissected or the student who may have been studying the image at the time. *This is death. This is dissection.* His figures lie slumped across dissecting tables, in some instances ropes tied around their wrists. In one sketch of a decapitated head, the dead man looks as if he is wincing in pain. There is absolutely no heart or respect for the dead, not that this bothered Bell, who in fact critiqued 'the subjection of true anatomical drawing to the capricious interference of the artist, whose rule it has too often been to make all beautiful and smooth, leaving no harshness ...' Come on John! Lighten up!

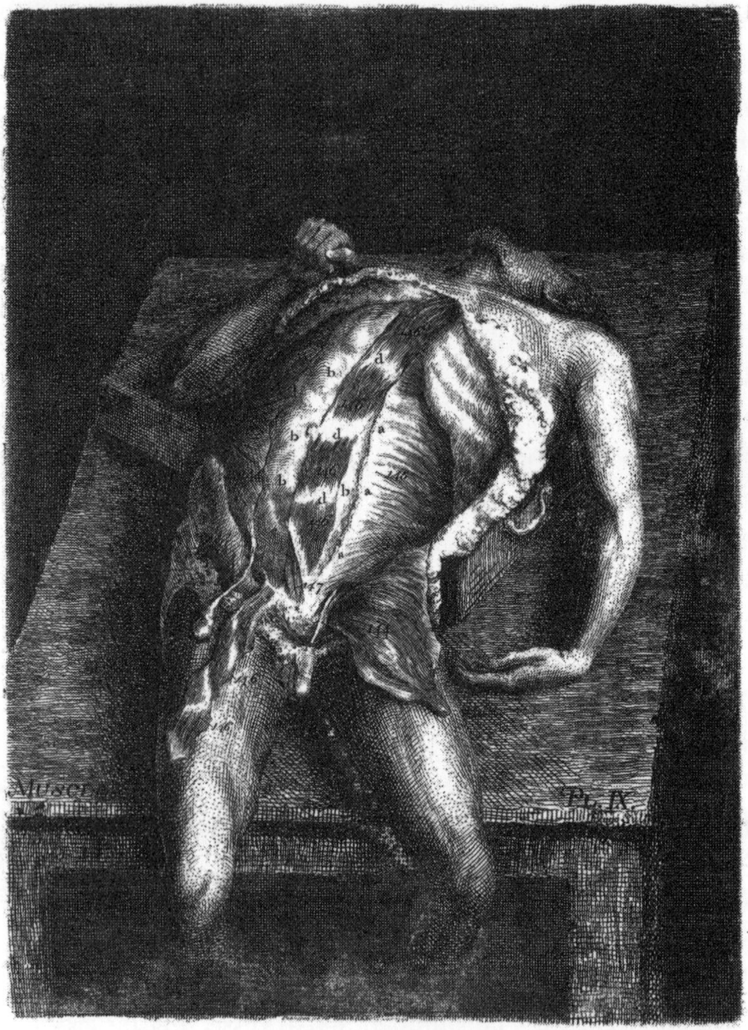

John Bell's somewhat gothic engraving from his 1794 book *Engravings, Explaining the Anatomy of the Bones, Muscles and Joints*. *Wellcome Collection.*

I ask Eleanor how she views the old works. 'I think, okay, so that shows the anatomy more or less successfully. What have they added that's not necessarily to show the anatomy but shows something else? And I think that's when the art creeps in.'

'So for example, those Vesalius figures—if you look right through the book in order, the artist is probably Johan van Calcar, who was a student of Titian [the Italian painter]—the physical poses of the less dissected ones are kind of heroic and classical. And as the figure gets more and more dissected, he starts to look sort of punch drunk and weak, and starts to buckle at the knees, and there's a real sense that the dissection takes it out of him. You can see him going from quite vibrant to completely exhausted across this suite of illustrations. That's not necessarily to show the anatomy—that's saying something about weight, dissection, and mortality. If anybody's ever tried to hold up a dissected body, it doesn't stand up for itself. It has that sort of punch-drunk floppiness that you see in those drawings. So there's a real physical knowledge in it that comes across to me—that's the art.'

Eleanor has spent hours in dissecting rooms dissecting and teaching drawing. As an artist, she has observed that various anatomy departments each have their own 'culture of dissection'. It reminds me of what Sophie Bolt, the body donor sage, told me about the labs in the Netherlands: 'They are their own small islands.'

Eleanor saw that the way the bodies are stored, what kind of embalming fluid they use, how the donors look is all a bit different depending on the school. 'The dissection room furniture is really fascinating and that varies a little bit from school to school as well. Whether you have the person's name and cause of death varies from school to school. They're all a little bit different.'

I'm piqued by this comment—again it's this layer coming off my perception of science as this hospital-white room humming with a generic and constant perfection. I know the French philosopher Bruno Latour wrote about this idea of communities of scientists creating facts in the 1970s but I suppose I've had to really trawl through anatomy in 2022 to get it myself.

Eleanor was commissioned to create a set of head and neck models for the Royal College of Surgeons so she was permitted to do a dissection course for a year at Guy's Hospital alongside other students. Fellow students knew she was a sculptor and assumed she was good with tools, so whenever a saw was needed to do a cut, she would get pushed to the front of the class to do it.

'I particularly ended up having to do a lot of what I would call the "carpentry of dissection". It was a real honour to do it and you have the sense of occasion because you think this person has given their body—what an incredible privilege. Here I am to learn it to make good teaching models. I better do this well—it's such a striking experience.' I watched a YouTube video from India of a man's skull being sawn off in a dissection lab and can see why students might have baulked at it.

Eleanor runs anatomical drawing classes for 'serious anatomy art students' in the London spring, which includes visiting the dissecting rooms at King's College upstairs from the Gordon Museum. 'Believe me, I read them the riot act about ethics and confidentiality. I don't want any jokey work coming out, or anything that a relative of a donor might not like. Everything has to be done in a respectful and dignified and humane manner.' She speaks with reverence and awe about the donors. It's a language I hear intermittently from people working in contemporary dissection labs—the dead are people, not specimens.

I say goodbye but Eleanor tells me there is one last thing she wants to say. It's a final word on donors.

'When I'm working with them in the dissection room, I have a sense that they are in a funny way still there and they are deliberately showing us things. So when I'm teaching, I'll go, "Look at this arm," and I'll turn it over and I'll go, "Look, he's showing you all his tendons here." I talk about it in terms of *he is showing you this*. And the students find this a bit odd at first, and then they realise it's actually true. This is what the person wanted to do.'

Chapter 22

I thumb my way through social media looking at famous women's bodies, and tap into articles about losing weight or how to dress for my figure. Why the fuck am I reading about what some influencer on the Gold Coast ate for breakfast? In a body-fixated society, I see I'm not alone in being disengaged from my elaborate, internal geography. We're all skin deep. Scrub that. I'm a little less skin deep. I now know about the jellyfish tentacles and trees that live on my tongue, I know about the snail trail and the seahorse in my head.

***

Part of my interest in what happened to Ruby and Julie is connected to my interest in dead bodies more broadly. I know other people who are into it—the Morbid Anatomy crew, my surfer friend Mike, the anatomists—but where exactly did my fascination come from? How come I've not been able to resist their magic like others seem to?

Throughout my life I have always been looking for the dead. If I'm on holiday, I'll often go check out the local cemetery. And where possible, I'll go looking for corpses or body parts too. In the Philippines, I went to Sagada to admire the hanging coffins. In Mexico, I spent the morning at the infamous Museum of Mummies in Guanajuato, where bodies from the local graveyard are on display after it was discovered that they were perfectly preserved. Going off the tourist track, I spent the afternoon with the local gravedigger, who believed the dead were in good condition as even though they were poor, they had led tranquil lives. By evening, I'd had a full existential epiphany. From Tierradentro to Rome to London to Vladikavkaz, I'd always relished the adventure of tracking down a cave, church or graveyard and then thinking about life in front of bones, a skull or a tombstone.

It's an inescapable lifetime interest, and one that began when I was eight years old and dug up the remains of my pet budgie Zazbut. He had been buried for about eight weeks in a patch of grass alongside our house in Dasmariñas, a fortified village in Manila, in the Philippines. Zazbut was a friendly little budgie. He spent a large amount of time outside his cage and Dad always predicted this would lead to trouble with the family cat, which it did. One morning at breakfast, the cat turned up with Zazbut in his mouth. My mother screamed and snatched him from the cat's jaws. Lying in her hand, his green chest punctured, Zazbut let out a final 'cheep cheep' and died.

With the frivolity that accompanies living expatriate life, my parents put on a large wake. The children cried and buried the budgie with full honours. RIP Zazbut. But for weeks after the funeral, I lurked by Zazbut's grave and wondered what his body looked like. I was old enough to know it was wrong to dig up the dead, but my curiosity persisted. So I dug him up … and was disappointed. All that was left was a pile of feathers. No blood. No guts. No bones. I took a feather and hurriedly buried my little green friend—again.

I'm not sure if other little kids were doing this but it's what I did. It wasn't a one-off—when we went back to Brisbane for a holiday one year, family friends had a slowly decomposing rat in a jar under the house and I remember being absolutely fixated and somewhat smitten by it.

Looking back, perhaps Mum and Dad spoke to each other about Ruby and Julie going to the dissecting room, and I absorbed it, took it in, mulled over what that all meant. Even if it was only a minor dinner table discussion, arriving in the Philippines aged six and growing up there undoubtedly got me into death.

How could I not be okay with it? First, it was Catholicism on steroids, dramatic, fervent. Mary was everywhere—gracious and calm. Jesus was everywhere—miserable and suffering on the cross or a smiling little baby. There were Santos everywhere: saints, angels, virgins, Our Lady of this, Our Lady of that, all made of ivory or a particular type of termite-resistant wood. Heaven, hell, purgatory, father, son and holy ghost.

My daily life was a blur of:

- elaborate Catholic festivals
- religious effigies in churches and homes
- people flagellating themselves in the streets at Easter
- crucifixes
- open-coffin funerals
- the front page of the newspaper splashed with images of dead bodies
- dead bodies on the nightly news
- opposition leader Ninoy Aquino shot dead on the tarmac as he stepped off the plane

It felt like we were perpetually at wild and spooky festivals. At Easter, most towns had a procession. Standing next to Mum and Dad, I watched thousands upon thousands of people walking the streets alongside floats with extraordinarily lifelike statues of the Virgin Mary and Jesus in elaborate outfits and poses. Jesus in the glass coffin was particularly evocative—there he was, with his crown of thorns, draped in lace and velvet, face serene. As a child, I wasn't sure if he was real or not, and I fantasised: Is that what the dead really looked like? So wondrous?

Each Easter, whole towns would re-enact Jesus Christ's path to crucifixion. Men would cut and whip themselves as blood dripped down their backs. Others would limp along, carrying heavy wooden crosses as a friend whipped them. Later, their hands would be nailed to a cross, watched over by a few guys dressed up as a Roman centurions and a woman playing the part of Mary.

It wasn't all necessarily religious either. My brothers and I used to sneak into horror films, which were often R-rated. So many characters in those films are as familiar to me now as the ones in *Sesame Street*: the tattered corpse in *Creepshow* which climbs out of a grave looking for a birthday cake, and the pale and striking-looking dead woman resurrected after being bitten by Dracula. I think we went to *Shocking Asia 1, 2* or *3* but I ran out.

I moved back to Manila in my thirties. Easter came around again. I watched the men flagellate themselves and get their hands nailed to a cross, and came home with specks of blood on my blouse. On my social media feeds, my friends would post pictures of themselves visiting their friends' graves—smiles and thumbs up. The images were never mournful. My friend Jude and I would visit various graveyards across the city as a weekend activity.

My parents came for a holiday. One of my dad's old friends died and we ended up at a large marble building which had little separate chapels for different funerals. We arrived for the 'work colleague' slot between 3 and 6 pm, and there, in an open coffin, lay a dead man, surrounded by an unrestrained collection of flowers. A lady was on a microphone, casually reflecting on her work friend, telling stories, making people laugh-cry. Soon they called on Dad to get up and say something. Dad hadn't seen the man for years but he got into the spirit anyway, telling a story next to the coffin. He passed the mic on to the next person. And so it went. Relaxed. Tearful. Friendly. Death.

Another element contributing to my interest is my mother. She has a medical background, having trained as a nurse at the Royal Prince Alfred Hospital in Sydney. At night, they would incinerate amputated limbs in the furnace and the sweet sickly smell of burning flesh would waft through their rooms. I don't know when she first told me that story but it was so evocative. It still is.

She also used to talk about William Clowes, my great-great-great-great-great-great-great-great-great-great-great-great-great-great-great-great grandfather, a barber-surgeon to Queen Elizabeth I, a specialist in war wounds and an expert in syphilis. Mum and I once tried to find his portrait at the Hunterian Museum in London but he wasn't there—apparently he's in a store room at the National Portrait Gallery.

Over the years though, I've frowned reading online PDFs of his various papers and books. In his 1591 work *Prooued Practise for All Young*

Chirurgians, I did manage to glean he was a Galen fan, and was yet to take on Vesalius' suggestions, but he certainly mentions the idea of anatomy. He tells the story of 'a certaine man that was thrust through his bodie with a sword, which did enter first vnder the cartilage or grisle, called of the learned *Anatomists, mucronata cartilago,* &c.' The sword went straight through the man's body and William pulled it out.

So can you see there is this jumble.

It's just what I heard and saw, and it all seems normal and natural to me—like getting dissected does.

Chapter 23

Again and again in the body donor studies, the overwhelming reason people say they donate to medical schools is to contribute to scientific research. At the 2019 London anatomy conference, you could get a sense of the expansive research that was being done in the poster room—anatomists discussing their work, some of them later tweeting happy images of themselves #IFAA2019, @IFAA2019, @anatsoc. Perhaps Ruby and Julie were studied by anatomists researching a particular part of the body?

I begin looking for research from the 1970s and the 1980s and can't find much, and sense either my beagle skills aren't that great or perhaps there wasn't much going on? Perhaps it was all teaching. I sit back in my chair and look at an elaborate brass pendant lamp I bought when I lived in Egypt and which I've never managed to hang up, and sense trying to find the research may be akin to looking for a new tomb in the Valley of the Kings.

If only I could randomly find a manila folder in a library containing black and white photographs of University of Queensland anatomists at a 1970s conference, sporting flared pants and minis, holding academic papers whose titles I'd read using a loupe. Were they researching back then? But I then find one portal called UQ eSpace and a few papers start popping up in which cadavers are mentioned—donor wasn't a term that was commonly used and still isn't.

One researcher was Nikolai Bogduk, who used donors to study spinal pain, and became a leading expert in the area, a professor, author and prolific publisher of academic papers. Another is Marius Fahrer, who wrote extensively about the hand. The first paper I can find dates from 1973 and I'm soon wandering the emporium of his work over the next decade, and beyond. While the research isn't conducted in the *exact* years Ruby and Julie were there it's a similar era, and I'm suddenly in the dissecting room watching. Some of the papers are a bit jarring, and a blue/green/blue/green flashes at me as I fall from the sky. Blue is for *yes this is science and this will help people* while green is for *this is what might have happened.*

In 1976, Fahrer and surgeon Raoul Tubiana in Paris studied the *palmaris longus*—the muscle in your forearm that some people don't have—and how it connects to the thumb. Five fresh cadaver forearms and hands were examined; I paused on this. I hadn't heard of donors being described as 'fresh' at the University of Queensland at the time.

The study looked into the best use of the *palmaris longus* muscle in the surgical treatment of the paralysis of the thumb, 'which is of constant interest to one of the authors', being Dr Tubiana in Paris. A dissection took place and a bit like a marionette, they got the thumb muscle moving by pulling at the *palmaris* at the forearm end. I think. I was finding this all very evocative and inspiring, particularly that there was a path to getting the paralysed thumb muscle working again. Look at what those Brisbane donors did! But then at the end there was an acknowledgement, which left me hovering around disappointment. 'The dissections were carried out in the Anatomy Laboratories of the biomédicale des Saints Pères Université, Director Prof. A. Delmas, Paris, France.'

A few years later in 1981, Fahrer and Peter J. Millroy wrote about the variation of the cute-sounding *abductor digiti minimi.*

They describe the variations in two real-life clinical cases and in seven instances in *400 hand dissections*—that's a lot of hands. In another Fahrer paper on the *palmaris aponeurosis*, my heart dropped a kilometre when I saw a photograph of a dissected hand, and the attack wasn't just because I momentarily thought it could've been Julie's, although I double-check the date and it says 1980. Our hands are so busy and grasping, and it often feels like they have a life of their own—a bit like Thing, the disembodied hand in *The Addams Family*.

We're quite lucky as a species that some of our members choose to take on a particular part of the body. Every anatomist I speak to had their areas they liked and didn't—Goran liked bones and muscles while Dr Claire Smith in Brighton found the pelvis interesting.

Fahrer was obviously into hands. In 1973 the renowned New York surgeon J. William Littler penned a highly technical but somewhat magical paper, which explored the extraordinary geometry and anatomy of the hand with gorgeous illustrations. In one proposal, Littler connected movements of the fingers to the *spira mirabilis*—the perfect logarithmic spiral that occurs in nature.

He also remarked that the curve of an eggshell also follows this famous pattern. Putting the two together, Littler found that the forces of the palm and the fingers are so perfectly distributed that it is impossible to crush an egg in the palm of your hand. I didn't quite believe this but it's true. Try this at home! Go the kitchen, get an egg and squeeze it as hard as you absolutely can—it will not break. I've tried. It's my new party trick. Inspired, Fahrer included the egg trick in a 1973 conference presentation, with a little autograph, 'Mf', attached.

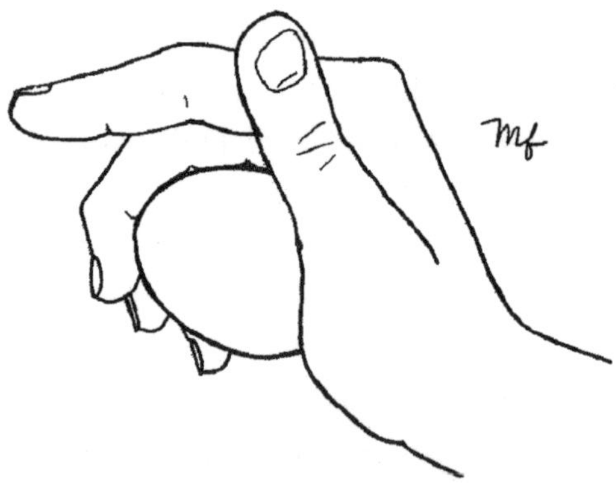

FIGURE 3
The curves of the egg shell are congruent with
the curves of the arches of the hand.

Fahrer's egg sketch in his 1973 paper 'Fingers Toes, Palmar and Plantar Arches', published in the *Australian Journal of Physiotherapy*.

Hoping that Fahrer might still be alive, and that we could discuss trying to crush eggs and the donors he dissected, I instead sadly find his obituary, written in 2013 by his friend and fellow surgeon Dr Pierre Chapuis.

Fahrer had an energetic, zig-zag life—he was a doctor training to be an orthopaedic surgeon but the communist uprising in Romania in 1955 thwarted his ambitions and he eventually fled to Paris. A refugee, he moved to Brisbane in 1963 where he landed a job in the anatomy department at the University of Queensland. The obituary mentioned that he had 'conducted the interview in some Latin and a little Italian … for this was the only means of communicating with the candidate who spoke little or no English'.

Aha!

Frank had spoken about a man who did his job interview with Professor Max Hickey in Latin! It had to have been Fahrer, who years later was to describe himself as 'one of the few surviving specimens of that now extinct species of surgeon-anatomists'.

I liked that Fahrer—who would duck back to Paris in the 1970s and 80s to be a visiting professor of anatomy—was researching, thinking about the *spira mirabilis* in the hand. I liked his drawing of the hand gently holding the egg. I liked that he was probably in the room when Ruby was there. By strange symmetry, months earlier, I'd spent hours with a much younger anatomist who also studied hands.

***

As I walked to my rendezvous at the University of Melbourne with clinical anatomist Dr Quentin Fogg one spring morning, I felt springless, weary and a bit over it, tempted to down scalpels on my anatomisation of anatomy. The constant weather changes matched my thinking: nothing felt clear, the field was too enormous (do I include zootomy? comparative anatomy?); my interests were too eclectic (theology of the bowel) and I didn't even know what formalin smelled like. I also was feeling bad that a family member of a donor might be absolutely devastated knowing there was a book out there about *what happens*. I sat down on a bench outside University House, momentarily drifting into the romantic and quaint 1885 buildings covered in vines, and the tinkle of the birds tweeting. But a weariness still hovered. In the way that cats can have the ins and outs—wanting to come in and then go out every five minutes—I also frustratingly had the ons and offs with my cardigan as I waited.

And then smiley Quentin Fogg arrived. With his striking, shaggy moustache and a blue and green spotty tie, an Edwardian air swirled about him, heightened by the Victorian environs. As we walked to get a coffee, I asked him about an enamel pin he was wearing—it had the word 'ally' and a rainbow behind it, and he explained it was for Minus 18, a charity he supports which helps young LGBTQIA+ people. He was so chatty, sparkly-eyed and instantly friendly that my dissection blues slowly wafted up into the blue and white sky above me.

When I left our discussion a few hours later, I felt like styling my hair into a contemporary bum-part, donning [insert latest Parisian trend made with organically produced fabric here], buying a delightful piece of anatomical art and bluetoothing a techno-sitar mix from my phone to a large amp: Quentin had ushered me into Anatomy 3.0, not just technically but emotionally.

***

When Quentin finished his PhD on the wrist in the early 2000s, he would rock up to international anatomical meetings and find hardly any younger people there. 'There'd be two or three people about my age—mid-twenties—and then a massive gap. There would be nobody in their thirties or early forties at these meetings … everyone was in their fifties and sixties,' he says. 'At this point, it looked like there was going to be a massive hole in anatomy internationally.' He says for this reason, these days, the upper echelon of the profession is quite young.

Where was everybody? Quentin says the surgical anatomy research that he is now doing had 'ground almost to a halt' in the 1960s.

'Everybody was getting into molecular biology and cell biology. That was the trendy stuff and that's where all the researchers went. There became this gap where there was no one that could really teach anatomy or no one wanted to research it because the money was all going into cellular research.' Medical schools resorted to bringing in retired surgeons and clinicians to teach anatomy, which in some ways persists today. The pool of anatomists doing specialist research remains small, as is teaching expertise in some areas.

I tell him about one surgical training staffer who mentioned there aren't really many people any more who can teach a whole-body dissection, and that most people only know bits. She'd said anatomy was hard, and if you don't use it, you lose it. 'Absolutely,' he says. 'I said this to someone yesterday that if I don't teach—as an example—the thorax—for a year, the detail starts dropping off. If I don't do it for two or three years, that detail will be largely gone. I can explain the basics to anyone but there's so much detail in there and the conceptualising of that detail is important. You need to be on it fairly regularly.'

Thus, back in the early 2000s, the anatomy field he came into was spartan and it wasn't too hard to find work. After training at the University of Adelaide, he taught on the tiny island nation of Sint Maarten in the Caribbean, and lectured at the University at Glasgow in Scotland and Monash in Melbourne, and has been at the University of Melbourne since 2018. In his early forties, the formalin must be agreeing with him because he looks young for his age. 'I look like I'm twelve, except for the moustache,' he laughs.

Quentin now specialises in hands and feet, and I ask him what he would say to the likes of the 'greats' like Andreas Vesalius and the Scottish anatomist and physician William Hunter if he walked into a room and they were there, and they asked him what was happening with anatomy.

'I'd say we're in a new anatomy revolution,' declares Quentin. 'My biggest bugbear is actually anatomists—other anatomists who go, "We know it all now" and I'm like, "Come on. Do we? Really?" The answer is we really don't.' Anatomy has long been plagued by claims it is 'over'—as far back as 1902 when it was seen as epistemologically exhausted with Dr Carl Hamann, a renowned Cleveland surgeon and anatomist, describing it as 'fixed and unchangeable'.

Quentin says the imaging revolution in the late 1990s and early 2000s with CT and MRI meant that scanning became so good that anatomists could see things they'd not seen before, and it shifted surgery—new techniques were invented, and plates and small pneumatic devices were planted in the body. 'Expectations shifted massively with the rise of the internet, and suddenly every patient's speaking to Dr Google first,' he says.

A patient would read a miracle story about someone running marathons after being told they could never walk again, and they would push their doctors for similar treatment. 'Because of everything getting more precise, we're realising that the anatomy knowledge we have is not precise enough,' he says. For example, Quentin is currently focused on really little tiny ligaments around the base of the thumb, which were first described in France in 1870 but through time have been forgotten.

In the past, where an anatomist would have just described it, these days they have to prove it is there. Body parts are now mapped with fine detail and evidenced with data. 'The classic surgical anatomy paper of the last fifty years has been "that ligament is there". But that's not science. That's you saying it's there. It's an opinion with some photos or a drawing. And so we've taken a very data approach so quantifying it—so it's all measured, it's all reproducible, it's over a sample size that's reasonable.' As part of his research, he looked at these tiny ligaments in up to thirty donors—he dissected and then used high-res photography, digital modelling and laser scanners to study them more closely.

Quentin advises surgeons. Say for example, a tendon has been pulled off in an accident. It needs to be reattached but it's not long enough. Quentin looks into what the other options are for transplant tissues in that area. 'How can you get enough length to pull it through? How will it change the function of other areas? It's using that area like a toolbox. Can you sacrifice a little bit of *that* to get *that*?' he says.

The University of Melbourne runs the only donor program in Victoria, getting about 200 bodies a year, some of which are shared with other institutions. They only take donors from within a tight radius around the university, 'because we couldn't handle any more'. Whereas dissection has waned across the world, Melbourne students—depending what class they are in—get a 'really big dissection experience' as Quentin describes it. The department also has a large collection of prosected specimens that students can work with.

Quentin tells me there are two paths I could take if I donated my body in 2021—embalmed or unembalmed. I could be dissected in undergraduate classes or professionally prosected and dissected. I could also end up in a six-month diploma in surgical anatomy. I joke to Quentin I would be happy if he had my hand to study and he stresses that I would need to donate my whole body and can't choose what it's used for.

He makes his lab sound like quite an inspirational place to end up. 'I really like the concept that the anatomy space is a transformative space for people. So you go in there and you come out a different person. The longer you're in there, the more different you become,' he says. 'Because if you engage with it normally it's not a macabre space—like you're not going in there thinking about death the whole time. But it's also not an easy space to be, and you have these moments where it can be really emotional.'

For some students, hands are an issue. I knew it! 'Hands are the things that most students react negatively to—you think it'd be faces but I think everyone's got an image of what the face looks like, but they don't appreciate how the hands will look, and you see them all the time.'

I mention to Quentin that there are lots of papers about how students handle dissection but there is little about how the anatomists feel. I'm quite surprised when he next tells me that he sometimes cries in the lab—not often but he does. 'I'll pull the student aside that's crying because they can't handle it on their first day. I'll often sit up in the corner and have a cry with them, and I'll say "It's actually pretty emotional for me as well. So let's just deal with it."' He stresses to the students that all the people in the room donated their bodies. They agreed to be there.

'I don't use the "C" word if I can avoid it,' he says at one point.

'What's that?' I ask, wondering how the word 'cunt' would come up.

'Cadaver—because that means "the fallen". It actually comes from the Latin root of something that is akin to someone who's died in battle. Most people translate it as "dead thing",' he says, adding that in his lab he uses 'donor' or 'body donor'.

Quentin feels like it's new age anatomy when he speaks like this but not in a *Power of One* sort of way.

Later, I ask him a question about using fresh-frozen bodies, he politely interrupts me.

'I try to get rid of the phrase "fresh-frozen" as well,' he says. 'I'm probably the only one that does this but I say "embalmed" or "unembalmed donor". I don't like the word "fresh" in there—it implies that the other ones aren't "fresh". It seems a bit crude to me.'

We discuss this tension around how to make anatomy more public. He knows of Gunther von Hagens but doesn't quite approve of elements of his infamous dissection TV series. 'I just don't like that presentation because it's this ritualised sensationalised dissection—he's dissecting with this flourish and passing the bits almost aggressively. All the aesthetics of it to me were wrong,' he said. 'The way that you mechanically engage with the donor is important, and that's not something that came through at all in that TV series.'

Quentin says von Hagens would argue that he cares, and that he's sharing it with everyone, but feels he doesn't understand the aesthetics.

I ask, 'When you watched it, you thought, "Oh, it's giving us anatomists a bad rap"?'

'I wouldn't say bad rap but more there's a lost opportunity to change the culture of what we do. I'm very much about when you interact with a donor—it's purposeful, it's respectful and appropriate for whatever your point is. But when you're doing something, it's a chance to show there is real care.'

Quentin was involved with a two-part BBC Scotland dissection series, and committed to it only because he had the power to stop filming if he wasn't happy with the way it was being portrayed. The only time he had to stop filming was when he took the skin off a donor's foot—the host nearly fainted and the crew went pale.

He wants to present dissection to the public but basically isn't allowed under current Victorian laws and policies. 'What we're missing out on is the opportunity to share and educate the public in something we can control,' he says.

While I've seen hundreds of drawings, etchings and copperplates of the dead, visited donors at a forensic facility, and watched dozens of people be cut up on YouTube and the historical medical dissection adventure movie *The Physician*, I still don't know what a modern dissecting room looks or feels like.

Am I a freak for wondering? In his wild book *The Body Emblazoned*, the historian Jonathan Sawday explores how anatomy in the Renaissance period created a 'culture of dissection', and became a theme in many plays, poems and works of art. Outside of scientific textbooks, anatomy was everywhere. Edward Ravenscroft's 1696 play *The Anatomist; or the sham doctor* featured a corpse coming to life and protesting against its own anatomisation. While Sawday describes the play as 'slight', it was popular because it tapped into the strange fascination and desire to know what it is like to be dissected. As he puts it: 'Imagining one's own dissection was a compositional device unique to early modern culture'.

Poetry of the period was also laced with dreams of dissection. I was taught John Donne's love sonnets at high school but sadly the teachers left off his dissection ones, which involve erotic and painful imaginings of being cut up by a lover. *Kill, and dissect me, Love*. Mr Donne, we've all been there.

It was a time when scientists, architects, poets and philosophers were all making sense of the human body. Centuries on, I'm still not clear why nowadays only scientists are allowed to engage with the dead. Why does most legislation not permit 'social science' or 'artistic' research? Why is it so difficult for artists and the poets to tell us stories about the dead? Why are there none working in anatomy departments? That said, some Australian medical schools such as the Australian National University in Canberra have a course for artists but the options are otherwise incredibly limited.

Tellingly, it was the art in *Gray's Anatomy* that drew Quentin to anatomy in the first place, when he found a copy on his father's bookshelf as a child. Decades later, he fell into an unusual project in Glasgow, which explored the idea of artists engaging with donors but it consistently faced authoritative opposition. The Scottish artist Christine Borland—who has long engaged with anatomical collections in museums as part of her practice—found two elderly women who wanted to donate their bodies but only if they could go towards arts research. There was no way it could happen.

I'm yet to visit an anatomy lab and when Quentin offers to take me on a quick tour of his, I'm probably a bit over-excited. I ask a few too many times if we should get started. We set off to the medical building, walking up a few flights of stairs and are soon standing in front of an old wooden sign above a door which reads ANATOMY.

Before we go in, Quentin explains he is going to use a live-action role playing or LARP technique on me. He got into LARP in Glasgow in 2013 after doing experimental work with an expert in the area, and seeing first-hand how there are often four different reactions to a dissecting lab and how he could have four distinct responses ready to help.

Thus, Quentin LARPs me, explaining what I will see. 'It's all very staged,' he says. 'You know what to expect so it's not a surprise.'

When we go in, I'm struck by how massive the space is, and how piercingly white-bright the lights are—you would not want to be stoned or to have just woken up, and I imagine the lights bring a particular tone to the donors. It's all as Quentin explained. Against one wall are thirty body donors, some in dark blue body bags, and others in pale blue, and I can just make out their shapes. There is a large yellow bin which says 'anatomical waste' and a chart on the wall listing causes of death.

'I wonder what my cause of death will be. It's kind of interesting, isn't it?' I say.

'You can go to some weird places mentally, which is part of our challenge working here,' says Quentin. 'Like we're often put in that situation where you've got to consider that sort of thing—somebody looks familiar or it's a bad time in other parts of your life and you've got to deal with being in this space.'

Quentin says it can be particularly hard in the lab when someone close has died.

'One of my best friends was an anatomist who I worked really closely with and every year around his anniversary, I really struggle in here.'

We head back outside and he starts telling him about his dear friend who died. They had worked together in North America and during classes, his friend—who was Māori—would often face the corner and say a mantra. 'It was him reconciling being in a place with deceased people,' recalls Quentin. 'He was really proud of his heritage and liked sharing it with all the North American students, and every once in a while he would be in the corner doing that. So every now and then I get a little click of that and imagine him standing in the corner here and I say, "Sorry guys, I need a few minutes." It's pretty full on for that sort of stuff.'

We are outside. I feel like throwing my arms around him and giving him a hug. It's not only to comfort him as he reflects on his friend but to thank him for teaching me his way of anatomy.

***

Months later, I emailed Quentin, asking him about Fahrer's hand papers.

Of course he knew him. 'He is considered by many to be a genius and highly impactful contributor to surgical anatomy,' he replied. 'Randomly, he was also a big fan (the only one??) of my PhD thesis (on the wrist).'

Still pondering what research happened at the University of Queensland in the 1970s—I suspect not too much?—I emailed Leo.

He replied that at the time the School of Anatomy was a sub-unit of the Faculty of Medicine and was primarily focused on teaching human anatomy to medical students, as well as physiotherapy, occupational therapy, dental and speech therapy.

'There was limited research using donated remains conducted during that time. In the early 1970s, the School of Anatomy was reassigned to the Faculty of Science and relabelled as the Department of Anatomy. There was then a move to encourage research by current and future staff, but not all teaching staff used donor material in their research projects. I remember both Marius and Nik and their research used donated material and was relatable to clinical conditions.

'Other researchers focused on physiological systems and used laboratory animals as subject matter. Wally Wood was dedicated to teaching human anatomy, mainly to medical students, but he also had an interest in forensic anthropology. He guided some of his postgraduate students in that field.'

Chapter 24

Some people like cakes for their birthdays. Some want to start the day with a yoga class. Others want to get drunk by a pool or do something adventurous. For my forty-ninth birthday, I was excited about visiting the Australian Facility for Taphonomic Experimental Research (AFTER), aka the 'body farm'.

I'd been told a mass grave excavation exercise was taking place, and I wondered about what that meant on the hour-long drive out to a secret location at the foot of the Blue Mountains.

I'd been invited to AFTER by Dr Jodie Ward, the director of the facility and a biological criminalistics expert who has a penchant for DNA. The facility is in the bush, surrounded by high fencing dug deep into the ground, trimmed with barbed wire and 24-hour CCTV. It immediately had an 'air' about it—and I could imagine Reddit threads with conspiracy theories penned by people who stumbled across it one afternoon and didn't know what it was.

The 'T' in AFTER stands for 'taphonomic'. Originally an area for palaeontologists and anthropologists studying decaying organisms and fossilisation, the word has recently been adopted by forensic scientists to understand the physical, chemical and biological processes that cause human cadavers to decompose. The first outdoor taphonomic facility opened in Tennessee in the US in 1981 and six more popped up over the decades.

While these sites revolutionised the science of death, the decomposition research results were unique to areas across the US. Thus, in 2016, the University of Technology Sydney opened up AFTER. Since then, teams of forensic scientists, biologists, pathologists, chemists, anthropologists, odontologists and police have headed to this location to study the dead in novel ways and do rare training exercises. There are now around a hundred donors on site. They desperately need more.

These sorts of facilities didn't exist in Australia when Ruby and Julie donated their bodies but it was difficult to not say yes when Jodie suggested I visit. If I was now inadvertently writing a history of body donors, their 'latest' fate was worth logging. Out in the bush. Open air. New science. Experimental. Also, I was sensing that I was never going to meet a contemporary body donor in a conventional anatomy lab. If Ruby and Julie had been alive and living in Sydney, they'd need to make a specific request to come here. Would they have?

I was met at the heavy metal security gate by Jodie, casual in cargo pants and sporting a nose ring I'd not noticed when we'd first met a year ago for a beer with the formidable Loren O'Keeffe, the head of Missing Persons Australia. Since that time, it'd been hard to catch up with Jodie—her work life is an intense seesaw ride between running AFTER for the University of Technology and trying to build a new national DNA program for the Australian Federal Police to help identify the remains of unknown people held in different legal jurisdictions.

I followed Jodie into a white shipping container and she explained a few rules as she made a cup of tea: absolutely no photographs and whatever shoes I wore in the field were NOT to be worn in the 'clean' shipping container area. Later at lunch when someone drops a grape on the ground and I quickly pick it up, offering to wash it, Jodie gives me a look and says: 'Nah. I know where our shoes have been.'

We walk into an open area cleared in the bush, and in the distance is a bashed-up car, a large pile of rubble, and people standing and crouching around a wide, shallow hole. It's obviously the mass grave excavation exercise site. Jodie introduces me to a 'Scotty from Vic Pol', who is overseeing it. He later gives me his business card, which reads 'Senior Sergeant Scott Harris from the Forensic Services Department from the Victoria Police'.

The diggers are mainly women. Dressed in white Tyvek coveralls, goggles, gloves, sunnies, hats and the odd pair of industrial-grade Blundstones, they crouch, sit or lean into the dirt, and methodically scrape away at the dense, black soil with trowels. A pale, face-down body is slowly being revealed. The odour is mercurial—sweet, tumbling to the odour of compost, dancing near sickening, back to sweet, darting to sickening. Nearby is a large marquee, buckets, a wheelbarrow, Australia's biggest sieve and an enormous mound of dirt.

'What's with the car?' I ask.

Jodie explains that in February 2020, AFTER ran a three-day mass-disaster exercise which simulated two terrorists driving a car into a building, which collapsed, and then blowing themselves up. The police arrived and had to deal with the situation. (This huge drama didn't actually happen on site but this was the backstory.) Six donors were placed under a large pile of rubble and the fragmented remains of two donors were hidden in the bush, which police had to find and recover. A temporary mortuary was set up where the remains and 'personal items' had to be properly documented, and pathologists, anthropologists and an odontologist conducted examinations.

By law, the facility can only have four bodies decomposing on the surface due to the odour, so four had to be buried. Jodie and Scott came up with the idea of using the buried donors as a mass grave training exercise for crime scene examiners, forensic anthropologists and archaeologists. Alongside the bodies, they placed SIM cards, mobile phones and fired cartridges from firearms. The scientists don't know any of this. They are looking for the unknown.

They are getting close to exhuming the first body, and a silence has drifted over the group. I lean towards Jodie and ask in a whisper if it's okay to ask her more questions, to keep talking or am I meant to be quiet—is there some particular etiquette around exhumation that I don't know about? I can feel something in the air.

'No,' she says, 'there's just a lot of anticipation.'

I look at the police and experts around me, looking into the grave—serious, quiet, watching.

All around is classic Australian bush, the type perfectly captured by the 19th-century painter Frederick McCubbin—gum trees toned green, pink, tan, cream, the sky a vivid bright blue. The quiet is broken up by the buzzing of a large black drone, which quivers in the sky down the bush track a little. It's a group from Australian Civil Air patrol, a charitable rescue, search and locate organisation. They are working on a separate project, using drones to test sensors which can help locate human remains.

Jodie suggests we check out the facility and as we wander into the bush, and the high grass, she lets out a small gasp.

'What?!' I ask, expecting something dramatic with a donor.

It's an animal. 'There was something slithery with no legs that went in there,' she says, laughing. 'Take a wide berth.' She then warns me about massive spider webs. 'So we just walk around like that,' she says, dodging a large web, 'or we walk around with big sticks.'

The donors rest in particular segments across the 12-acre site. Nearer to the fence are donors who are in graves that may be exhumed as part of ongoing experiments. 'We want to prevent any stickybeaks that are looking through the fence to actually see any of the donors. Out the back here,' she said, pointing deeper into the bush, 'we have all the donors that are on the surface. That's kind of in the centre of the property.'

We soon come across donors lying in large metal cages, open to the environment and safe from scavenging animals. Some are skeletons. Some wear worn cotton t-shirts. Some are naked, their soft tissue now their only cloak. Some jaws are ajar, as if screaming. But what is uncanny are their colours—they are the exact tone of the bush. Rich red and brown skin blends in with the fallen leaves while patches of vibrant green mould growing on their skulls and bones match the grass and trees.

It's bucolic—in a deathly sort of way. I'd be content knowing my body was lying in the bush like that forever, sinking into the earth, the sky above me, known just by a four-digit number. But by law, donors can only stay on site for four years, with a possible four-year extension after that. The remains are then meant to be interred.

The raison d'etre of the facility is multi-disciplinary and all the forensic disciplines are represented—it's not just about time of death and decomposition. As Jodie pulls out bits of grass, lamenting how high it is at the moment—and joking that maybe they need a goat—we pass different cages, and she discusses the research that has gone into them. Often, they will be used for two, sometimes three projects. Off in the distance, Jodie points out a car. She says there were two donors sitting inside it for six months as chemists analysed their odours. We are near an area where cameras were set up to study a donor decomposing over a period of time.

I later look up academic papers which feature AFTER: how tattoos change, how bodies move (just slightly!), different odours in different seasons. The 'E' stands for experimental, after all. While a lot of taphonomic work is now quantified with high-tech cameras and elaborate measuring systems in labs, critics say there are still biases and limitations to this sort of whole human cadaver research and what is needed first is a suite of global baseline studies using pigs.

In a crime drama, conversations often go like this: 'When did he die?' says the rugged detective.

'Last Thursday between 5 and 9 pm,' replies the earnest scientist in a lab coat.

Crime shows give the impression that the 'time of death' question can be precisely answered but the science is more fraught. In 2005 Mary Megyesi and other researchers developed a 'total body score', which attempts to measure decomposition over time, also taking temperature into account. Her chart shows decay's colourful and busy journey. Take my head and neck, for example. In the early stages of decomposition, I would be pinky-white with skin slippage and hair loss, and then some gray to green discolouration would appear, then shades of brown. Fluids would purge out of my eyes, ears, nose and mouth; my flesh would go brown and black. The insects come in these early stages—but not always.

At AFTER, the scientists have come to see how donors' lives shape their afterlives. If someone had chemotherapy or was an illicit drug user, the insects steer clear. 'Even the bugs know not to go near this person—just for now,' says Jodie. 'We go, okay, well, something weird is going on—this body is not behaving like the other bodies. When we go back and try and find out some further medical information, it all makes sense.'

The facility has also reshaped thinking on decomposition: if you are left to the elements in this part of Western Sydney, you are more likely to mummify than if you were in the US. 'Many of our donors are still covered in mummified tissue because they don't kind of transition through the stages like you would expect and by expect I mean what we've seen in other sites,' she says, adding people would decompose differently in other parts of Australia, say in the alpine areas or in tropical North Queensland.

Professor Dame Sue Black, a well-known Scottish forensic anthropologist, anatomist and something of a celebrity in this space, has been critical of taphonomic centres, including for this very reason—people decompose differently in different climates. Says Jodie: 'The critics out there will say that you almost need a facility in every possible climatic zone in every country to able to draw any real inference about the accuracy of the technique.'

We keep wandering. Jodie says she gets strange calls from people wanting to visit the site, including a monk who wanted to sit by the dead. While she rolls her eyes at this, I chew my lip. I sort of get why they'd want to. There is an intense energy exuding from the donors, and I feel very alert and animated. Or perhaps I'm just over-excited and my imagination is laying the boot into my senses.

Jodie is on a mission to use DNA to identify missing persons and one of her jobs is program lead for Australian Federal Police's National DNA Program for Unidentified and Missing Persons. There are around 750 sets of unknown remains sitting in mortuaries, labs and police stations around Australia which can hopefully be identified. Perhaps some of them will match up with some of the estimated 2500 long-term missing people. As we speak, she points out skeletons that date back to the faux terrorist exercise in 2020. While four donors were buried, four were kept above ground to decompose. All of these eight donors have been slowly skeletonising—either above or below ground—and will now be used for DNA research in PhD projects.

'I love that one donor has now been in an exercise and trained up to fifty police in disaster victim identification,' says Jodie. 'It's now been in that mass grave, and now training another group of police. And it's now being used in two PhD projects, the results of which I'm using in the national missing persons program.'

The PhD students will compare the accuracy of different identification techniques. 'For example, a forensic anthropologist will examine a set of remains and try and infer what the ancestry of that person was. We now have new DNA techniques that can tell us what someone's genetic ancestry and hair and eye colour are—so we want to compare these two different tests, which can tell us what someone's ancestry is.'

'What? From a skeleton, you can tell what someone's hair colour was?'

'No! No,' says Jodie. 'So . . . if we just focus on the ancestry component.'

'So you can tell if they're Swedish or something?'

'Yep,' she says. 'We want to determine how accurate and what the efficacy of these techniques are that we're using, because we don't usually have the ground truth to tell us what the answer is. Whereas with these donors we do.'

After lunch, the team is back at the mass grave, and I ask Scott about the intensity, the anticipation in the group that I saw and felt before. He says it happens at real crime scenes too. Being here has given me a slight inkling of the pressure police would feel exhuming a real grave—not only is there the psychological element but police would be so wary of making any mistakes or missing something as they slowly trawl through the dirt.

'I guess this is why something like this is kind of quite incredible that you can practise in a sort of—not a relaxing environment—but a . . .'

'It's a safe environment,' says Scott, finishing my sentence. 'The risk of failure is totally different if you do something incorrectly. It's not the end of the court case, or a homicide investigation or something like that. It's a good place for that training and how the procedures hold up.'

As I drive home on that birthday afternoon, I contemplate the world the donors go into. They go into 'science'—a place of reason, rationality, forensics, measurement—and let loose a wild, cosmic code to be deciphered. When I check my notes at home later, I can see I've underlined ODOUR a few times. I then remember that it was related to the donors seemingly being used for quite a few odour projects. I make a mental note to look into it and then step in the shower to wash off a feeling—real or imagined—of death before celebrating my birthday.

***

I'm back at the facility months later, and feel a sense of familiarity—the green fencing surrounded by wire and security cameras, parking nose-out in case a bushfire suddenly tears through the surrounding eucalyptus woodland. Once inside, the feeling continues—signing in inside the demountable office, and a different set of shoes for the field. But I hear the sound of a machine, of loud beeping, and suddenly it feels different.

Prisca, a technical officer who works in the anatomy laboratories at the university, advises me to put on a protective suit.

'Are you okay with what is out there?' she asks.

I say yes but I don't know—I don't actually know what's out there this time.

'How long have these donors been placed here?'

'They've been here for two weeks.'

'Only two weeks?' I ask. For some reason, I thought they studied people for much longer. 'Just put under lots of rubble?'

'Yes. The donors were placed on the concrete and the bricks were placed on top of them.'

Out of the demountable, in the distance, are a group of women in white coverall Tyvek protective suits collecting bricks from a large pile of rubble, and throwing them into smaller piles. The beeping is coming from a small, bright orange loader which is picking up heavy concrete blocks and moving bricks.

Prisca and I walk past a series of sheds, including a large one with four brown cardboard coffins lined with plastic—they are plain, simple, and the sort of style I wouldn't mind for myself actually. Prisca explains they are going to coffin the donors and send them to the crematorium directly. These are the first donors to have left the site since AFTER opened in 2016.

I stop to watch the women, all in sturdy boots, chucking bricks into piles. I don't recognise anybody but suspect one of them is Dr Maiken Ueland, a forensic chemist and deputy director of AFTER, who is a little bit older than the other women and looks Scandinavian (i.e. blonde), and who in an interview with the venerable *Chemical and Engineering News*, published by the American Chemical Society since 1923, listed her favourite molecule as dimethyl trisulfide, 'one of the key volatile compounds released by humans'. I've returned here to follow up on my ODOUR note, which is basically seeing what Maiken is up to.

She and the team are standing on a large slightly raised concrete platform next to piles of metal beams, concrete blocks and pipes, and bricks, which have been placed to simulate a building collapse. Underneath the rubble are four donors who were taken from freezers at the University of Technology campus in Ultimo, thawed for a few days and then placed at the site fifteen days ago in what is essentially a faux disaster situation. Maiken and the researchers have been watching how they decompose and making various measurements for different projects.

The first is related to their smell. When we die, and if we are left out or not found for a few weeks, our lipids, proteins and carbohydrates break into compounds—methane, ammonia, sulfur dioxide hydrogen, hydrogen and carbon dioxide. Hanging over the disaster area are two very small field stations covered with sun shields and fitted with four tubes, which for the past two weeks have been collecting volatile organic compounds

(VOCs) in the odours coming off the donors as they decompose. The tubes have a coating inside that collects and traps the VOCs which make up the scent of the site. Maiken has done the long drive from Sydney every day to change them. She puts caps on the tubes, wraps them in aluminium foil, places them in glass jars and drives them back to the lab.

Aside from the field stations, Maiken had earlier been using NOS.E, a portable electronic nose, to see if it could detect the smells from the donors. It had been programmed to pick up specific compounds. Maiken is hoping NOS.E can be used to locate victims in mass disasters alongside detection dogs.

This is the third time Maiken has done this novel study on donors, which is the first of its kind in the world.

One donor has already been uncovered: a man lying flat on his back in a very decayed state, an unusually beautiful horror. He looks like he is wearing the remnants of a suit but on closer inspection it's a dark t-shirt and pants. Flies buzz everywhere. At this stage, the smell, while important to the researchers, is *sort of* okay for me, and I'm privately acting cool with it, particularly as the women are in the thick of it, talking, the constant chink of bricks hitting each other in a pile in the background. At one point someone screams out: 'There's a huge spider!'

A blue gurney rests against a gum tree. 'Head' is written on one end. More bricks have been cleared away and the women are now getting ready to move the donor's body. I'm not sure how they will do it—he seems very sludgy and soft. But Prisca appears unperturbed, confidently advising the group how to do it.

'If you grab his shoulder and his hand, and if you grab the hips and the legs. Then we roll that way. Ready one, two, three. Up.'

He is in fact very stiff and they easily, gently roll him on to the stretcher. The five women then discuss where they should stand so as to best carry him over to a nearby makeshift outdoor morgue, which is essentially a marquee with a large blue tarpaulin for flooring.

'We need three people up here,' says Prisca.

'You are putting the old people at the end,' jokes Maiken.

They arrange themselves around the stretcher.

'From the ... what are they called? Knees?' says Prisca. The women erupt into laughter.

'One, two, three, up!'

They carry the donor across to the morgue and place the stretcher on to the tarpaulin.

Maiken and Alicia, a student studying mummification, then begin a methodical process of using long needles to take samples from the muscle and fat in the upper arm, the torso and the thigh. The tissue is then dabbed into small plastic tubes, and will be analysed against samples taken on day one. The donors are thus being used on a second project, which looks into decomposition over a period of time—the holy grail of time of death. Maiken explains that the tissue that is collected will be processed in a certain way, and run through an instrument which tells them exactly what it's made up of—it's a chemistry-based approach. 'It's a major challenge in a lot of investigations because it's so hard,' she says.

Maiken and Alicia are also using sterile cotton swabs to collect hair, toenails and tissue samples for Jodie for DNA analysis.

Initially I stand quite close studying and watching the women but the smell slowly pushes me away 5, 6, 7 metres. Within ten minutes, I realise I'm 15 metres away. But the scientists stay close. For the rest of the time I'm there, they will move three more donors from under the rubble, place them on the tarp and collect the samples. They will coffin them and close the lids. Throughout that time, I do not hear absolutely one moan from anyone about the work they are doing and in fact it's the opposite: they seem content, absorbed, methodical.

'It's interesting it's all women here,' I remark.

'Are you surprised?' asks Alicia, her white suit covered in what they call 'decomp'.

'Our research team is ... we have?' ponders Maiken.

'Eighty per cent women,' says Alicia.

'I wonder why that it is?' I ask.

'It's dirty work and women are better at it?' muses Maiken. 'Less sensitive in terms of smells and stuff? Forensics is very female-dominated in general.'

Bridget, a young PhD student with a nose ring, chimes in: 'We talked about something in one of my forensics classes called the "Scully effect". After Scully became big in *The X-Files*, there was a big influx of women into forensics and the police as well.' I never became hooked on the show but do recall FBI agent Dana Scully—played by Gillian Anderson—was a cult figure in the late 1990s.

Others attribute it to the crime show *CSI* or Patricia Cornwell's novels. Maiken, originally from Stavanger, Norway, was reading local crime writer Jo Nesbø; while he inspired her to want to be a detective, she knew it had to involve chemistry. 'I wanted to use science to help solve criminal cases,' she says.

It's not all women—there's a PhD student named Zach, who is there but not doing brick work. And there's Mohammed Shareef or 'Mo', an anatomist and head of University of Technology Sydney's body donor program. He's been sitting in the demountable office working and has come out to check on proceedings and say hello. A committed Muslim, he sports a thick beard, which is nearly two fists long and not one that appears on any of my beard charts. He's instantly into joke mode, stirring the team, prompting silly spars and jibes. I later ask Mo about his joviality and he remarks: 'Ours is not the easiest job in the world. You have to keep the mood light.'

The hours pass. The donors are methodically taken out of the rubble. Samples are collected and photographs taken. They are wrapped up, placed in coffins. I watch, taking notes, sometimes staring at the blue sky, listening to the hum of the bush and decide even though it would be chilly in winter, I could totally donate my body to this place. Projecting my future dead mute self, aside from the serene bush setting, I like the women, the research, their banter, their collegiality, their professionalism.

Andreas Vesalius, in his black doublet and stockings, is watching too. He leans against a tree, staring at an upside-down science 500 years on from when he revolutionised the study of the human body. It's all women, wearing white plastic suits. Their research is based on the bodies of humans willingly given and will in part go towards solving crimes.

Where he had knives and dissected in front of a throng of feisty students in halls, these women use boxes to capture smells and temperatures in the open air. He walks closer to look at the dead. *Nosce te ipsum*, he wrote on page after page of his great tome *Fabrica. Know ourselves.* A sense of familiarity strikes him as he looks at these people who gave their bodies to science. Ah. *Know ourselves.* The dead still have so many stories to help us do this.

I've spent so long seeing intricate patterns in our inner world in anatomical textbooks—the leaf-like lobules in the female breast, the way the *atria centralis retinae* in the eye is like a crack of lightning in the sky—but these donors seeping back into nature help me know myself, help us *know ourselves*, in such a radically new way. We are brown, burnished red, black, mustard, bright yellow, tan, green. We are mottled, stringy, mouldy. We are centipedes, cockroaches, maggots, flies, fungus. *This is who we are.* I mention this to Maiken later on as she helps me find a hose to clean my boots.

'Yes,' she says, smiling, nodding. 'It is very natural, isn't it?'

I remark to Maiken that it's a weird space with the donors—this shift between objectivity and subjectivity. I think they were a person and now they are science.

'We always need to remember that it's a person. I think it's really dangerous if you stop thinking of them as a person,' she says. 'I always encourage everyone to think this is someone's loved one, this is someone who has given us an absolutely amazing gift of coming here and letting us do this type of work that is really is going to help, it's already helping case work, it's already changed the research sphere as well. It's going to mean in the future we can solve more cases faster, we can help get answers for family members a lot quicker.'

Occasionally Maiken learns bits of information about the donors. 'It's really nice to get those back stories,' she says.

That night, I keep waking up. The film set inside my mind is filled with images of the donors in their psychedelic state—all those chaotic colours and patterns—and my brain is attempting to compute, cleanse, mull over, jiggle around, wash the extraordinariness of the scene. I walk my son to school in the morning, a tad weary, and on the way home, see myself lying on the earth, and melting into it. I now sense how intrinsically 'in' the world we are.

The Australian environmental philosopher Val Plumwood—who famously survived a crocodile attack—long argued that humans seeing themselves apart from nature has had all sorts of dire consequences, and that we 'stand apart from it as masters or controllers'. But I saw no mastery in the bush that day, just a mutuality—and a slow vanishing. *We are in the world* as all else is.

***

It's a few weeks later and I'm in a generic meeting room at the University of Technology in Ultimo with Maiken, who in a shirt and slacks looks quite different out of her white Tyvek suit. Ironically, while I had permission to go to AFTER and visit the donors, I don't have clearance to go to the labs here.

The donors are making a massive contribution to odour research, which initially started because of rhino horns. In 2015 Kyle Ewart was an AFTER researcher based at the Australian Museum in Sydney. He was drilling holes in a rhino horn to take a DNA sample and he noticed that it smelled a bit funny every time he did it. 'The thing is, when things smell, they call us,' says Maiken. She and others started running experiments to try and capture the smell coming from the rhino horns. This soon triggered a larger project where they looked into collecting the smells from illegally traded wildlife horns and their fake counterparts.

They would heat the horns a little to generate smells, which were analysed on a large instrument that can identify VOCs. They discovered fairly quickly that based on smell alone, they could tell the difference between seized, illegally-traded wildlife items. For example, black rhinoceros horn had distinctly different VOCs from the white rhinoceros horn. 'We can actually use the compounds coming off to say what they are,' she says. They looked at all sorts of wildlife parts—water buffalo ivory, different types of whales.

The researchers soon turned their attention to the blue-tongue lizard—in particular the shingleback, which is one of Australia's most frequently illegally traded native animals. It's a dismal world where you have losers capturing, duct taping and mailing these sweet, docile and colourful reptiles overseas to become exotic pets. To counter the problem, PhD student Amber Brown travelled across Australia collecting shinglebacks, and putting them in a small chamber for a few minutes to capture their smell. She would then let them go. They are in the process of finalising the key compounds to look for in the reptiles and working out the NOS.E's sensors.

Seeing the potential, Maiken decided to turn NOS.E to smelling humans at disaster sites. We're all losing our jobs to AI and algorithms, and when I first told my partner George about a new e-sniffer, he was worried about whether sniffer dogs were losing their jobs.

So I ask Maiken: 'Is it putting dogs out of work or are there just not enough dogs?'

'There's not enough dogs, they're expensive, and you can't put them everywhere,' she explains. 'If you take a disaster, for example, if you have a plane crash, there are dangerous fumes, there's all this other stuff going on. So it's dangerous to put the dogs in too soon and that's where an electronic nose could come in. It's not going to put any dog or human lives at risk.'

Volatolomics is an emerging scientific field and is used for a whole range of things—one can chemically smell different corals, drugs and even diseases such as certain types of cancer or cystic fibrosis, which are picked up through studying the VOCs in the breath.

Aside from the body donors informing Maiken's research into search and rescue, she also works on time of death. 'There is a lot of work out there but there is still the misconception that time of death is easy,' she says. 'If it's very early, it's a lot easier to determine time of death, and the pathologist will be really good at that. And then once you get to a couple of weeks, the insects are really good—the entomology is also quite precise. It's still being worked on but quite good. But then once you get beyond that, it gets quite, quite difficult. Once it's weeks to a month, it gets very difficult to get a very precise time. It's more like you get ranges and the longer the time goes, the larger the ranges. So if you find like a skeletal sample, the ranges could be really large.'

It feels like whenever scientists find a skeleton in a pit and they're wearing an amazing crown and an incredible ring, they know exactly when they died. I ask Maiken if they are more likely guessing. She thinks they might be assessing the artefacts. 'In terms of skeletons, it's quite challenging for anything that's like ten, twenty or thirty years,' she says.

I tell Maiken that when I was at AFTER that first time, the police were ribbing the forensic scientists about time of death. 'It's a very challenging thing. Some methods are based on observations, which means that you can have human error. So we're trying to get methods that are going to be a lot more objective than relying on a person saying, "I believe it's been this long,"' she says. 'I'm also one of these people that says, "It's been this long" but what we're using to identify that is colour changes and things like that—there's always a subjectivity to it.'

I remark how at AFTER the colours of the donors were quite striking. 'There's a lot of colour changes due to different chemical reactions in the body,' she says. 'It's really useful for times of death, up to the point where you have those colour changes. It's when all of that goes away, it gets challenging.'

Maiken is fine about donating her body. 'I'd like to do something after I'm gone, like leave something behind, and if that can be my organs, or something that people can work on to further the field, I think that's a nice thought.'

'Death isn't scary—that's another thing,' she says. 'Probably if you have an illness leading up to it, of course, that's incredibly scary—if it's like this uncertainty. But I think death itself, I don't think is a scary thing. It just is.'

But while she's confronted death, she tells me she still has a lot of questions. For one, she wishes dogs could talk.

'What would you ask them?'

'A lot of times I would ask—why are you stopping here? Like, what are you smelling? Or what does that smell like to you?' she says, laughing. 'A human body has like thousands of smells, and I just want to ask "What is it that's attracting you to it? Why can you find it? What is that smell?"'

Chapter 25

Wobbles of nausea and unease hit me on my first visit to the J.T. Wilson anatomical museum at the University of Sydney, my brain shielding my body from the radical sight of human heads and dissected feet in jars. But once the nausea passed, I could see why the early anatomists were prone to invoking a higher power when it came to the study of the human body. Oh my, I thought, look at this palace we are; this palace filled with trees, spiderwebs, soft corals, roots of plants, honeycombs, a flat muscle appearing exactly like a horse's shimmering coat. How do I classify what I can see? Specimen? Parts? Objects? Bits of human? Art pieces? For years, the university has run an annual dissection prize and the winner's human remains are placed in the museum. It's a shame the remarkable technique in these dissections is so hidden.

Nursing a mysterious groin injury, I gazed at the dissected legs on a wall, earnestly tracing the fan shape of the *adductor longus* and the flat, triangular *adductor brevis*, the pain now making more sense. The Zoroastrians could see the universe in the body, penning in their scripture: 'The skin is like the sky, the flesh is like the earth, the bones are like the mountains, the veins are like the rivers, the blood in the body is like the water in the sea, the hair is like the plants, the hairier parts are like the forests.' I limped out of the museum transformed and informed, and in hindsight naive about aspects of the collection and many like it around the world.

***

Covid-19 meant I never made it to the unromantically but efficiently named Integrated Pathology Learning Centre at the Royal Brisbane

Women's Hospital, its exhibits starring old specimens from the University of Queensland's pathology museum. The space is open to the public through booking, and to school groups, and I imagine that among some of those little girls and boys, one will become fixated on one particular specimen, like I did with the crusty convict fingertips in the little bottle at the Old Commissariat Store in Brisbane I saw as a kid.

I also partly baulked at checking out the new centre as I worried parts of the collection might include bits of Ruby and Julie. I didn't know. Dr J.V. Duhig collected specimens that helped found the original museum in 1950, which was named in his honour. It was the museum that Ted, the obstetrician I interviewed, used to walk past as a student and feel strange about.

The museum went through various iterations until the 1990s. Collecting waned, teaching relied more on digital imagery and the museum space was reallocated. Specimens were packed away in boxes. In 2006 activism in pathology circles saw the collection saved from obscurity and reopened at the hospital in 2010.

I'd been left slightly altered for the better by the J.T. Wilson because I could objectively appreciate it but I wasn't sure if I'd feel that way in the learning centre. I didn't want to think that my grandparents might be in there. Would it be weird? A source of pride? A way to learn objectively? Sadness? Nothing? Anatomical museums seemed so scientific and ordered but I would soon come to see them as yet another complicated, politically charged and emotive corner for the dissected.

***

After I spent time with the anatomist Quentin Fogg, he walked me up a flight of stairs to the Harry Brookes Allen Museum of Anatomy and Pathology, which is, to quote the blurb on their website, 'one of Australia's largest collections of human tissue specimens, comparative anatomy specimens and historical anatomical models'. Like many anatomical museums, it is not open to the public and is predominantly used as a resource for medical students.

I'd been inspired to go to the museum for a few reasons. For starters—I could get in. While I'd been to the J.T. Wilson, the other major anatomical museum in Sydney was The Museum of Human Disease at the University of New South Wales but it had been closed since the pandemic.

Various characters at the University of Melbourne were engaged and keen to chat. First, there had been Quentin. Second, Dr Ross L. Jones, a historian on the management committee of the Harry Brookes Allen, had all sorts of stories. He'd not only written a history book about the university's anatomy department but in the spirit of archaeologist Howard Carter and Tutankhamun, had stumbled across the 'Cadaver Books', a set of huge, old leather-bound volumes, which had been kept in the basement of the anatomy building alongside plastinated body parts. The books contained the names and some details about bodies that had come into the department from 1898 onwards, and were about to be thrown out when he found them. Earlier archives starting from the 1860s had been destroyed in the 1980s.

I thought there may be some answers in the books. Ross had done a preliminary study and found that body donation picked up in around the 1950s, and that a lot more women started donating in the early 1970s.

At this stage, I was yet to get a grip on the social forces that brought about body donation. One theory was that in the US, Jessica Mitford's 1963 bestseller *The American Way of Death*—an exposé of the funeral industry's excessive fees—raised awareness about body donation by suggesting it as a way to avoid funeral costs.

Ross had warned me it would be difficult to access them—they were tightly held in the bosom of the anatomy department to maintain the privacy of the people listed in them. I would need special permission if I wanted to have a look.

Either way, I was also keen to meet Rohan Long, the museum's curator, and visit the plastinated body parts—a new fate for donors, a radical technological shift in the history of body preservation and something I'd never seen in reality.

I'm met at the door by Rohan, thirty-something, upbeat, bespectacled, in a plaid shirt and sporting an elegant silver wristwatch. He describes himself as someone who has been hanging around museums his entire life but with a more 'animal background', having previously worked at the university's Tiegs Zoology Museum. He's been curating the Harry Brookes collection since 2018 and his glass-walled office looks out on to a large room filled with specimens, skeletons and models.

I don't know if it's deliberate or accidental—the memories of my nausea at the J.T. Wilson Museum telling me to be cautious—but we instantly jump into talking about a kitsch-looking 1960s plastic dummy at the main entrance. Its head is half carved away to reveal a skull and its torso shows all its organs. It reminds me of my Officeworks man but larger and much cooler. 'This is such a University of Melbourne thing. That is a pre-unification German model, probably worth quite a lot of money and it was in a meeting room upstairs,' says Rohan. 'I was like "Guys, I think it's time to transition this from a thing that hangs around the meeting room to exceptional museum object."' He says there is all sorts of valuable material sitting in cupboards and in shelves. 'Many things we look at we think—to quote Indiana Jones—"that should be in a museum."'

Rohan leads me towards two glass tanks containing abdomens which have been plastinated. The ribs, the guts unfurling and the dull brown, meat tones look as if this section is about to breathe. It's also exquisitely rendered: you can see where the saw has struck neatly through the bone. While it's a teaching tool, people in the university's in-house anatomical services team have obviously made aesthetic decisions, choreographing death into something I can't quite define.

'Do you ever see the bodies upstairs?' I ask Rohan.

'I do. Not heaps but yeah.'

'Are the colours pretty similar?'

'Similar. It's funny but a lot of people ... we all think about the colours of these things. It changes. The colours of a living tissue or organ compared to the colour of a deceased tissue organ compared to an embalmed one compared to a fluid-preserved one—all these things change depending on how the body is treated.'

In a nearby glass box is an arm and part of the chest suspended with wires.

'This arm was lying on a shelf in the next room. I was like: "That is a gorgeous thing—that is a gorgeous specimen that is just sitting there on the shelf. We should show it off."'

I see the person it once was, about to fly.

'You could see it at the Guggenheim.'

'Yes. Absolutely. I love the aesthetic of it but the structural anatomy is also there. The arm is being supported by the shoulder and you get an idea of the way the muscular system works.'

We move towards the most dramatic person in the room, the latest addition to the museum, added in early 2021.

It's a plastinated head sitting on a pillow.

'That was my aesthetic choice to put a red pillow under there,' he remarks. 'I thought that had to be done.'

The pillow adds a touch that is partly elegant, part David Lynch. I lean over the glass box to take in what happens to a donor in the hands of a master dissector. The facial skin has been peeled away. At the scalp, they have gently made graduated incisions, which look a bit like a set of stairs, to reveal five separate layers, each with their own distinct colour and texture. The eyebrows have been left and stand out as two distinct thick strips. The lips remain too, looking like lipstick as the rest of the face has been carefully carved away.

Rohan is effusive about it all and the people who created it, and ponders whether von Hagens' *Body Worlds* has had an influence.

'Most people in anatomy—more so than in other sciences—are very open to that intersection of art with their practice. I guess it's that long, long history of anatomical art,' he says. 'That's the thing with the plastinates—they are absolutely gorgeous but they are only as good as the dissection that is being preserved. There are obviously incredible dissectors in this department.'

We head into the main area and the rows and rows of neat white cabinets instantly conjures the 'white space' feeling one gets in museums or art galleries—but instead of art or old Etruscan pottery shards, there are body parts in little perspex rectangles. They used to be in glass jars or 'pots' filled with Wentworth Solution, a formalin-based preservative commonly used in medical human tissue collections but in the fifties and sixties, Rohan says there were 'some absolutely heroic efforts' to put everything in perspex rather than glass. After seeing the plastination, the perspex-preserved specimens seem almost quaint.

I admire two blocks with what look like vibrantly coloured, elaborate root systems and ask Rohan what they are. He explains they are corrosion casts from the 1960s, and involved injecting the organ with silicone and a plastic resin and letting it harden. The tissue was then destroyed, leaving perfect casts of an intricate vascular network—in this case it is a brain and a liver.

I remark to Rohan that it feels very museumy, and he says this is the plan. 'These days, those of us in university museums want to treat these collections with much seriousness and as much professionalism as you would at a state museum.'

The medical historian Dr Ross L. Jones arrives and I feel a flutter of kindred spirit upon meeting him. I'd met Ross via email and on the phone a few months ago as he's part of a tiny posse who have closely studied elements of Australia's anatomical history. He's particularly interested in the dark turn the science took when the 20th century anatomist Richard Berry was a professor at the University of Melbourne.

Ross has also looked into many other uncomfortable episodes in the late 1800s and early 1900s: the university's anatomists pressuring mental asylums into handing over their dead, students holding 'meat fights' with body parts of the poor and unclaimed.

I haven't had an easy time getting some anatomists to speak to me so I imagine he is pissing some people off in the Melbourne establishment by dredging up past horror stories. His history of the anatomy department might have been uncomfortable and difficult in parts—the eugenics, the thousands and thousands of people dissected without consent—but the transparency is laudable.

'Melbourne decided they wanted to do this because they had such a bad history. They thought, "Let's be the leaders, let's clean all the cupboards out and let's start again,"' says Ross. 'So the anatomy department has been very much like that too. I think they want to lead.'

The cupboard needed airing as the university had long housed Indigenous skulls and bones collected by amateur anthropologist George Murray Black, and separate Indigenous material studied by the eugenicist Richard Berry. According to the Aboriginal Heritage Council of Victoria: 'The Murray Black and Berry collections at the University of Melbourne alone comprised over 1600 Ancestral Remains and were just two of the many collections in Victoria. Ancestral Remains from the Murray Black collection are known to be between eighty to 14,000 years old.' Ross says all the known Australian Indigenous remains have been repatriated, and the only ones left from the Berry collection still at the university are not Australian.

As Rohan puts it: 'We want to treat these like proper museums and in museum culture today ideas about repatriation and decolonisation are *so* prevalent—it's just what's happening.'

I excuse myself to absorb the collection but there is too much to take in, and I'm hungry to the point that I'm a bit weak and shaky. For some reason I stop and study a pancreas for quite a while. I'd never thought what it looks like—maybe a bit like Java on a map? Here is a very dramatic-looking torso—a woman's abdomen spilling out, her breasts looking a bit squashed, sections of her skin pale and lumpy. I see some death masks. I read later that the infamous bushranger Ned Kelly's death mask is there but it wasn't obvious. Upper limbs. Bones. Brains. There is so much.

I go back to Rohan and Ross, who are standing in front of a portrait of Harry Brookes Allen, the professor of anatomy and pathology the museum is named after.

'Was Harry an okay guy?' I ask.

'He hasn't been cancelled just yet,' says Rohan.

'He wasn't into collecting Aboriginal remains,' pipes in Ross, in reference to Richard Berry. Harry also wrote poetry although Ross isn't a fan of it.

'He must've been quite cool. He had daughters who went off to do extremely progressive things,' says Rohan. One of them went on to become a famous painter in the US.

A new train station is being built literally outside the large window. Due to worries that the vibrations from the construction would damage some parts of the collection, including Victorian-era anatomical models made from wax, plaster and papier-mâché, they have moved these items down to the basement.

Rohan asks if I want to have a look. Sure, I say. Ross is also eager to see a particular specimen.

We head down a few flights of stairs, Rohan taps his security pass, and we are soon in an old-school area which feels like it's not been renovated for decades, and walk along a corridor with a low roof.

'I find the body parts less spooky than this creepy corridor,' says Rohan.

We go into a small room, known as the dry store. 'This is models, bones, casts, all sorts of wonderful things,' says Rohan, pointing at shelves lined with all sorts of beautiful and eerily rendered medical displays, including a striking wax model of a baby with its guts spilling out, a placenta attached. 'Ross, if you want to see the dissection—it's over there,' says Rohan, pointing to a bottom shelf.

I study the anatomised baby. Meanwhile, Ross and Rohan are animatedly discussing a particular object so I take a closer look. Sitting on a bottom shelf is a very large perspex rectangle, in which is a 3 cm or so slice of a pregnant woman. Face-on, she looks as if she is asleep, her eyelashes at rest. Side-on is her whole body: her brain, her spine, her organs and her very small baby. I'm momentarily startled.

Ross explains that Richard Berry and his offsider William Preston did this section.

'This person would not have given permission,' says Ross.

'No,' says Rohan.

'She must've been itinerant. She's obviously very poor—look how tiny she is. She would've been very poor or in the benevolent asylum in North Melbourne,' says Ross sadly. 'Every body part in this place before the 1950s was not donated and was taken. Even up until the 1960s and I think the 1970s maybe, they were using parts from people in the mental home.'

I look at this poor young girl, trapped in this perspex for eternity.

'I didn't realise it was as thick as that,' says Ross, looking at the girl, who was preserved in 1910.

'How do you know he [Berry] did it?' I ask.

Ross says, 'Because they talk about it—it's all in his papers, and it's always been known as "Berry's section".'

Rohan adds, 'A lot of these potted specimens do have a little plate sort of saying "This was dissected by so and so in this year."'

Ross tells me, 'This one's famous because it's ...'

I say, 'It's quite sad ...'

Ross replies, 'It's so sad. They developed a supposedly new technique, they got a special saw made.'

I ask, 'How did they cut it like that?'

Ross says, 'They had a bandsaw.'

Rohan adds: 'Frozen and then they bandsawed it.'

I'd heard the University of Melbourne had an *Anatomical Venus*, a prized wax made by the Italian sculptor Clemente Susini, so I ask if it's here. Ross says there was one in the early museum but he thinks it's been lost.

We leave the dry room and head into a much bigger room filled row upon row of storage compactors, their shelves lined with thousands and thousands of specimens, models, casts, papier-mâché and waxworks with little bar codes on their sides. In some of the specimen containers, the fluid levels are low and there is a layer of yellow fat. Rohan explains that they need maintenance. 'They need a bit of love but it's just me to do all this stuff,' he says, looking at the shelves. 'It should not be yellow like that. It should be beautiful and clear, and it should be topped up to the top. And that's not that difficult to do.'

While all these objects are meant for teaching, some of them are mesmerising. On one shelf rests a man, strangely handsome and poetic-looking. *Tramond a Paris* is written on his chest—it's a well-known anatomical supplier from the city in the late 19th century. He is so life-like he looks like he could sit up at any moment and ask for *un café* but for the fact he is made of wax, a torso and dissected. The collection was recently valued at millions and millions of dollars, in part because some of the models are considered artworks. 'But then in terms of insurance value, if you wanted to replace 10,000 human tissue dissections, what cost would that be?' Rohan asks.

I ask Rohan if has any idea who any of the people in the collection might be.

'If we did some detective work, it's theoretically plausible,' he says, explaining that some of the pathology specimens came from the hospitals so they have detailed information about the person's age, condition and location. The oldest 'known' specimen probably dates from the 1960s but for the most part the collection is anonymous. There is still so much more to examine and explore but I'm about to faint from hunger.

I head to a cafe and find that I can't stop wondering about the pregnant young woman trapped in perspex, feeling blue/green/blue/green as I fall from the sky. Who was she? Who will ever advocate for this poor unknown woman? How can I honour her? Perhaps I am by writing her down now.

***

In 2015 David S. Jones, a medical historian at Harvard, and Dominic Hall, who curates the Warren Anatomical Museum at the same university, gave a lively talk on 500 years of dissection history. The pair charted the different ways anatomists got bodies over time, a slow and controversial journey from using executed criminals and resorting to grave robbing to the process becoming highly regulated. As Jones pointed out, students do not have to bring their own bodies to class any more. They ended on the latest controversy about the rise of body brokers in the US.

At the end of the talk Jones made a quip which got a chuckle from the crowd: 'Everyone knows that it's very difficult for pre-medical students to get into Harvard Medical School. But it turns out this is true for dead bodies as well. Harvard Medical School has a wait list not just for pre-meds but also for cadavers.'

I wanted to find out if this was still true so I got in touch with Jones, who suggested I speak with Dominic Hall at the Warren, which I was to realise is one of the oldest surviving anatomical museums in North America, dating from 1847. It's filled with thousands of items—human tissue, old dissection kits, plaster casts of heads, 19th-century crutches, watercolours and paintings. They have the skull of construction worker Phineas P. Gage and the long iron rod that went through his head, a case considered a unique medical mystery as he survived for twelve years after the terrible accident with a different personality.

I had images of the Warren being a grand ye olde wood-panelled Harvard museum. But when I phoned Dominic, he explained that it was no longer a bricks and mortar space, that much of the collection lived in boxes, and this was actually the fate of many anatomical collections around the world—they had either shrunk or closed. The Warren first opened to the public in 1860s and peaked around the 1930s and 1940s, the crowds drawn in by a natural curiosity about the body. But not long after, it was dismantled and stored. In 2007, Dominic, a museologist and historian, began working at the museum and has been slowly reconstituting and researching the collection. It is now largely a research facility housed in Harvard Medical School's Countway Library of Medicine.

I was a bit taken aback by our conversation—I wasn't at all expecting to hear that this venerable museum and many like it had such troubled backstories and potentially fraught futures.

Dominic says the Warren and many anatomical museums across the world began to wane in the mid 20th century as anatomical practice changed dramatically from an interest in the macro to the microscopic. 'Museum collections and medical schools in particular start to lose some of their teaching utility, and they take up a lot of room,' he says. Downward pressure meant a lot of museums either closed or their collections were just put into storage, which is what happened to the Warren.

He says another factor—'this is me editorialising in some way'—was the Nuremberg Trials of members of the Nazi Germany leadership, which were held just after the Second World War. 'What captured the American psyche—and probably around the world—are the Nazi medical atrocities, some of which are very anatomy based,' he says.

'Then there are all these stories about making specimens out of people that are attached to Nuremberg—these stories of lampshades, for example, and shrunken heads, and I think even stories of things like curtains. Some of might be apocryphal, but a whole new tissue ethics comes into being.' Dominic sees that human subject research started to really change after the Holocaust and then in 1968, the Uniform Anatomical Gift Act was introduced in the US. Spurred on by organ donation, it also controlled whole-body donation, which changed the way whole bodies were sourced, and subsequently treated.

While people have long asked questions about anthropological museums, Dominic says they are also now turning their attention to medical collections across the US and elsewhere. 'I think people are very uncomfortable with thinking about these collections,' he says. 'People are all of a sudden having a moment of reckoning where they're really thinking about "Okay, so we have these collections. Where did these collections come from? Who are these people?"' he says. The answers, sadly, are tied into narratives about race and poverty because these are the people who end up in collections. 'Very few well-off people end up in medical museums.'

Dominic has studied US dissection history, which begins in 1641 with the first law allowing for doctors to anatomise executed criminals. Since then, dissection has long meant the practice was 'highly criminalised' and also included people who died in prison and weren't claimed. 'There's always been sourcing from people who have committed some sort of criminal offence,' he says.

It continues into the modern age, and he raises the issue of Joseph Paul Jernigan, the thirty-nine-year-old executed man whose body was scanned as part of National Library of Medicine's Visible Human Project and who I saw floating in London. I didn't know that his body was in the Anatomage table, one of which is at the Countway Library. Dominic tells me that he has placed a provenance statement next to the table to give context to the origins of the images 'to best inform users'. I found this impressive.

The Warren has detailed records about the majority of the specimens—the person's name, their hospital records, age, cause of death and other elements of their life. Dominic says it varies but you can also end up accessing different sources to tell the story of that person. They might have been collected because something was significant and articles were written about them.

'So then you're always stuck with this ethical question of like, how much of the story do we tell? There's this balance that no one's really figured out. In this historic anatomy world, the balance is between restoring somebody's humanity and protecting their privacy. It's almost impossible. But that's a tension that colleagues and I talk about all the time,' he says. 'Some people are very much "give me every piece of information that you have, tell me their entire story" and then others want to be more careful.'

While Phineas P. Gage's mother donated his skull, Dominic says there is little consent behind the specimens in the collection. Most people died in a hospital unclaimed or had an organ removed and the museum somehow acquired it. As he puts it: 'When I think about publishing somebody's name, I'm always thinking that with very few exceptions, that person didn't choose to be here, that person didn't choose their kidney to be here.'

He says the other difficult question is what constitutes an individual? 'Most of the Warren—there are no full skeletons. And I think that's true of a lot of anatomy museums, it's like pieces. And so is someone's teeth—is that them? It's a very interesting thing. There's a lot of ideas of personhood that get very difficult to work through.'

I hung up from Dominic feeling a bit strange, having been knocked over by the tsunami of ethics he'd just flagged and questions of whether my tooth or my kidney was really me. Spring was beginning in Sydney but I was still cold, so I walked outside to stand in the sun and warm up a little. Here I was thinking that a way to restore humanity to the dissected was to tell their stories but now Dominic was telling me that some people think this is wrong. I don't know.

I keep leaning towards this idea that we need to do something about the taboo of dissection in the first place, and we do this by talking to the ghosts. The small woman in the perspex in Melbourne comes back to me again. Do medical students really need to study her? Should she be buried? But what about her baby—there is genuine value in scientific study of her embryo. Perhaps a provenance statement? I don't know.

A few days after we speak, Dominic emailed the answer to the question about whether there was a waiting list to get into Harvard as a body donor. He'd spoken to the Harvard Anatomical Gift people. 'It turns out the rumour isn't true. There is no waitlist. They accept body donations based on need and their needs are met each year.'

***

You can read Google reviews of Museum Vrolik in Amsterdam because incredibly, alongside the Wellcome and the Hunterian in London, the Mütter in Philadelphia and the Muséum d'Histoire Naturelle in Paris, it's one of the few anatomical museums open to the public.

Stefan: 'A bit cold inside, so bring a jacket.' (5 stars)

Chrissy: 'Vrolik is such an awesome museum. You can see a large amount of medical wet specimens, body anomalies, human and animal osteology… a must see for lovers of the curiosities and anatomy world. ♥' (5 stars).

Sara (translated from Arabic via Google): 'Unbelievable views that are not beautiful to the human soul and harmful psychologically (the honour of the dead is burial in the dirt) and to not be put in bottles for other people to see. What I have benefited from? Nothing from visiting the museum and I do not advise to visit. There are natural scenes worth visiting and contemplating more.' (1 star)

Cokyoi: 'Very unique and objectively amazing collection. It was a lot more confronting than I was expecting. It kind of upset me :/ If you have an interest it's worth seeing but it isn't…fun.' (3 stars).

The anatomist Gerard Vrolik (1775 to 1859) and his son Willem (1801 to 1863) put the collection together and it was later sold to the Athenaeum Illustre, the predecessor to Amsterdam University. Vrolik had a particular interest in teratology, which is the study of congenital abnormalities, so alongside skulls, animals, skeletons and human heads, there are cabinets with rare stillbirths and odd skeletons.

Dr Laurens de Rooy is the current director and curator of the museum and has worked there since 2002. We catch up on the internet, where he speaks to me from his home, a bookshelf and large palm in the background, which at times makes me think that he's speaking from the tropics and not Amsterdam. He sketches the collection, which was put together between 1750 and 1950—25,000 items, 5500 of which are human remains, including lots of bones. Little is known about the majority of the people in the collection, which includes heads floating in jars, and babies with extreme deformities, including Siamese Twins and one with cyclopia, a rare, fatal condition where the brain doesn't split into right and left hemispheres, and the foetus has a single eye. With such visually arresting material, Laurens co-edited *Forces of Form*, a 2009 book featuring striking (or repugnant for some) photographs of the specimens and a series of essays.

The Museum Vrolik lay dormant until the 1990s, when the *American Journal of Medical Genetics* rediagnosed the congenital abnormalities in the collection and put it back in the spotlight. Its uniqueness also lies in the fact that it's a bit of a wild 19th-century jumble. Or as anatomist Antoon Moorman wrote in the book: 'Never again would congenital abnormalities, pathological specimens and comparative anatomy be brought together in the same systematic way.'

But what's not unique is the way Laurens—like many anatomical museum curators—is now grappling with its past. Dating from a time when the Dutch were colonisers, Museum Vrolik has material—largely bones and some foetuses—which were taken from Indonesia, Suriname and other parts of the world. Laurens is currently focused on this aspect of the collection, liaising with colleagues in Indonesia to access archives with the hope of being able to repatriate them. They are also looking into the animals. When shipments of human skulls were sent back to the Netherlands, they also included primate and other animals' skulls. 'It's all part of colonial practice,' says Laurens.

Museum Vrolik began slowly opening up in the 1990s and was made fully public around 2000. 'At some point, if you want to become a better museum, in the sense of more meaningful and contextualised, we needed to address these questions of provenance of material, and also talk about it. When you have a museum that's not open to the public, you can't talk about those historical elements in your museum that deal with inequality and racism,' he says.

Laurens, who in moments reminded me of the blond Matt Berninger, the lead singer of The National, says they will also look into studying the provenance of the material that comes from Amsterdam, which is largely made up of the poor and vulnerable of yesteryear. 'Eventually you want to determine what is of value—why is it of value to keep certain human remains within a museum and relevant to not keep others?' he says.

'We hope to achieve eventually a kind of taxonomy. In the case of this [preparation of human remains] we will decide to do this. In the case of that, it's anonymous but it's a relevant part of a human remain because it shows a specific disease that doesn't exist any more so we at least keep it in our collection. Further on, you can decide what you will show the public and what not.' Over time, Laurens imagines that some specimens will be repatriated or reburied, and it's part of the dynamics of the collection. 'They tell us something about how such collections develop and change in that sense. It's not static.'

Museum Vrolik, which is housed in the university's medical faculty, has some of the more confronting anatomical material I've seen online and it says something about Amsterdam's culture and its medical community that it is public. Laurens and I talk about how in many parts of the world, it is only the medical establishment and medical students that are allowed to see this material. 'I'm not fond of Gunther von Hagens' shows but they show that people are interested in looking at human anatomy,' he says. 'People are so busy with their own lives, and looking at their own health, at their own bodies and their mental health and they are also interested in how they look from the inside. There is this interest in the human body. I think the interest is genuine. I don't think it's going for a freak show. Why wouldn't we want to?'

I tell Laurens that in speaking to the anatomical community, some see the desire to see a dead body or go to a von Hagens show as partly being about 'entertainment'. Laurens counters this by saying that many doctors themselves are interested in abnormalities: 'They are simply fascinated in the same way that other people are fascinated by normal bodies.' I also tell him about Dominic's conundrum at the Warren about whether to identify people, and Laurens sees it a clash of cultures. 'In that sense, medical ethics is in a way opposing museological ethics, right?

Museological ethics says that you need to do your best to find out whereas medical ethics say you do your best to keep the body parts and people anonymised. That's interesting.'

***

I'm not expecting anatomical museums to fling their doors open on Friday evenings to let DJs in to do sets for young people clutching Aperol spritzes—although that would be fun—but it does feel elitist and paternalistic that in many instances, only the medical caste are allowed in. I've seen body parts outside of anatomy museum contexts—St Thomas' scrawny index finger in the Basilica Santa Croce in Rome, the hundreds of skulls and bones lying haphazardly in an enormous cave in Sagada in the mountainous north of the Philippines, and the mummified people exhumed from a graveyard in Guanajuato in Mexico—and they got me intensely reflecting on my insides, my skull, the eternity of death, my fate, all the people who lived before me, how exquisite it is to be alive.

Do I think there needs to be some discussion and lessons learned around the young woman in the perspex? Yes, and I'm sure the responses will be as varied as Maclise's thirteen different branches of the aortic arch.

Months later, I emailed Leo to ask him about the Duhig museum and if that is where specimens from the anatomy department went. He replied that he didn't know anything about the Duhig and that the pathology department was quite separate to anatomy.

'Specimens for pathology were generally retrieved from autopsies conducted by pathologists identifying abnormal/diseased conditions. Teaching specimens for anatomy were retrieved from normal donated remains used to demonstrate particular normal anatomical features,' he wrote. 'I doubt that there would be any possibility of any material from your grandparents being in the collection.'

Chapter 26

Glass of wine in hand and just back from Melbourne, I was in Mum's all-purpose room trawling through her meticulous family history folder when I stopped at one page: a list of DEATHS in the District of Beechworth in the State of Victoria. *Beechworth.* This sounded familiar somehow. Maurice shared the large page with four other dead men, their endings detailed in little boxes in flourishing cursive.

The first column was 'When and Where died' and it listed *Hospital for the Insane* in Beechworth.

Okay.

He is described as a farmer, and a male who had died at the age of seventy-six. His 'Cause of Death'? *Disease of the brain and heart, The result of a magisterial inquiry held by John Armstrong, Justice of the Peace on 31st August 1906.* He was listed as 'Married', but there was no further information about who his wife was, or his 'issue'.

What was a magisterial inquiry?

***

Maurice Snr had long been a difficult man but he first appeared in petty sessions records in 1867 in the small but successful town of Sale in regional Victoria. He would spend the next few years in court attempting to resolve his ongoing disputes with his neighbour Patrick Geogegan. The pair were neighbours in nearby Maffra, where they fought over stock and disagreed about fencing. Their fighting eventually spilled into assault and battery.

In 1875 one of Maurice Snr's disputes was documented in the *Gippsland Times.* At the hearing, son John told the court that Patrick's horses were running loose on the family grounds so he drove them off, and furious, walked over to tell him of the trespass, and that there were fees to be paid. According to John, when he arrived, he found the family in the milking yard and was left stunned when Patrick immediately jumped him, violently striking him three times with a stick, and then a spade.

'I'll murder you and cheerfully hang for it!' screamed Patrick.

Well, that was one side of it. Patrick, his wife and sister said things unfolded differently that day. No blows had been thrown or threats made and in fact, the opposite had happened—John had threatened and assaulted Patrick, and Maurice Snr had pulled a gun and threatened his wife, and later struck her. She had begged: 'Give me two minutes to die!'

These fights between farmers must've been a nightmare for the Bench to sort out. In this case, the warring neighbours were told to keep the peace for six months. But it didn't last long. There were more disputes, more charges of assaults, cases dismissed, and the Twomey sons were slowly getting dragged into it. Maurice Snr faced court for unlawfully and maliciously breaking down a fence and blocking off roads. There were allegations of dodgy contracting work for the council—a bridge was built at Heyfield and the Twomeys were accused of putting in dummy bolts.

Warily, Sarah watched her husband's descent, and could only hope that something would shift for her and their children. She and Maurice had left Ireland together when they were just kids—she was nineteen and he was twenty-two when they sailed into Melbourne in 1852. Neither of their parents had signed their marriage certificate—perhaps they didn't approve of their Protestant daughter marrying a Catholic agricultural labourer or perhaps they were dead.

Maurice Snr's violence turned to Sarah and in 1888 he faced Sale Court for assaulting her, and was jailed in Melbourne for three months. He was bailed out and for the next four years he became more and more terrifying until finally, on 24 November 1892, under the Lunacy Statute, he was officially deemed a 'lunatic, and a proper person to be taken charge of and detained under care and treatment'.

Sarah and their son John took Maurice to see two doctors in Melbourne to get the legal paperwork to commit him, their terror at living with him and his completely broken mental state seeping through the 'MEDICAL CERTIFICATE TO ACCOMPANY ORDER FOR RECEPTION INTO AN ASYLUM'.

Under a section titled 'Facts indicating insanity observed by myself', Dr W. Hall Owen has written: 'Loss of memory. Incoherent conversational powers. Excitement in manner. Thinks his wife is plotting against him to even the extent of murdering him. Thinks she is casting him off for a lodger named "Holster". Has suspicion of everybody trying to injure him to get him out of the way. Says his wife is a mistress to the said "Holster", which statements I learned are utterly unfounded.'

There is a second section: 'Other facts (if any) indicating insanity communicated to me by others'. Here Dr Hall Owen writes:

> Sarah Twomey his wife says that he is violent towards her, threatening to kill her, and only the other day attempted to strike her with a piece of wood. That he secretes knives and hammers about his persons and in bed. That he comes up to her with excited violence and the other day took a chamber pot and attempted to throw the contents over her in the presence of a stranger. John Twomey (son) states he talks to himself, hears voices and raves about his mother being unfaithful, and has seen him trying to kill her more than once. Goes about the house at night and also partially dressed in the streets in an aimless manner. Gave himself up to the police the other day for protection against his family and others whom he said were trying to kill him. Patrick Mahoney police constable states he has had to go across to Twomey's house many times to quiet him down when violent, excited and violent in his behaviour to his wife and children.

They travelled across town and recounted the story to another doctor, who reports more mental sickness, and trauma for the family. A Dr Diash writes: 'Abnormal loss of memory. Excitability. Incoherence. Suspicion of all around him especially his wife and family whom he accuses of ill treating him and throwing him out of the house.' Maurice told the doctor that up until five months ago he was bridge-making but as Sarah and the children knew, he'd not worked in years. Mother and son had to recount to the doctor again what had been happening all those years, how dangerous he had been, trying to poison her with 'Spirit of Salts', his foul language, threatening death, and nailing up windows so they couldn't escape his rages.

He was admitted to Kew Asylum that same day. Sarah signed the paperwork herself. Later there's a page from the asylum's 'Case Book'. He is number 163:

> Form of insanity: Delusional
> By whom brought: Friends
> Duration of present attack: Six Months, coming on gradually for seven years.
> Supposed cause: Drink.

Over the next year, there are various notes on Maurice's file and at one point—six months after his admission—Sarah was obviously worried that he might be released. 'Mrs Twomey his wife called and stated that he had previously tried to poison her by secretly putting copper filings in her tea and on one occasion, changed some medicines she was taking to Spirit of Salts, which she drank in his presence. She is very much afraid of him and wants him not to be discharged. She also says that he has not worked for 30 years and once tried to stab her with a pitchfork.'

There are only three more brief entries about him in the ensuing years. He is quiet and works in the ward. He does not express delusions. 'I regard him as dangerous to wife,' writes someone unknown. 'Bodily health good. Demented.' In 1903 he was moved to Beechworth in rural Victoria, an asylum where the chronic cases ended up. At this point, most of his family were far, far away in the deserts of Western Australia.

It's such a miserable record of violence, fear and vulnerability. I didn't know any of it. I didn't want to put this on the page; nor did I want to leave it out.

But I couldn't believe what I was about to realise.

***

Gazing at his death page, seeing that Maurice died in Beechworth mental asylum and with no relative to claim his body: he had to have been *anatomised.*

It had been law since 1867 that the unclaimed in asylums, prisoners and people who died in public institutions were sent to the University of Melbourne for dissection. While the death certificate didn't mention the university in any way, someone had cut him open, as how else would they determine that he had died of a disease of the brain and the heart? I could see the other men on this page who died in Beechworth had also undergone a *magisterial inquiry.*

The historian Dr Dolly MacKinnon has documented how between 1850 and 1900 postmortems were regularly performed in Victorian mental asylums under the auspices of a number of laws which dated from 1838 to 1896, and that the inmates were largely dissected for medical research into the pathology of madness and its possible treatment. As she puts it: 'Asylum doctors knew their patients inside and out.'

While Maurice died in 1906 and MacKinnon's work only examined up until 1900, I can get a gist of what was happening to mental patients at the time.

Maurice's cause of death is listed as 'disease of the brain', which was a generic label for mental illness. But as MacKinnon says, from the mid-19th century onwards, terms such as 'softening of the brain' as a cause of death had no basis in pathology. Still, asylum doctors published numerous papers on the causes of insanity, and were part of prestigious international organisations also studying the problem. Inmates' body parts were also kept as specimens for further study and in one instance in 1887, Dr James Neild showed off to the Medical Society of Victoria a German silver dinner fork that he supposedly found in the body of an inmate during a postmortem.

Some of the stories about how bodies and parts were treated in Victoria asylums are unpleasant. At an 1862 Inquiry into Yarra Bend asylum, attendant Samuel Wainwright said when he went into the keepers' room, 'in the pannikin there was a man's brains, brought from the dead-house and left there'. He said he was looking for a pannikin to drink with 'and reaching this down, smelt what it contained'. The attendant Mr Goode told him it was 'old So-and-so's brains'.

Claims were also made that body parts were left hanging in trees on the grounds of the asylum. Former patient Mr Robert Coats said, 'the stench was so sickening and offensive that we could scarcely bear the place ... There were skulls and portions of skulls lying about the garden. They were afterwards taken, and put into the dead-house, and that box was subsequently taken away.' Dr Robert Bowie, the man in charge of the asylum, vaguely denied the claims. The attendant Goode also dissected bodies in what was called 'the dead-house' even though by law he wasn't meant to. MacKinnon documents how in 1910—just four years after Maurice died—strict regulations were brought in, setting out what morgue attendants were allowed to do, which included 'the cutting of the scalp and sawing of the skull in preparation for the doctors to remove the brain for examination'.

The law allowed that if a family could not be contacted within twelve hours, then the inmate could be dissected. In a few recorded instances, dissections went ahead even though family members made efforts to keep in touch with the asylum to make sure it didn't happen. But with old Maurice's paperwork saying he had no family and with them far away in Western Australia, possibly not wanting to anything to do with him, what was to stop it happening?

This felt too bizarre: that my great-grandfather was one of these unclaimed people I'd spent all this time reading about.

Is this how Ruby knew about dissection? Mum says she never mentioned it and perhaps the family never spoke of his fate.

Chapter 27

All this time I'd been stumbling along, fixated on trying to find out Ruby and Julie's fate in the dissecting room.

But as I swam through ghost dissecting rooms, beavered through old papers, transported by lecture notes dating from 1540, I could see that I had a standard view of anatomical history that wasn't quite right. The biggest ghost was how left out of history the dissected are, how dishonoured and dismissed they have been—even today not many scientific papers mention their dead.

But I also began sensing all these other unexpected elements to Anatomy's story. People had dissected all sorts of people for all sorts of wild reasons—not just in the name of science.

The anatomists weren't necessarily all dreadful either. It wasn't all dark. It was lots of disconnected adjectives: brave, private, revolting, competitive, focused on cash a lot of the time, amusing. Being history, there were so many gaps, and in some instances I felt like it needed a bit of rewriting, and it was only the psychopomps who could take me there.

Curiously, there is one place they kept dragging me back to again and again too, and one that I kept diving into and swimming through. It was to the very beginning of Anatomy, actually. The foundation story.

***

A man crouched in the king's jail, weary, rattled. A cup of milk and a loaf of bread sat next to him, untouched. Still but restless, his mind buzzed from the reality of the sentence meted out by the henchmen around King Ptolemy I Soter. He mulled over the efficient Alexandrian *phylakitai* coming to his home, armed with a petition written by the scribe. He was soon arrested, taken to jail under armed escort, and just days later stood before a steward, who heard details of his alleged crime.

The trial was so quick, the man cannot recall much, just his wife sobbing, and the sentences. Each one uttered was followed by one far worse. The first sentence was the seizure of all his property, a financial death in itself—if he were to live, his life would have been impossible. In 300 BC, what is a man without his property? There were fines too—100 drachmae of silver, 3000 drachmae of copper. There was more, including a fine for hubris, but he cannot remember the details.

But then the next sentence came—that he was to die in a most unimaginable way. The Greek rulers did not usually mete out such a punishment so he was at first taken aback. Now, months later and languishing in jail, he had come to accept that his life was over. He had known his friends to die from drunkenness, in accidents, from painful disease or in war but his manner of death was too unbearable to contemplate. By the order of the court, it would not be possible for him to meet Osiris, the king of the dead and the forty-two assessor-gods. Anxiety surges through his body every time he contemplates it.

***

Herophilus clutched the mast and inhaled, attempting to calm his excited jitters. He could smell his fate in the sea air and see it on the flat blue line of the horizon. He had finished medical school on the island of Cos and spent the ensuing years mastering his craft. But he had been restless. He and his friends had spent hours on sandy beaches, drinking wine and pleasantly rambling about the world. They argued about where intelligence lay. Was it the heart or the brain? And where was the soul? They romanticised all the wondrous things they had heard about Alexandria, the city founded by Alexander the Great and transformed since his death, and since his general and close friend Ptolemy I Soter had taken charge.

Now, here was Herophilus, on the deck of a ship after two choppy days at sea, nearing this city whose opportunities had been ringing in the ears of young men across the Mediterranean, including his, for decades.

It was said it had become a place to turn any man's head and heart. And what an opportunity Herophilus had—he was to be the personal doctor to the pharaoh himself in the city where the body of Alexander the Great was now resting in a gold coffin.

But his curiosity was also piqued about Egypt's somewhat strange medical practices. They were sophisticated and steeped in history but prone to incantation, amulets and magic. *Welcome remedy, welcome, which destroyeth the trouble in this my heart and in these my limbs. The magic of Horus is victorious in the remedy.* Alexandria was the place where Helen of Troy laced a wine with a herb that banished all care, sorrow and ill humour. Here was the place that had been fixing head and spinal injuries for nearly 2000 years before him.

Herophilus, with his Old Dutch beard* and hair long, as was the fashion of the day, eyed the spectacular Pharos filling the sky. The forty-storey lighthouse was topped with a huge statue—maybe it was Zeus, maybe it was Ptolemy, he couldn't quite tell. He'd heard that at night, its fires reflected against large metal mirrors which pulsed light out to sea.

As his boat pulled into harbour, he felt discombobulated at the vision before him: he'd never seen so many ships, so many people buzzing around huge warehouses filled with grain, so many traders yelling and screaming about plants, elephant tusks and ebony in the cargo.

Alexandria was still under construction but a new library had been built, filled with scholars attempting to collect every book in the world. Crews on one boat scurried around as a captain handed over scrolls and books to a group of serious-minded men carrying ledgers. A fellow passenger on the trip from Cos had told Herophilus that whenever any boat pulled into port, the librarians would search the boats and take all the reading material. They would keep the original in their library and

---

* I imagine it would be like this on the beard chart.

hand back a copy to its owner—the building now housed anywhere up to 700,000 scrolls.

Herophilus threw his bag over his shoulder as he stood at the dock, unsure of what to do next. Leaving Cos, and his mentor Praxagoras, had been an impulse, which he felt wary about. But how could he resist such an invitation from the king himself? He took a deep breath and pulled out the map of Alexandria he had been studying for months, his finger following a grid pattern and stopping at the large Royal Palace complex.

As he wandered the wide streets, he felt his stomach rumble and decided to stop at a busy market, where after handing over two copper drachma, he snacked on roasted goose, sacred corn bread and a cup of beer.

He watched people to-ing and fro-ing in the busy streets, an old lady fastidiously cleaning the steps of a new temple and men in army boots and cloaks loitering. He knew these people would soon be his patients: Egyptians, Greeks, Jews, Arabs, Nubians—cultures from all over the region.

He hoped the gods would bring him a good fate working for the king. Herophilus had spent most of his life on the island of Cos, his days either at the famed medical school founded by the great physician Hippocrates or in the vicinity of the sanctuary to Asclepius, the god of medicine. Sick people had long flocked to Cos for treatment but in recent years, the school had waned due to the medical debates that were ricocheting among philosophers and doctors throughout Greece. The biggest one was about understanding the seat of human intelligence. Praxagoras believed it was the heart but Herophilus thought it was the brain.

As he drank his beer, he recalled a night when he was drinking on the beach with his friends, and a visitor came, claiming to know Egyptian secrets. He told them the doctors there kept hidden many things they knew about parts of the body, including the pulse. He also went into great detail about the manner in which they treated their dead, and Herophilus was privately desperate to witness these strange practices for himself.

There was no way Herophilus would've been allowed to cut open a dead body back at home. He'd grown up surrounded by endless purification rituals for the dead, who were seen as polluted and polluting to those around them. He'd watched his mother and sisters laying olive branches and leaves around his dead father, sprinkling sea water and lighting a new fire in the home. For days, weeks and months after, whenever they visited their father's grave, they became polluted again, and had to stay away from shrines.

But in Egypt, the response to the dead was the opposite: it was a hands-on preparation for the afterlife. If you had money, you could pay for an intense process of mummification which took seventy days. Priests would gently use special iron hooks to take brain tissue out through the nostrils, careful not to damage the face. The dead body would be cut open, the organs taken out and the empty cavity rinsed with palm wine then filled with myrrh, cinnamon and frankincense. Next, the liver, lungs, spleen, kidneys, stomach, intestines and pelvic viscera were placed in different canopic jars, and then the body wrapped up, and further dried out with natron, a type of salt.

Herophilus finished his beer and set off for the Royal Palace, passing public baths and a theatre. He spotted a crowd of people and stopped to see that they were looking at young men wrestling. But soon, he found himself distracted by a group of pretty, well-dressed young women also watching the fight. So it was true what they were saying about Alexandrian women—there were more of them than the stars in the sky, and their beauty could compete with that of the goddesses.

As he walked the streets, how unaware of his fate he was, that he was about to become a central actor in what is considered a stunning moment in the history of science. He would found a Greek medical school. He would pursue his passion for the pulse, a fashionable issue across the Hellenistic world. His younger colleague Erasistratus, who trained at Cos, would work with him, seeing the heart as a pump and coming very close to working out how blood circulates. King Ptolemy I—both cultured and a military strategist—and his entourage at court would grant the men permission to dissect in a climate in which learned men were breaking literary, political and scientific frontiers. Herophilus would systematically cut into the bodies of dead men, and would make discoveries that would be written of for thousands of years.

***

The man in his cell was increasingly sleepless. Few people were put to death in Alexandria—the Ptolemies and the pharaohs had long been reserved about the death penalty. He'd heard other prisoners discussing the grain seller killed for using false weights and measures, and the businessman who was executed for cutting dishonourable deals which undermined the Royal monopolies. Their fate? They died by *apotympanismos*, a horror the man had never seen but his friend had told him about. Chained to a post, the prisoner was beaten to death with a cudgel.

All the Egyptian doctors in his village had been good men who only cared for healing. He had read a report of a man in Memphis sentenced to death for violating codified therapeutic prescriptions, but he generally trusted doctors. However in recent years, stories had spread of two Greek doctors who had come to enact a new form of death, which the man could not fathom how he would endure.

For he knew that at any moment now, 'he was to be taken from his cell and laid open while still alive, and while still breathing, the doctors Herophilus and Erasistratus would observe his parts which beforehand nature had concealed, their position, colour, shape, size, arrangement, hardness, softness, smoothness, relation, processes and depressions of each, and whether any part is inserted or received into another. With various kinds of disease happening inside the body, it was difficult to apply remedies if one was ignorant about the parts. It had thus become necessary to lay open the bodies of the dead to scrutinise their viscera and intestines.'

***

The way the dissected are left out of history is strange. I spent so many hours looking at the exquisitely rendered people in anatomical art. I looked at the organs and the legs in the museums. Again and again, I kept circling back to this: who were all these unknown midwives of medicine? We know about anatomists like Herophilus and Andreas Vesalius but who actually are these people whose bodies helped make them great? The men, women and children in the books and the museums are as much Anatomy, Surgery and Pathology as the anatomists, surgeons and pathologists are.

These significant characters in medical history largely remain nameless. There is no 'we honour the dead' in any of the old textbooks. There are no stained-glass windows in hospitals memorialising them. In the sweeping histories of anatomy, they rarely pop up as part of the story. Some social historians have had a crack. Ruth Richardson, the doyenne of dissection history, tried to find out who the dead were in *Gray's Anatomy* but had little luck.

Even dead, they don't have fixed names. They've been called corpses, cadavers and criminals. In 18th-century Vienna, they were called free-of-charge corpses, study corpses and failed corpses. Perhaps in some instances the dissected were absolutely unknown but a fair few of them were taken from hospitals, prisons, poor-houses or asylums, which more than likely knew who they were.

Admittedly, things have been looking up for them in contemporary anatomy—in some anatomical schools they are known as the 'donor', 'silent teacher', 'great body teacher' or even by their first name.

So I start hunting the Dissected—all of them. I begin looking out for these silent teachers, whose hearts, lungs, thoraxes, nervous systems, arms, brains, sciatic nerves—each with their own variations—who birthed medicine. One way to counteract objectivity, said Andreas Winkelmann, who looked at what German anatomists did during the Nazi regime, is to go back in time and give people an identity.

At first, it seems like they are all 'criminals'. The first named dissected person I could find is a Chinese man named Wang Sun-Qing, a rebel who was captured by the imperial army of Emperor Wang Man in 16 AD. As recorded in the *Han Annals*, the biography of the Emperor:

> Measurements were then made of the internal organs and bamboo rods were inserted into the blood vessels in order to discover where they begin and where they end for the purpose of a better understanding of how to cure diseases.

For the next nearly 2000 years or so, it's all criminals, undesirables, the poor and 'low lifes' getting dissected so *ipso facto* it's a 'bad thing'. Somewhere between 960 and 1127 AD, the robber Ou Xi-Fan and fifty-six of his followers were dissected *en masse* by the coroner Wu Jian. In 17th-century Europe, the notorious thief Cotula was dissected and found to lack certain muscles in his hand. A woman called Sancta was sentenced to death for suffocating her newborn twins and was then dissected.

I began wondering about these criminals' charges. What did the criminals in the Alexandrian jail really do? What did Cotula steal? Was Sancta evil or did she have postnatal depression? Regimes have always banged the law and order drum to shore up their power—whether it be in their own interests or to get the community on side about a non-existent danger from a certain political or ethnic group.

There was a spell in 1700s Britain when people got hanged for petty theft. Some men were hanged for having sex with other men. When I lived in Alexandria, Egypt in 2003, spending my days writing and reading donated textbooks in the rebuilt Great Library, people were put to death for all sorts of crimes, including being a 'terrorist' or making and selling drugs.

But then I also start to see it's not all 'criminals'. Yes, the King of Anatomy, Andreas Vesalius, trudged around gallows in Leuven and

Paris, finding skeletons in graveyards and dissecting all sorts of people sentenced to hanging—in some instances tragically arranging with the judge to do it at a suitable time. But Vesalius also dissected people from all strata of society, some of them privately done at the request of the family looking for a cause of death.

He conducts an autopsy on a girl from the retinue of the Duchess of Egmont and while the family thinks she's been poisoned, it seems likely her corset was far too tight—her abdominal organs and thorax were severely constricted. He dissects an old lady who died from starvation, a stonemason who fell to his death and men killed by cannonballs in warfare. We also have quite a few names: the Prince of Orange, a patrician from Florence named Prosperus Martellus, Lord of Halluin, Lord of Immerseel, Ferrante Gonzaga and King Henry II of France. Vesalius later skeletonises a French priest and an eighteen-year-old man, and constructs the skeletons of a six-year-old girl, a thirty-six-year-old nun and a deformed seventeen-year-old girl.

Andreas' student Realdo Colombo, who went on to become a professor of anatomy at Padua, was also busy dissecting all sorts of people, including one unusual Venetian, who didn't appear to be a criminal—'Lazaro the glass-eater', who Realdo wrote about in his 1559 book *On Things Anatomical.* It is worth quoting this wild and rare dissection story in full:

> ... what caused me the greatest astonishment was inspections of Lazaro, commonly called the glass-eater, whom all the patricians of Venice, indeed all Venetians and all those of Ferrara, knew by sight. While alive, Lazaro has had no sense of taste, no pleasure or displeasure in eating; he did not distinguish insipid, bitter, sweet, fatty, salty, acrid; he ate glass, stones, rocks, wood, live animals, coals, fish drawn still wriggling from the fishpond.
>
> He ate mud, linen and wooden clothes, hay, straw, and in short whatever men or living things ate, whatever was offered him and he was told to eat he would devour for a price. Among others, Martini

> the spice dealer at the Sign of the Angel in Padua is a witness that he ate a little bag of charcoal which was offered to him, and the bag as well. When Martini saw this he paid Lazaro what he had promised and warned him not to come by his spice shop any more since he feared lest the man eat the shop and its contents.
>
> Therefore, when this monster of nature had to be dissected by me, I began, insofar as it was possible, to seek carefully the cause of such a thing, and I believe that with God's guidance I discovered it in the special structure of that person. For the fourth pair of nerves, which in other men had been extended by nature for the sake of taste, in this Lazaro the glass-eater crept neither to the palate nor to the tongue but were reflected to the occiput*.

Many dissections were done privately, and involved women, like Bartolomea Rinieri, who died at forty-two in 1486. As her husband wrote: 'She died of a diseased womb; this caused a flux which had lasted about eighteen months and which no doctors could cure. She asked me to have her autopsied so that our daughter or others could be treated. This done, and it was found that her womb was so calcified that it could not be cut with a razor.'

The bustling dissection history scene has had a tendency to focus on men dissecting at universities for male students, and the criminal element. While this happened, medical historian Katherine Park suggests that early anatomy in medieval and early modern Europe grew out of more private and domestic practices at the time, such as embalming, autopsies and obstetrics, and that women were at the heart of it. Cutting often had nothing to do with medical school either. All sorts of people were embalmed and autopsied, Christian figures were chopped into parts which were used as relics and women who died in childbirth had their live baby taken out so it could be baptised. (I am not clear if the babies went on to survive.)

---

* The occiput is the back part of the head or skull.

Yes, they were often thieves or murderers or both, like the tea smugglers Thomas Henman and Benjamin Harley hanged in 1776 at Tyburn for killing a customs officer. But they were also young women, struggling to get by in London. Sarah Ashton, twenty-four, was a servant who suicided by swallowing poison after her cad boyfriend Richard Sutton abandoned her when she was four months pregnant. 'Charlotte Burton', a twenty-two-year-old sex worker in the East End died giving birth in secret without medical help. They both ended up at the Dead House at St Bartholomew's. Burton was sold to the medical school by her fellow lodgers.

But poor, criminal, stonemason or lord—they were still *people*, central to the story of anatomy.

***

Chiara had long been known for her feverish virtue. She read the minds of her fellow nuns and was prone to intense visions. She ate rotten apples, wore a hair shirt and slept on the floor. Considered wise, people would come to speak to her through the grille in the door of her nunnery in the walled city of Montefalco in Umbria. She had lived there since she was six and became abbess at twenty-three, although she never wanted the job.

In the lead-up to her death in 1308, she kept telling her sisters she was not afraid of what was coming. 'Why?' they asked. She told them she carried the crucified Jesus in her heart. When anybody tried to put a cross in front of her, she would say: 'Sister, you need not place the cross there for me, for I have the cross of Christ in my heart.'

Another nun from a different convent came to pray and had a sublime vision of three little blond boys, one of whom she believed was Christ. He told her they were on their way to Chiara and that 'in her body will be found three things like precious stones'.

Chiara died seated. She was just forty years old. As the superfluity—the collective noun for a group of nuns—held a vigil, they discussed what to do with her body, which they saw as having been a living temple to the Holy Ghost. Perhaps she should be preserved? As she was a virgin, and had never been touched by a man while she lived, they decided one of her fellow nuns should open her body.

But who would do it? Sister Francesca agreed she would, and that sisters Helen and Illuminata would help embalm her with the herbs given to them by Tommaso di Bartolomeo, the town apothecary.

A decade later, an inquiry to have Chiara canonised heard what happened next. Sister Frances, one of 400 people to speak recalled that she and the nuns cut open Chiara from the back, 'took out her viscera and put the heart away in a box, and they buried the viscera in the oratory that evening'. Her hagiographer Berengario says that later, when the nuns were using a razor to cut into her heart, which was 'as big as the head of a little baby', they came across 'the cross, three nails, the spear, and the reed, and on the other side, the pillar, the scourge of five cords, and the crown'. Dramatically, the cross in her heart had the contours of a crucified body.

Three biggish stones were later found in her gallbladder, 'each as large as a medium-sized nut or a woman's thumb ... Form, number, Likeness, and colour all suggest the Trinity of divine persons.' What is curious here is that he says 'physicians and experts in the natural sciences' also had a look and thought they were formed by divine power.

I rented a small cottage on the grounds of a large school in Alexandria in Egypt from nuns, and these women were autonomous too—as well as charming, money-hungry, cordial, tough and benevolent. I can totally see them having the nous to dissect a body.

Days after Chiara's death, villagers—many of them cynical about the items found in her body—lined up to have a look. Berengario reports this was when the long list of miracles began: a man long limping from severe leg pain was cured, a bricklayer chuckling at his wife for visiting Chiara hit by a brick, a priest relieved of a toothache and children regaining their hearing and no longer fitting from epilepsy.

You can visit the Santuario di Santa Chiara della Croce in Montefalco today—Tripadvisor has given the monastery 4.5 out of 5 as a tourist site.

I watched an interview with a bespectacled old nun standing behind a cross in which bits of Chiara's heart are supposed to be stored. The nun points to the fleshy-looking bit of cross found in her heart, the three balls which are meant to be the signs of the holy trinity, and some heart nerve. Chiara's preserved body is also on display.

***

So you have this holy anatomy, you have women dissected privately to find out their cause of death, you have 'normal' dead people being studied. But I think part of anatomy's image problem is that it supposedly starts off with criminals being dragged from jail and vivisected, the sounds of Bach's Toccata and Fugue in D Minor on organ ringing through history. But there is actually another possible starting date for dissection.

The ancient Indian surgeon Susruta, who is believed to have lived anywhere between 1000 and 600 BC, wrote *Susruta Samhita*, a manual with all sorts of advice on surgery and what tools to use. He was the first person to do rhinoplasty in India but crucially, also endorsed human dissection. Even though in Hinduism the body is sacred in death and not to be touched, Susruta got around these laws in crafty ways. As people over two had to be cremated, he took to dissecting children under that age, which was technically legal.

He also came up with a method of dissecting grown-ups that did not require touching them directly. A dead body would be wrapped in grasses and barks and placed in a cage in a slow-flowing river out of sunlight for seven nights. The person had to be someone 'who had not died due to poisoning, but not suffered from a chronic disease (before death), had not attained 100 years of age and from which the fecal contents of the intestines have been removed.' They were then rubbed with a small broom, which took off skin and flesh without needing to touch the body.

I don't know why many of the accounts of early anatomy don't mention toddlers or a dead person lying in a wooden cage in a bucolic stream, and then patted with brooms of fragrant plant roots, hair and bamboo. Perhaps someone being hauled from jail and vivisected alive is more exciting?

But the more I look into it, I really don't think the man in the king's jail suffered this horror. I find it more likely that Herophilus and Erasistratus were just dissecting and in the ensuing centuries, the Roman writer Celsus warped the true narrative and started the vivisection rumour. He's the one who wrote that fateful paragraph all those centuries later, the one that suggests that the man, the criminal, the first dissected, was pulled from the king's jail and cut open while still breathing.

The philosopher and historian of ancient science G.E.R. Lloyd thinks Alexandria had the culture for vivisection. Even though the ancients respected the dead, they were open to desecrating corpses, torturing slaves in court to get evidence and trying out poisons on convicts. So it's a possible from him. But the British neurosurgeon and historian Jeremy Ganz is doubtful, largely based on his experience in the operating theatre. He sees it as 'not so much improbable as downright foolish'.

'Any surgeon will know that during an operation under general anesthesia, if the anaesthetic becomes lighter or the muscle relaxants used to keep the patient still during survey begin to wear off, even a little, the patient may start to breathe against the ventilator. This increases central venous pressure and the consequence is that the operating field disappears under a sea of blood. It is believable that if a criminal's body were open to be incised and opened against his will, the criminal would protest.'

Ganz also doubts that someone would lie still and relax while being cut open (as do I). They are more likely to scream, shout and struggle, which would mean 'central venous pressure and haemorrhage into the area being demonstrated'. I see my man in the king's jail doing this.

Contemporary anatomists have told me they can get lost in dissecting. They will begin dissecting a body part and will eventually look up, check their watch, and suddenly realise that hours have passed. This sort of experience has been dubbed 'flow', a term the Hungarian psychologist

Mihaly Csikszentmihalyi came up with in 1975 to describe people in a highly focused mental state. He named it after interviewing people who said the feeling of absorption in a task was like flowing along in a water current.

As Andreas Winkelmann told me: 'I don't think anatomy is horrible. I wouldn't do it if it was horrible. I think it's fascinating. If you step back and look at it, of course, it can be nauseating to have a body on the table, with all the fat and everything but when you start following a small artery or nerve and see how intricate it is, and how nicely everything is in place, it is fascinating, and you can actually forget about the rest and focus on the beauty of the human body.' He sees that for the early dissectors it was 'heroic'.

I see Herophilus too got lost in dissecting, and later, colleagues and patrons would listen eagerly as he relayed his findings. He would tell them of a man who had a cavity in the cerebellum which reminded him of the nib used in a pen back in Cos, and so he called it 'calamus scriptorius'. Another man had a depression in a section of his skull which was just like the trough of a wine-press. All this life in death.

Chapter 28

One dissected person I feel has been missing a little from all this has been Julie, my grandfather. I remember him so vaguely. I have nothing firm: it's shimmery, like a hot day at the beach, and you can see the world hazy in the distance. I remember the feeling of him more: that he was kind, that he wasn't in any way a scary grandfather.

His back story gives no indication of why he would donate himself to science. He certainly grew up in a tough environment. Born in St George in Queensland in 1903, he came from a family tree filled with convicts, all transported from England and Ireland for stealing, robbery, break and enter, and manslaughter. It was far from illustrious. Even when my relatives got here, were freed and settled, some went back to crime and were put in jail. Julie was only seventeen months old when his father, a saddler, died. His mother Bridgit was left to raise eleven children.

He is mysterious, and I can't quite piece him together. I have his lovely old lowboy wardrobe with some of the original wooden coat hangers, and it's a reminder of how few things people had back then. I know he was into looking stylish, as Mum says he was always well turned out. She also says he wasn't around much, and did his own thing. My Aunt Lindy recalls he might have had some sort of head injury, and that he was often grumpy, remarking that he had some sort of scar on his head. My dad doesn't say much, just that he was into sport, and they went on camping holidays as kids. Julie seems to have always been very physical: tennis, football, cricket, dancing, table tennis, rugby league. This energy pops up in the Brisbane newspapers, like a story in the *Truth* from 1931:

> **KEEN ON TENNIS**
>
> The only man on the electoral roll with such a Christian name is Julie Kelly Dent, well known in Toowoomba and other places as a keen tennis player. One on occasion he broke his toe just before starting an important singles match in Brisbane but played through in spite of the pain and won well.

A few years later, in the *Telegraph* in 1934, he's mentioned in 'DANCE NEWS AND GOSSIP' for—weirdly—not dancing: 'Mr Julie Dent, an old stalwart of the Trocadero, has been missing from the floor in recent months owing to illness. We wish him a speedy recovery and hope to see him back again in the Trocadero shortly indulging his favourite pastime.' An article a few months later in the column welcomes him back after his illness. 'Mr Dent has a wide circle of friends in Brisbane's dance world who are wishing him many more nights on the dance floor.'

He married Ruby in 1936—their nuptials delayed by a law at the time that if a woman married, she lost her job as a teacher.

But I can't really say what his motivations were except that he did what tends to happens with body donation—it runs in the family. He died suddenly of a heart attack when he was seventy-eight, and while he wasn't religious in his life, mum and dad found a request in his will for a Catholic service. In terms of his afterlife, he was obviously content to spend part of it in the dissecting room.

Chapter 29

I'm sitting in the office of the engaging and busy-minded Professor John Pearn. He's a senior paediatrician at the Queensland Children's hospital/Emeritus Professor at the University of Queensland School of Medicine/historian/author of thirty books and 200 academic papers/ former Surgeon General of the Australian Defence Force/knower of obscure and important historical facts.

He is wearing a colourful tie with cartoon-like drawings on it, which he describes as his 'kids tie'. I wouldn't know where to put John if I had to categorise him. His interests are everywhere. He could've popped up in every chapter of this book and been able to elegantly riff on each topic. His desk reflects these interests—there are folders and books and papers piled up everywhere.

Cases in point:

When I mention how the forensic facility in a location I can't name moved me, and how beautiful the skeletons were, how I would be okay with that fate—left to the elements, green mould growing on my skull, my bones the colour of the bush—he points out that there was once a belief that the moss of a dead man's skull had potential curative powers for some infections.

Months later, when researching the death of poor little Maurice from appendicitis in 1928 in a private hospital, I email him to ask for advice on how to find information about medical care at the time. He calls me back and generously goes through the system back then, what would have happened to Maurice, including details on nursing care.

John studied at the University of Queensland from 1958 to 1964 and dissected in the old US army huts in his second year. 'It was a feared subject because it was a huge curriculum,' he says, adding that conscientious students felt they needed to know the whole of *Gray's Anatomy*.

The style of medical degree that John and all the other doctors I spoke to has long gone. Anatomy has always been central to doctors becoming doctors and he points out the University of Queensland's student medical society has a skull as it's logo. But these days, it is not studied in the way it once was, to much debate. In 1997, most Australian medical schools followed a shift in education that was happening all around the world, a completely different model of graduate-entry four-year programs with a focus on self-directed learning. John goes into great detail about how the degrees changed, and more broadly how technology shifted medical education.

'Is the old way better?' I ask.

'That's a crucial, fundamental question,' he says. 'We have no way of measuring what is a good doctor, there's absolutely no measure, no way it can be codified.' He uses the hypothetical but unexpected example of an imposter who set himself up as a doctor and goes to court. During sentencing, a number of former patients come forward to say he was the best doctor they'd ever had.

'Some doctors are very careful, very skilled, and very accurate, very caring but they're not necessarily popular with patients. As most clinical medicine is a very confidential, one-on-one interaction, there's no other way of quantifying it,' he says. 'Most of medical education is a series of good ideas, but not underpinned by any fundamental science. And, frankly, there've been enormous changes from time to time in medical education, but they are experiments.'

John says there are 10,000 applications for 800 places in medicine each year, and the people who get through are elite. 'Elite students tend to do well whatever they do,' he says.

***

To dissect or not to dissect—this is the question. The issue of how much was enough, who should do it, kept popping up. Was what Ruby and Julie went through a waste of time?

In fact, it was Marius Fahrer, the hand surgeon, who began lobbing bombs about dissection and the need to restore anatomy to the curriculum. One such bomb was in 2001 when he wrote a short editorial in the *Australian and New Zealand Journal of Surgery* with the provocative title: 'Art Macabre: Is anatomy necessary?' In it, he remarked that gross anatomy and dissection had been 'deleted' from modern medical schools:

> Is dissection of human cadavers still necessary for educating surgeons today, when cost-effective clean, odourless and timesaving 3-D electronic simulators are available? As one of the few surviving specimens of the now extinct species of anatomist-surgeons, I continue to stick to the obsolete concept that surgeons operating on a patient must literally have the anatomy of the relevant area at their finger tips: the only way of acquiring the necessary tactile as well as visual 3-D knowledge is through dissection.

His short missive sparked a flurry of replies, agreeing, disagreeing, agreeing, sort of disagreeing.

I only found out about Fahrer's dissection activism after speaking to his friend Pierre Chapuis, who serendipitously finished his medical degree at the University of Queensland in 1969 just before Ruby arrived.

Now Professor Emeritus of Surgery at the University of Sydney and largely retired, he spent much of his career treating and researching colorectal cancer. And instead of talking about his youthful days at the University of Queensland, he's keen to discuss what he describes as the 'existential crisis' facing anatomy, and one that he believes has been brewing for some time. Some anatomists may disagree with what he says but he certainly has a take.

According to Pierre, the crux of the problem is that since medical degrees switched from a traditional six-year course to a four-year one, fairly detailed knowledge and study of anatomy has collapsed. Students now have to do another degree before they get into medicine and during their Graduate Medical Program, the amount of anatomy they're exposed to is almost negligible.

For those wanting to get into surgery, they need to pass the Royal Australasian College of Surgeons exams. 'You've got these young doctors coming through with very little foundation having to pass a pretty stiff exam in anatomical knowledge set by the college, and unfortunately, it's proving more and more difficult for them to reach that level of knowledge that is required.'

I'd heard so many mixed views on the value of dissection from the old doctors. Too much. Too little. About right. Waste of time. Would rather learn from a book. Too much. Too little. Pierre agrees there was probably more than was needed in the old days. 'But to go from too much to none at all, or very little, is the other extreme, and that's not really solving the problem. It's just compounding the problem—and it's not just gross anatomy, it's also the knowledge of embryology, histology, and so on.' Pierre says it's a worldwide trend.

He says another issue is that most anatomists these days do not have a medical background—they come from the sciences. In the past, it was a tradition for young doctors to leave the hospital, go back to an anatomy department and teach one or two years full time, and prepare for their college exams. This is what Pierre did himself. I know of one contemporary young surgeon teaching anatomy but he was too busy to speak with me. Pierre recalls in the 1970s and 1980s at the University of Queensland—when Ruby and Julie were there—at least a dozen surgeons and trainee surgeons were lecturing in the dissecting rooms. He says across the world it's not the case any more. 'I can remember ten, fifteen years ago when I went to the Department of Anatomy at the University of Paris and most of the senior anatomists were practicing surgeons. If you go there now, you may find one or two perhaps.' I get it.

Why would a surgeon bother teaching anatomy when they could be making the money they can earn from surgery—one of the highest paid professions in Australia?

Pierre says some trainee surgeons return to universities and teach anatomy but many cannot afford to. There are various courses, 'some of them are pretty good and a lot of them are hopeless'. They are expensive and trainee doctors in hospitals don't have the time, and often resort to weekend courses. 'It would take me hours to explain to you all of this,' he sighs.

'Basically, today, it's teach yourself medicine,' he says in summation.

Pierre is part of a group putting together a White Paper to have a national approach to anatomy at all the universities. (I was surprised when he mentioned that he was working with Quentin Fogg on it. All these random connections.) 'That'll take some time and a lot of debate, and it won't happen overnight but we feel concerned enough that you know, that we reached a sort of a crisis point,' he says.

I felt as if Ruby and Julie, and all the other donors, and people who had been dissected, had been kicked to the kerb when I'd first heard that dissection was waning. Had it been for nothing? All this time—this seems so bizarre to write—I'd somehow been in dissection's corner. I suppose I'd wanted their donation to science to matter.

Of course, I had my quarrels with the fact that it was only the scientists and the surgeons who were given access to a deep knowledge of anatomy through dissection, and that they were the sole storytellers of our bodies. But I could see too that yes, while we could replace the study of bodies with sophisticated computer software, what would happen 200 years down the track when the lithium ran out, and anatomy software glitched?

From what Pierre was saying, what had happened to Ruby and Julie and the donors mattered.

I found Pierre's clarion call auspicious, particularly as in the coming weeks, I'd finally been invited to a dissection workshop with surgeons.

Chapter 30

Q. Can the young practitioner be expected to possess the necessary courage in performing a difficult operation on the living if he has not already been taught to perform a similar operation upon a dead body?

Sir Cooper: He must be a blockhead if he made the attempt; and the practice of the most sensible and most expert surgeons in London has been to visit the receptacles for the dead, for the purposes of performing the operations which they were about to execute upon the living, if the operations were in the least novel.

Q. Can a student know where to cut with freedom, when with caution, and when not at all, if he has not an intimate knowledge of every part of the human body?

Sir Cooper: I would not remain in a room with a man who attempted to perform an operation in surgery, who was unacquainted with anatomy, unless he would be directed by others; he must mangle the living, if he has not operated on the dead.

– The British surgeon Sir Astley Cooper's appearance before the Select Committee on Anatomy in 1827 in London which looked into how bodies were being acquired for scientific purposes.

***

In the weeks leading up to attending the St Vincent's hospital head and neck dissection course, I became paranoid that I was going to faint. I kept thinking about Quentin Fogg's LARP technique before I went into the University of Melbourne anatomy lab, how he'd explained what I was going to see. The clinical anatomist Sven Kunkel had invited me to the course, so my plan was to do makeshift LARP on myself and make sure he told me what was in the room.

Sven had said on the phone I would fine if I'd been out to the AFTER facility. But still. I kept thinking *don't faint, don't faint, don't faint* as I arrived on the grounds of the historic Sydney Hospital and Sydney Eye Hospital on a stunningly pretty Saturday morning and walked around trying to figure out where to go. The workshop was being held at the Sight for Life Foundation Training Lab, an anatomy facility on the top floor of the historic hospital—if you stand next to the famous bronze boar *Il Porcellino* out on Macquarie Street and look up, you can see the space. The foundation regularly hosts weekend courses for surgeons and those in training who need to practise their skills on body donors. During the week, the not-for-profit runs pro bono classes training for ophthalmology and hand specialists, registrars, and doctors and nurses at the hospital.

I'm met by Sven, who looks more like a sportsman than a scientist. He's wearing a bright blue sports t-shirt, a lanyard which has *2015 Boston Marathon* written on it, jeans, sneakers and has a raver-style haircut—shaved short on the sides, long on top. Instead of taking me straight to the lab, he first wants to effusively and admiringly point out a few features of Australia's oldest hospital, including a series of stained-glass windows, which feature the anatomists William Harvey and William Hunter, and the staircases, which were built wide so people could be carried between floors in their beds.

We walk through a glass hallway and a short distance away is a large, old room, where I can see people in pale blue surgical gowns and white caps standing around tables. I think I can see a donor's head but I'm not sure. But before we go in, Sven takes me into his small office to meet his daughter Jonna-Susan Mathiessen, twenty-six, who is sitting behind a computer, surrounded by paperwork and wearing a polo shirt which says 'Sight for Life Foundation Training and Research Foundation Lab'—she's the manager here and also the anatomical licence holder. Evidence of Sven's sportiness stretches to his office, where running bibs and medals from the 236 marathons he has run—Paris, Kyiv, Okinawa, Luxor, Melbourne, New York etc—completely plaster one wall.

I confess to Sven and Jonna that I'm nervous I'm going to faint and be sick, and ask him to tell me what I will see. Sven, who is German, doesn't pussyfoot around. He says I have picked one of the hardest workshops to come to. 'It's the face after all,' he says. 'You will see faces.' Thanks Sven!

He takes me into a spacious and high-ceilinged, tan-coloured room, which is known as the wet lab, and Sven remarks this used to be a ward for children. There are five tables in the room, and resting in the middle of each is a donor's head, lying on its side. Standing around the heads are two trainees and one senior consultant. Wearing face masks and black Vortex head torches, the trainees peer into the sides of the donor's head, their hands busy with scissors, scalpels and retractors as one dissects and the other acts as an assistant. The mood is one of total absorption, and they are speaking Anatomy and Surgery, which I do not understand at all.

I stand near one table and can see the donor is an old man, and he has a white absorbent material wrapped around the top of his head, a code written in red pen on the side. He looks real but then he doesn't—I keep switching between the two perceptions as my brain settles into what it's seeing. I look around and see all the other donors are old people, their heads swathed in white turbans.

Sven is keen to introduce me to ear, nose and throat (ENT) specialist Dr Julie Crawford, a co-convenor of the workshop and one of eight doctors volunteering their time over the weekend to help the trainees. 'The importance of today is that you are operating in a setting where it doesn't really matter if you cut something important,' she says. 'It gives you a better conceptual idea of where important structures of the head and neck are.' The course is only run once a year and the students here—they all look to be in their late twenties and early thirties—need to do it before they can be an ENT surgeon. There is also a radiologist who has come to learn more head and neck anatomy.

Julie explains that today the trainees are practising a parotidectomy, an operation where the parotid gland—a salivary gland which provides your baseline saliva plus the saliva you secrete when you eat—is removed because of tumours. In Australia, the most common cancer to get in the parotid gland is skin cancer. When doing this operation, the most important structure to preserve is the facial nerve.

'It's the nerve that provides movement to one half of the face,' explains Julie.

'Wooah,' I say. 'You don't want to . . .'

'You don't want to cut that,' she says. 'If ever you see someone with Bell's Palsy, that's what would happen if you cut the parotid gland.'

On the other side of the room are rows of red chairs arranged theatre-style and that morning, the trainees had watched a talk and presentation on how to do this procedure, and four others. They are now putting the lesson into action, setting off on a journey into the head to find the facial nerve, which has been known to momentarily paralyse surgeons themselves as they know the ramifications of cutting it. To get there, they identify structures—which are like little signposts—on the way, which helps them to find where the facial nerve comes out at the base of the skull.

I stand next to one table and watch as one trainee meticulously and slowly cuts and picks away at a gash in the side of a donor's head, just below the ear. Their scalpels gently slice through the donor's fascia, a thin whitish tissue that forms a soft stretchy web connecting, enclosing and supporting each part of the body to the other. They also cut through what I think is fat, which has slightly different shades of yellow depending on the donor. Julie says if it were a normal operation there would be a lot more blood.

It's very slow and I recall Frank, the amusing maxillofacial specialist in Queensland, lamenting how laborious dissecting was.

'You can see how time consuming it is,' I remark to Julie.

'You can take your time. That's part of the beauty of being able to dissect the cadaver,' she says.

Julie explains the donors today are all American and were incredibly expensive to transport into Australia—they usually have sixteen dissectors, but they had to limit it to ten due to cost. The trainees pay $2500 plus GST for the weekend.

I wander between the tables and can see the donors are four men and one woman, and some have their teeth missing; some have no eyes. They have been frozen and then defrosted, and for this reason they look quite fresh in their own dead way.

My thoughts zig-zag between studying the donors' faces, contemplating whether they travelled to Sydney when they were alive, and observing the meticulous cutting and picking, and listening to the senior surgeons speak Anatomy and Surgery. *Sacrifice the anterior. Jug. Follow that anterior border to the SCM. Release some of the superficial stuff. You'll have a better idea of the digastric. You'll set yourself up to find the nerve.*

I move between thinking *oh my, we are so meaty* to silently cheering the donor, *Good on you–you seriously are training surgeons! This is amazing!* At times, there are six blue-gloved hands clutching at a medley of tools that pull, stretch and hold the sides of the donor's faces into various positions.

The language around the tools and the supplies is a bit more understandable. The retractor aka the 'cat's paw' hooks under skin and pulls it back into position. A bigger version is known by some as the 'tiger's paw'. The donors are resting on large sheets of absorbent material, which are known as 'blueys' as they have a blue underside absolutely no connection to Queensland's beloved cartoon blue heeler. At one point a bluey slips away and I can see the head is resting on a small tyre, which makes ergonomic sense.

I head back into the office to talk to Jonna and Sven, curious about the pair but also mindful of how serious the session is for the trainees, and not wanting to bother them too much.

Sven's mind works quickly and he loves talking but I feel like I need to be quite strict to get him to answer my questions.

'How did you get into anatomy? You're German obviously,' I ask Sven.

'I can answer this question. I told you before I was into horse riding,' he said.

'Yes, but you said I wasn't allowed to record you. So now I'm officially getting this all down so I don't get it wrong. So you were a horse rider?' I ask.

Sven was twenty-one and a professional rider, competing in dressage and showjumping just outside of Hamburg. He was riding a horse which belonged to a woman whose father was Bernhard Tillmann, a Professor of Anatomy at the Christian-Albrecht University of Kiel or Kiel University. The marks to get into medicine were, as always, very high, and Sven says the professor had a theory that you didn't need to be a high achiever in school in order to become a good doctor and to study medicine. Encouraged, Sven enrolled in medicine with the provision that he'd never become a real doctor, 'so I'll never be unleashed on real patients'.

He did all his pre-clinical classes—embryology, histology, biology—and ended up in clinical anatomy and surgical training. 'You need people who can talk to the surgeons to understand what they're operating on,' he says. Sven says Professor Tillmann started the first surgical training centre in Europe around 1987 and they worked closely together. 'My first workshop was actually an ENT workshop like this,' he says excitedly.

Sven worked in universities in Hamburg and moved to Australia in the 1990s, where he was a dissector at various universities, and says he later pioneered using 'fresh-frozen' donors for surgical training in Australia. In 2007, Professor Frank Billson, the ophthalmologist who founded Sight for Life, a not-for-profit aimed at improving eye care, approached Sven to open a wet lab to run microscopic surgery workshops for ophthalmologists and hand doctors.

Jonna has been around labs all her life, and shows me a photo of her as a little girl smiling as she sits in a large transport box.

'Is that to ship body parts?' I ask, incredulous.

'No,' says Sven. 'This is a knee replacement navigator.' He points at a large black object in the photo.

Jonna has over the years replaced Sven as lab manager. 'It's such a high-stress job,' he says like he's stressed.

Jonna has a lot going on. Not only is she the anatomical licence holder, she juggles the logistics of putting on classes, has her own anatomical services business, works as a part-time lawyer, is doing a Masters of Health Law and will have moved on and be working as a judge's associate at the Federal Court by the time this book is published. Long-term, she says she would love to work for the World Health Organisation. Sven brings up her plan to go to Germany to do what he sees as a 'proper' medical degree and to open up a tissue bank, and Jonna looks on smiling. I can't quite tell if it's her plan or his plan but the pair see there is a need for private tissue banks.

The lab is springing back to life after Covid-19 largely closed it for nearly two years, and all sorts of local and international specialists, universities, medical device companies and the like are using the space. During the week eye specialists and other medicos at the hospital can take pro bono classes to treat eye problems like glaucoma, and by using a pig's eye they can simulate trabeculectomy surgery.

Doctors work using a virtual-reality technology which simulates cataract surgery, and will also dissect on 'orbits'—which is a quarter of a donor's skull—for ocular plastics training. The hand doctors work on chicken marylands—the drumstick and thigh with skin on—as they have a vein that is very similar to one in our hand. On weekends, Jonna and sometimes Sven run the surgical classes for all sorts of specialities.

'Every day is something new. You're always working with doctors who although they are sometimes difficult, they're highly intelligent. We're doing ENT [this weekend] but last weekend we were doing orbital compression and trauma,' says Jonna. 'There's always new technology. You are always at the forefront whilst with law it's almost the opposite.

You're always trying to catch up—what are the problems? Okay, now we will find the solutions, but this is the other way around.'

Workshops can take anywhere from three months to one year to plan. Aside from sourcing donor parts from the US and locally, she needs to make sure the surgeons from each discipline have their unique tools.

They are known as 'cadaver kits' and they are often flown all over the world to different workshops—and it can take time and patience getting the right one to Sydney on the right date. It is industry practice that once surgical tools have been used in an anatomy lab, they cannot go back to a hospital operating theatre.

Jonna also needs to make sure doctors stick to what they are meant to do as the donors are often used by other disciplines. 'The difficulty can sometimes be when you have, for example, a dental extraction workshop where they're very, very confined in what they do. They're meant to be extracting teeth. But then you might have a dentist who thinks this is a great experience, I can now start dissecting up around the face and look at the facial nerve. But we've already dedicated those specimens for a particular workshop.'

It seems like logistical hell and I can see why Jonna says she sometimes doesn't sleep before a workshop as so many things can go wrong—the audiovisual system might not work, the wrong instruments can arrive and the donors might have been operated on when they were alive, which can create a problem in the workshop. But she says she likes the challenge.

I'm naturally interested in the donors, particularly as they are American. Jonna says they came from Science Care, a company in the US, and I later look them up and find they are a large body broker owned by Northlane Capital Partners, a middle market private equity firm. The donors sign up themselves and in return, their bodies go to science and their families do not have to pay for their cremations.

The company organises death certificates and paperwork, and then in some instances dismembers the bodies or keeps them whole, and they are then shipped around the US and internationally for medical education and research. It's legal in the US to donate your body to a for-profit organisation, but this is a controversial development that some anatomists have major ethical concerns about.

Jonna says they need to bring donors in as there aren't enough local ones for their surgical workshops. The main reasons? Australia's small population and people don't know they can donate their bodies. She says sometimes she can access donors from universities but not always.

Sven chimes in: 'I told you. It's the demographic. You don't have Muslims or Māoris to donate their bodies . . .'

'Because they need to have a specific burial,' says Jonna.

Sven says Science Care has been around for a while, and he knows the former CEO. 'They are very well-looked-after people. They are not from the streets. You can tell by their bodies,' he says. Jonna remarks that some of them have gold teeth and she can see from their medical histories that some have had plastic surgery. She says even though Science Care can be more expensive than other brokers, she prefers to use them as they are reliable and the donors' tissues are well preserved.

I'd noticed that some of the donors didn't have teeth so I was thinking that perhaps this was a sign of poverty, and that their families had donated their bodies to save on cremation costs. Some see this as a broader issue for all body donation, whether it be to universities or American for-profit companies—that it is the poor who tend to donate. But before I raise this, Jonna remarks that these donors had already had teeth pulled by dentists in a dental extraction workshop, which helped balance out the enormous costs to bring them in. Ophthalmologists had also taken out some of their eyes.

'It reduces costs because it allows the cost to be shared between different specialities, different courses, different people,' she says. 'It increases the access to cadaver training and ultimately promotes education.' In 2022 they cost even more due to a variety of factors—rising courier fees, the Australian dollar and the added expense of getting donors Covid-tested.

All the donors were Anglo and I wonder about the brewing issue of diversity in all forms in the dissecting labs. Jonna says they do get African American and Hispanic donors and occasionally get comments about them being poor or not donated, which she sees as an unfortunate stereotype.

***

Most of the trainees have headed outside for lunch except for two tables, where a few remain hunched around their donor, focused on dissecting. Jonna remarks that sometimes the students get so absorbed they forget to take breaks. The two tables soon head outside and once they are gone, I watch Jonna walk around the room and gently place the blueys over the donor's heads. She says she always does it. 'I don't know why, I just do,' she says. 'It's a matter of respect.'

I need to leave to go to a fiftieth birthday party at the beach—forget death!—but before I go, Sven says I have to see something. I ask if it's specimens in jars in a museum. 'No!' he says. We walk through the rabbit warren of the grand old hospital, and he continues to speak effusively about it, clearly affectionate about this historic space. We head outside on to an outdoor walkway, and he points out the roof of the next-door building, explaining there used to be a skylight in it so the surgeons could see while they were operating. It's since been covered over. We then head downstairs, upstairs, and into the old Chapel of St Luke, a spacious area with stained-glass windows, wooden pews and plaques on the walls.

'Basically, they operated upstairs and here they prayed for these people being operated on,' says Sven pointing above him, admiring the ceiling, the space, the story. He then points out a plaque on the wall honouring Anita Cobby, a young nurse who was horrifically raped and murdered by five men in 1986 in a crime that is seared into Sydney's DNA. 'You might remember that story?' he asks. 'It gives you the goose bumps.' I hadn't known she had worked at the hospital.

***

It's a Sunday morning and I'm back in the top-floor lab. Jonna has taken her first day off in sixteen days and Sven is behind the computer, wearing a sports shirt advertising a marathon in Abu Dhabi and showing me one of his 'masterpieces'—it's a dissection of a man's spinal cord system which took him six months to do when he was at the University of Kiel.

It's on the university website and he seems chuffed that it's still on display at their anatomical museum. As he points out and explains various nerves near the base of the skull that I'm trying to keep track of, it reminds him of a case. An avid cricket fan—a game was playing on his computer screen with the sound down when I first arrived—he says he was devastated when the young cricketer Phillip Hughes died after being hit with a cricket ball in 2014, and asked his doctor friends what happened. Sven points to a general area on his old dissection and says while you can't see it, there is a vertebral artery which goes into the brain and creates blood supply. The cricket ball hit this artery at a weak point and it burst, and he likens it to the lights going out on a whole city.

'That's the whole purpose of dissection—I could probably talk for two weeks on this dissection,' he says pointing at the screen. 'Once you get interested in anatomy and functional anatomy and clinical anatomy, anatomy becomes very fascinating.' He also says it means he often doesn't go to doctors because he's scared of the diagnosis—he knows what's behind it. He tells another story about a professional surfer friend who got hit by a surfboard in the back of the neck in Indonesia, and was left paralysed. Luckily, he still had sensation in his ulnar nerve, which runs through the palm of your hand near your pinkie. A German hand surgeon transplanted this functioning nerve to his thumb, which means his friend can now drive a car by wiggling it.

Sven shows me a slice of knee in perspex, which is another one of his dissections. He is obviously proud of it—it's so fine it looks a bit like a shaving of parma ham. I ask him how he feels about plastination and when he calls it 'gummy bear', I get the sense he's not a huge fan of the process.

Back in the wet lab, the donors on the tables today are all old Australian men, and have come from different universities. They have been cut off just below the shoulder, and are resting on the blueys. Some of them have lines drawn in blue on their neck, where they will be cut into.

Like yesterday, the trainees are in their blue gowns and head torches, and are in a state of utter focus and absorption. I'm drawn to a table with two young women dissectors. Again, I'm loathe to bug them too much so I ask Dr Richard Gallagher, a head and neck surgeon at St Vincent's, and co-convenor of the course, what they are up to. He explains they are doing a neck dissection, which involves taking out lymph nodes. 'This is a very pure operation,' he says. 'You are taking out the lymph nodes and fat, but you are leaving behind the important cranial nerves. There is a bit called the accessory nerve which goes down to your shoulder, there's a nerve that goes to your tongue, there's a nerve that goes down to your larynx. There are all these important structures like your carotid artery.' It gets more complicated.

As one trainee holds the neck flesh back, the other goes in deeper and deeper, cutting out what looks like fat but is apparently a lymph node. I'm reminded of the anatomical illustrator Marie Dauenheimer and how she used to spend evenings in the library studying surgical procedures to get a sense of what was going to happen in an operation.

I can see why. It looks fleshy and red and I can't tell what they are doing but they are talking about the accessory nerve and heading to Level Five. As Richard puts it: 'Essentially surgery is all about landmarks—it's like a roadmap. And it's a matter of understanding how that map works, and what the variations on the map might be, and you can only get those things by experience and doing and looking and training on specimens.'

It's quite noticeable how aside from learning through haptics—the sense of touch—the trainees are also picking up other tips like different ways to hold a retractor or approaches to take into the neck. Richard occasionally offers a tip speaking Anatomy and Surgery. *I don't always routinely just go straight across. Once upon a time I did–put a silk on it to relieve it? But I suppose I'm a bit more ... I try to be a bit more discreet about the dissection, so identify the Supraclavicular...*

On the table next to the two women rests a number of tools, and I eye a 'cat paw' which has a handle with a circle in it. I ask what it is.

'That's called a Langenbeck retractor,' says Richard.

'Is it named after Mr Langenbeck?'

'Yes,' says Richard.

I mention there is an issue in anatomy with the body parts being named after men but I hadn't seen anything about a push to change the names of blokey surgical instruments. Richard points out the names of other instruments—the Senn retractor (Nicholas Senn), the Crile forceps (George Washington Crile) and others. I wonder if anyone is lobbying to give them new names—perhaps it will take a generation to change as, particularly in surgery, you don't want confusion when you ask for a particular tool.

I wander off and sit on one of the lecture chairs, and suddenly sense that the nuns of Montefalco are next to me, watching, murmuring, wondering if the trainees will find any signs of Jesus Christ in the dead. Vesalius sits down on my other side with a sigh and putting his soft leather shoes up on the chair in front of him, ponders if they will later dissect the larynxes of any of these men, who all seemed to be in such good condition, and how did they get five all at once? He's also in awe that the students are in there dissecting too. He nods agreeably.

My little team of psychopomps arrive next, dancing around the tree, laughing, smiling, almost gloating. *See! Look where we led you!* Yes, indeed. Look where you led me.

Sven and I are sitting on the balcony at lunch and he is wearing a bright yellow jacket advertising a marathon he did in Seville, Spain. I ask him how many sneakers he owns, and he pulls out his phone and shows me a photo of what looks like around twenty pairs neatly lined up in three rows. He says he has more pairs in other parts of the world.

I'm telling Sven how studies have shown that some students struggle with dissection as they believe in the soul, and how various religious beliefs play out in anatomy labs and with body donation on the whole. I ask him if he's ever had a weird sense of *something*.

He says: 'I grew up in mortuaries which had 200 cadavers, and I walked through them at two o'clock in the night when all the chillers were going, and the rattling—no.' He knows of someone else who freaked out, though. He recalls one of his friends at medical school once lay on the table in the dissecting hall and when a cleaner walked past, he grabbed her leg. Oh. The poor woman.

He then recalls another strange story. Sven has enormous respect for retrieval doctors, specialists 'who have a rucksack, fly into the outback, and open up the rib cage and do heart surgery or brain surgery on the spot with a Swiss Army knife'.

'They are hardcore guys,' he says. 'They are the Most Amazing in my book. They are cool as ice. These are the ones if you have a severe injury like you've cut your arm off, they are the first ones to help ...' He says if you get stabbed in the street, they can cut you open, cut the diaphragm and manually palpate your heart and hopefully keep you alive.

Sven hosted a workshop for the retrievers with two donors who had come from a university. When retrievers arrive somewhere, they usually use a machine to test if someone is alive. This day, when they put it on the bodies, it began to work.

'You should have seen all these people looking at each other,' he says. 'So they looked at me and I looked at them. We looked at all the machines—they told them the donors were alive.' It turned out much higher levels of carbon dioxide were detected in the very-dead donors when intubated than normally expected, and that subsequent research was needed. In that one moment, he saw these awe-inspiring people lose their cool.

***

As I take a final look at the trainees dissecting and the donors on the tables, I sense I'm somewhere between a parched walker chugging down a glass of water and a scholar who has stumbled across a theory that explains years of work: I'm satisfied and finally get it. There's nothing quite like being in it—for both the surgeon cutting into the body and me as a writer *trying* to understand it.

I walked through the grounds of the hospital on my way to Hyde Park, and think maybe when I'm older—which is when people usually do think about their deaths—I'd be fine to sign up to be studied by ENT trainees, dentists and ophthalmologists. Perhaps by then my irrational fear of the cold in the afterlife will be gone too. I now know that if I need an operation, the surgeons will be following a map armed with cat paws.

It's extraordinary how a few years after that first Christmas drink conversation, the psychopomps led me to the American donors, and ultimately my grandparents' fate. It's all so strange where I have been, the sleepless nights and the conversations with scientists. But it reminds me of the French medievalist and historian Philippe Ariès—the man who wrote an extraordinarily playful 1000-year history of death—who saw the interest in anatomy as being much more than a rational quest for knowledge, that it corresponded to 'an attraction to certain ill-defined things at the outer limit of life and death, sexuality and pain.'

***

A few days later, I call Jonna to say hello and check a few things. I also ask if she really wants to open a tissue bank or is it more her dad's dream? She says, yes, she sees a need for something like Science Care as it would cater to the body shortage she consistently experiences, and reduce costs. 'You could give more access to the smaller, regional and young universities who don't have the means that Sydney, Melbourne and Adelaide do.'

I email her 'Bodies R Us', a paper written by Thomas Champney, Sabine Hildebrandt, Gareth Jones and Andreas Winkelmann, on the emerging growth of for-profit willed body companies in the US. The group argued that there should be no commercialisation or commodification of willed bodies.

It's a topic that leaves me personally wading through an ethical swamp:

- the donors consented to be there
- your approach to privatisation depends on your world view and I personally am not into it
- the surgeons need to practise
- if it is mainly poorer people donating, how does body donation become egalitarian? Do we get celebrities to donate? Do we start a #Iamwholebodydonor hashtag on Twitter?

Jonna emails the PDF back with all sorts of comments a few hours later. She's now thinking of writing a paper about it.

Chapter 31

The anatomy hall was and is still a mystery to me. Yes, Quentin walked me through one. Yes, I have watched a lot of dissection videos and spoken to lots of people. I know a little about embalming and how parts are chopped up. But day to day—bar getting a job in an anatomy lab—I will never really know what happens. I found that when I raised the issue of anatomy being 'a bit secretive', some anatomists pushed back a little, as if I was a behaving a bit QAnony. I would waver around suspicion and began thinking *what are the anatomists hiding?* I would lurk near outrage, scowling at yet another unanswered email. I was definitely ashamed and a bit paranoid at times, sensing that part of this curiosity was driven by me wanting to see a dead body.

In 2021 people paid up to US$500 a ticket to watch a retired professor of anatomy dissect David Saunders, a ninety-eight-year-old man, at the Portland Marriott Downtown Waterfront hotel as part of an Oddities and Curiosities Expo. He had donated his body to a private company but his widow had no idea it would be used in such a way. Would I have gone to that? I rang my death friend Mike—a mellow Northern Beaches surfer dude—and we agree we would have been tempted.

I kept returning to this idea: did Ruby and Julie know what they were signing up to? Do contemporary donors know? And if not, why? If you look at some anatomy school websites, there is a certainly a vagueness to the language about what happens.

My instincts that anatomy was a bit closed to the public were confirmed when a Brisbane friend told me that a book written about body donation at the University of Queensland anatomy school had been pulped a few years earlier.

In 2015 the acclaimed Brisbane journalist Andrew McMillen spent a year at the anatomy school and wrote about his experiences in *Skeleton School: Dissecting the gift of body donation*. But on the eve of its publication in 2016, its launch was cancelled, and the University of Queensland Press issued a statement that said it was not able to publish the book and that it was through no fault of Andrew's.

It read: 'The University is now of the view that the publication of any book on the issue of the Body Donor Program, however sensitive, may upset some families and friends of participants in that program. There is no suggestion that this decision reflects in any way on the quality and standard of the book, which met the expectations of UQP.'

I could understand this fear of upsetting family members—it has stalked me too and I was cognisant of my dad and Uncle Maurie, particularly when some of the older doctors went into intricate detail about the dissecting process, which at times left me squirming.

But then I finally came across *The Silent Teacher: The gift of body donation*, an inside account of what happens in a contemporary anatomy lab written by Claire Smith, a professor of anatomy and the Head of Anatomy at the Brighton and Sussex Medical School in the UK.

I was stunned at Claire's openness detailing how when using the bandsaw, human heads are frozen first to get a clean line through the middle of the nose or how on occasion, it was like playing Jenga as technicians tried to get legs attached to the hip and pelvis into the freezer. But the book was also very straightforward—details like people who are too tall or too emaciated cannot be accepted for donation, or how mould can form on a donor through a small spore that was already there or through a student or staff member sneezing.

I liked how amusing and British it was too. Claire included pictures of herself and colleagues in gas masks, as they prepared to clean up a phenol spillage, as well as stories about her dreams. In one, an overseas donor comes to life on the table and Claire and her staff frantically call the police to try to work out what to do with a reanimated corpse, whose lover had also sneaked over in the shipping container.

So late one evening, over Zoom, I asked Claire why she had been so open and decided to write a sort of anatomy memoir.

'I think it just came about because I was fielding a lot of questions from the public and from the sector. We are not allowed to advertise so I was going to events—older age forums, or Death and Dying Week,' she explains. The Human Tissue Authority and various universities had information about donating on their websites but she sensed people wanted more. 'I wondered if we as a sector were too afraid to give too much detail because we'd put people off? So I thought I'd just do something,' she says. 'If people read the book and it puts them off body donation, that's not my intent, but that's also fine because I feel that informed consent should be as informed as that person wanted.'

Claire's total transparency about her dissecting room (or DR as she calls it) is unusual. 'I think some people have a slightly rose-tinted notion of donating,' she says. 'Some people think that "Yeah, we're going to help science and we're going to help learning," which they do but I think there's a reality side of it, which means that it's a bit brutal at times to be chopped up, and to be opened and dissected and have trauma surgery undertaken on them and things like that. I think that side of it—what we do to the body—is quite hidden, I think because we maybe are a bit worried that might put people off. But the more I have spoken to people, actually people just want to know.'

She says part of the reason anatomists aren't explicit is logistical. At the moment in the UK, there are three types of consent—for anatomical examination, for retention of body parts and for use in images. 'But if we said, "Oh, would you be happy if your arm is chopped off? Would you be happy if your organs were removed? Would you be happy if you had trauma surgery done to you? Would you be happy if we broke your leg and then fixed it again? Would you be happy about all these other things?"' she asks.

'To give a higher level of informed consent, we would never probably be able to match incoming body donors with actually what we were doing.' Donors are very carefully matched with whatever activity is going on in the department, whether it's undergraduate medical teaching or surgical teaching in a particular timeframe.

She and social psychologist Tom Farsides looked into the concerns people had around body donation and found striking differences in how they conceptualise their dead bodies. While the anatomists themselves may have ideas about a 'top-down' approach to body donation and what is important, donors saw themselves in different ways. For some, they were 'just meat' while others believed they were 'sacred gifts', to be used only by particular people in particular ways. Another study she did found that while donors felt comfortable with their bodies being used by medical, dental and allied health professions, they were less excited by the idea of artists, beauticians and yoga teachers having a go. (I quite like the idea of wearing Chanel lipstick and having my head sketched.)

Claire writes of the particular awe students hold for the brain. I recalled to her a conversation with Andreas Winkelmann, in which he said when dissecting the brain you still cannot understand anything about the person. Even though someone's name is somewhere inside, from the outside, you can't find it out.

'Does the brain have some sort of power over people?' I asked.

'It's amazing how when you look at it, when you take a fresh brain out—I'm taking some brains out next week—it's just this kind of gloopy substance. When it's fixed with formaldehyde, you can very clearly see the white and the gray matter of it, and you can slice it and you can see the different tracks and things but you're still quite amazed about how on earth does that make my body function? How does conscious thought happen from a series of cells and electrical connections? It is intriguing.'

I'm not sure what makes Claire so transparent but perhaps she is just generally open. She had an interest in the body, which was borne from illness when she was young—she suffered from epilepsy and struggled at school. 'I was on quite a lot of meds,' she says. She got into dancing, and started doing sports science. 'Because of my own health or because of what I was doing—I was just fascinated with the body.' She was later 'amazed' to discover that she could study anatomy at university, which she did. Once she'd finished, she wasn't sure what she was going to do. 'It never occurred to me to be an anatomist,' she pauses and laughs, 'despite doing an anatomy degree.'

She worked in operating theatres, thinking she wanted to do medicine, but the hospital environment really put her off. She started teaching anatomy to surgeons, and later to nursing students, but realised that she 'missed her dead bodies'. She started working at St George's Hospital as an anatomy demonstrator. It just carried on. 'Each anatomist has their own lovely story,' she says.

Her openness meant that I learned about all sorts of nooks and crannies of her DR. For example, I'd told her about how I'd become interested in the different mixes embalmers used and their secret recipes, and she soon cracked open a new world, discussing with affection the respect she held for her embalming colleagues. As she puts it: 'I think this is beautiful. I think this is the side that's about craft and an art. It's about embalmers that take pride in their work. They know the work the anatomists are doing, they know how the anatomists like that tissue to be fixed or not fixed or movable. Over time, they have their own recipes.'

There probably was secrecy, she said, but people do share information—more likely informally, over a pint at the pub.

'I quite like it when my technicians are free to do what they want, and they use their skills. So if a brain isn't quite fixed, and they know that brain is going to need to be sliced to show the different structures in the brain, then they might finish an embalm, and do a little local inject through the orbit without disturbing the eyeballs, just to put a little bit more fix in where it might not be fixed.

'Different bodies take differently to each and every embalm. You can use the same fluid, the same chemical formulas but because of the amount of fat or the time since death or the storage, each body will take differently. So the embalmers have to be very skilled to adjust what they're doing—that's probably why they've got their own kind of mixes and fixes because they're just adjusting.'

Claire is dissecting nearly forty years after my grandparents' bodies were at the University of Queensland but she is still embedded in an old tradition. Of course much has changed. Her lab is high-tech—temperature-controlled freezers, air-conditioning, CCTV, hand-washing sinks that operate via infrared sensors to stop contamination, and powerful bandsaws.

Her bodies are donated and if they need other parts, they can be shipped in from the US. (She recently sent back a body part that was from someone who had been executed.) We talk about how what she does is so extremely different to how her predecessors worked—quickly, by candlelight, in winter.

'It's never pleasant getting your head inside a body, whether they're fresh, whether they're embalmed. After about day three or four when they've been out … it's not pleasant at all,' she says but adds everybody learns ways of handling it.

'I learned in operating centres to breathe through your mouth when you're doing prostate shavings, or you're doing an operation where you've got burning skin or flesh smells. So, we learn to put Vicks on your nose or have mints in your mouth. So I suspect they had their own similar types of things—they used to smoke cigars when dissecting. I wouldn't have been allowed to—being female—and it was a very white male-led profession.'

But there is also something so elemental—the pleasure of dissecting itself—that she shares with the anatomists of old. I wonder if this is what it was like for Marius Fahrer when he studied the hands of the donors. Or Vesalius when he looked into the thorax.

'I guess when you're trying to find something, you've got your head in something, you actually just care about that structure, and you just care about dissecting it. Hours can disappear when you're dissecting and you're working or you're teaching or operating on something. I guess that's a very common part that we share with my predecessors —the focus and awe of the anatomy, and you can lose and forget everything else that's around you. You forget you're working on a dead person. You forget that it smells because you are just so focused.'

Claire likes teaching either head and neck or pelvis. 'Head and neck because it's really complex, and the bones—things like the sphenoid bone—are just really beautiful. There's lots of nerves, lots of kind of exceptions to rules. And pelvis? Yeah. Pelvis I just like as well. I don't really like feet or hands particularly—bit boring.'

I hung up from Claire feeling like some of the mysteries of the dissecting room had dissipated into the part of my brain marked LESS MYSTERIOUS AND TERRIFYING. Other anatomists might not have agreed with me that anatomy is secretive but I felt like Claire exonerated an instinct that I'd thought was off-kilter. This veil around what happened to bodies was there for any number of reasons: a form of power, protecting grieving families, fear of people not donating if they knew the ins and outs, paternalism. But Claire made me realise what happens when you open the door—all of us are welcomed into the world of medicine.

Chapter 32

When I met John Pearn, we bantered about history and I mentioned that I've been reading about Christmas dissecting celebrations in the Netherlands in the 1600s, where up to 600 people would wander the botanic gardens and watch dissections in a magnificent hall. He too had a historical story: 'I did a secular pilgrimage to Pergamon and walked in Galen's footsteps,' he says, in reference to the influential and prolific ancient Greek anatomist.

I told John I had wanted to do a pilgrimage to Iran to visit the grave of the Persian polymath Avicenna aka Ibn Sina but Covid-19 knocked out the plan.

'It's very interesting when you and I looked out at the river earlier, those mangrove trees that we see there are *Avicennia marina*,' John says, referring to the view from the hospital out on to the Brisbane River. 'He lived in Hamadan in 1000 AD, so a thousand years later his living memorials are crucially part of the ecosystems here in Brisbane.'

Avicenna?! Here? WHAT?! I'd fallen into a love of Avicenna's works after watching *The Physician*, a RARE movie for a) featuring an anatomist and b) featuring dissection. It's an epic, kitsch, medical history adventure movie about Rob Cole, a young Englishman in the 11th century who treks through the desert to reach Isfahan in Iran, where he is apprenticed to Avicenna, played by an austere but thoughtful Ben Kingsley. Rob studies under the great physician but is consistently frustrated that religious lore bans them from dissection until he meets a Zoroastrian who asks that his body be left out for the vultures to devour him.

'So you care nothing for your body?' asks an astonished Rob. Hidden in the depths of a stony basement, Rob turns into a dissector and when eventually caught, he and Avicenna are sentenced to death. 'These men trespassed against Allah,' a henchman to the Imam declares. 'Desecrated and defiled a corpse, making the sin of necromancy!' I won't tell you the ending but the message in this film is consistently blunt: faith and superstition get in the way of science and progress.

While this movie borders on fantasy, the arguments over 'did he or didn't he dissect' continue to pepper academic papers about Avicenna, but he did make original findings for his time, leading some to stand in the 'he did dissect' corner.

The real Avicenna's mind wandered everywhere—poet, philosopher, physician and pharmaceutical studies. I particularly love how in his *Canon of Medicine*, he wrote about someone with a broken heart, in what some believe is the first documented case of a stress-related condition:

> A cachectic patient was brought to me with a plethora of chronic and debilitating diseases and prolonged fever, all of which were related to the love disorder. By reaching his sweetheart, I was amazed at how quickly he became reenergized. So, it became clear to me that human health is obedient to and under the control of the mind.

But outside of anatomy, Avicenna, who apparently wrote some of his books on horseback, was also a philosopher who spent a lot of time thinking about the soul.

Ah.

The soul.

I have no perfect way of writing about it. I might as well write *Soul = ?* in red lipstick on the back of the door in the unisex toilet and come back a month later to see what people have said in follow-up. The answers could be:

- soul = separates from body at death goes to God
- soul = are you kidding?
- soul = misty
- soul = how an egg grows into a chicken

- soul = that which animates, cadaver by definition does not have one
- soul = DJ night coming up in April
- soul = body must be whole for soul to get resurrected and enjoy party in afterlife

The fact I don't want to donate because I think I would be cold—does that possibly mean I do believe in a soul? Others might think it bullshit but whatever your entry on the back of the toilet door, the soul has lurked around human dissection for millennia and still does. It was a mystery I kept bumping up against. If science is objective and about testing truths, why was it that the soul still lingered around the dissecting room, even in the so-called secular West. But also, it was absolutely extraordinary to me how ideas about the soul and the afterlife played out in the anatomy lab in such contradictory ways.

***

In 2011 the anatomy department at the University of Otago in New Zealand did a number of curious soul studies with medical students. Helen Martyn and other researchers surveyed second-year students and found that 50 per cent believed in the soul, and that this belief contributed to stress in the dissecting room. In another study, interviews with sixteen students found they also had very different reactions to dissecting certain parts of the donor's body, particularly the brain and the heart. Some students considered the brain as the 'seat of the soul' while others thought it the heart.

As one student said of dissecting the brain: 'It was just like I was taking away all of their memories and all of their life away from the rest of their body and it wasn't them any more. Yeah it just … taking away their whole soul, it was just really odd.' Another said of the heart: '… holding the heart was like holding the seat of the soul … there was some kind of aura involved in it.' Curiously, none of the doctors I talked to spoke of a glow around the kidney, the tongue or the stomach.

But it's not just the students 'feeling something'. In 2011 anatomists from twenty-nine different countries at an anatomical conference in Turkey filled out questionnaires about dissection and whole-body donation, and when asked about the afterlife, 39 per cent of them believed in it, while 19 per cent weren't sure. There was also a pattern with non-believers being more in favour of donating their bodies or parts.

So if the people in the room buzz with a sense of soul and the afterlife, it makes sense that this stops millions of people from donating themselves. In 2020 anatomist Brenda De Gama and a team of researchers—including Gareth Jones, who did the world's first ever study into body donors—wanted to find out why the Zulus, one of the nine main ethnic Black groups in South Africa, weren't donating their bodies to science. African researchers held discussions with Zulu custodians of culture—traditional leaders and healers—and hauled up epic themes, a constellation of ideas about death, burial and ancestors in the afterlife which clashed with 'science' and the idea of body donation.

In Zulu culture, the most common way to describe death is that it's about 'going home'. Before a man dies, a cow will be slaughtered and its hide will be used to cover the body for burial. When a woman dies, she is covered in the grass mat she used to sit on when she was alive. Death is not considered the end, and there is a strong belief in the ancestors. 'When they get buried, they become themselves but in spirit form. For me, they are not dead because I see them and talk to them,' said one traditional health practitioner. 'I have never heard of body donation. We as Zulus know that a person passes away and is buried. We are thereafter able to speak to them. The story of the body going to be studied, how will we ask for things from them?' asked a traditional leader. Whereas in the scientific model death is seen as the vital organs not working any more, the African perspective is that death is a transition to a supreme, ancestral level.

From the study, De Gama and the team saw body donation as a likely impossibility. 'It is not up to anatomists to attempt to cajole a

Black African population, such as this one, into donating their bodies, since that would amount to a domineering, arrogant scientific attitude,' they wrote. And thus, they continue to use the unclaimed bodies of strangers.

But the reality of these cultural beliefs aren't easy to manage, particularly when you are trying to teach anatomy to medical students and have no bodies at all.

***

Many Western anatomists can switch the lights on in their laboratories each morning knowing that their students will have bodies and body parts to study, and that an administrator is making sure new ones arrive. As they dissect an arm or explain an artery in a prosected torso, they can do so with a clear conscience, knowing that the person on the table sat down and inked paperwork giving themselves to the university.

The Turkish anatomist İlke Ali Gürses operates in an entirely different universe—the dissecting room is empty of both donors and unclaimed bodies. 'The situation is dire,' he sighed when we spoke over the internet in 2022.

It's been dire for years and has actually worsened since İlke was a medical student at Istanbul University in the early 2000s. Back then, unsavoury as it is, on the few occasions he had to dissect, he and twenty other students worked on the 'unclaimed'—the person had either died at a state hospital or a psychiatric institution in another province, and more than likely had not consented to be anatomised. 'Most of the patients had no relatives. They had for example, chronic schizophrenia or some really incurable or terminal mental illness,' he recalls. 'When they died, the hospital sent their bodies to the department.' But in recent years, the hospital has stopped doing this.

In 2006 İlke was made a resident in the anatomy department at Istanbul University and for the next five years only dissected unclaimed bodies. At the time, they were getting about ten bodies a year so he estimates he worked on around fifty to sixty people who hadn't consented to being there. They had no choice—he estimates the school had *one body donation* in a decade. Two other people signed up but they never arrived. Just recently he's worked on unclaimed body parts in the Istanbul University's vast museum collection. 'Nearly all the specimens are unclaimed,' he says.

Over the Turkish summer in 2021, İlke moved to Koç University, a not-for-profit private institution in Istanbul, where luckily they have two donors who had given their bodies the year before. They are shared between ninety students. 'We actually let the students dissect but only a limited number of them can do it,' he says. 'Three or four students dissect a forearm, and another group of students dissect the hand. So students will only probably have a chance to dissect two times on the body in different regions, different systems. It's not going to be constant. It's not going to be continuous, but at least they will have the experience.'

The problem exists throughout Turkey. İlke says larger, more venerable medical schools in Istanbul are bequeathed around six bodies a year to teach around 400 students. Many newly established schools have no donor programs so rely on the handful of unclaimed bodies that do arrive at their universities or import them from the US at great expense. Other schools have one or two bodies, which they have used for up to twenty years. 'They are not in good condition but they use them anyway,' he says.

Having no willed *or* unclaimed bodies is reminiscent of the situation European anatomists were in hundreds of years ago, and İlke says some anatomists in the West understand the dilemma, and support him as he tries to find ways to increase donations. Others find the use of unclaimed bodies absolutely unacceptable. 'They cannot fathom the necessity of using any human bodies in that manner,' he laments.

'And do you feel a bit judged at times?' I ask.

'Yeah, of course. Yeah, I feel judged.'

I ask what it's like to work on an unclaimed body, how he feels about it.

'I actually feel … how should I say it? The exact word is not guilty, but I feel as if I owe them something because I know I use their bodies in research and education without their consent,' he says.

He says the situation has been so bad in medical schools that in 2014, the Turkish government passed a law allowing bodies to be imported. Anatomists now often spend up to US$15,000 to import a body from the US, a country which allows companies to profit from the distribution of bodies and body parts. A person will donate their body to the company, which will cover the costs of cremation. The companies then ship body parts or whole bodies around the world to be used for medical and research purposes. İlke is wary of some of these US companies, and suspects some of the bodies are either unclaimed—a homeless person for example—or were donated by family members. He's not confident they are direct donations from the individual.

One of the obvious hurdles İlke faces is religion: around 96 per cent of the population identify as Muslim, and therefore hold strong beliefs about the sanctity of the body after death. For centuries, during the Ottoman period, it was forbidden to dissect a Muslim person—even if they were unclaimed or an executed criminal. In 1841 however, Sultan Abdülmecit gave permission for the bodies of non-Muslim prisoners and those executed at the Maritime Arsenal to be used. İlke says, however, that in the last decades of the Ottoman Empire during the transition to Turkey becoming a republic in 1922, it became acceptable to dissect unclaimed Muslim bodies from state hospitals.

Organ donation faced similar religious restrictions until a group of transplant surgeons sat down with Islamic scholars at the Department of Religious Affairs in 1981. For a week, they argued about whether organ donation was permissible in Islam. A fatwa was later issued, essentially giving permission for it to happen. In 2020 the same department published a statement saying they supported body donation—it's not quite a fatwa but İlke says anatomists can send the link to potential donors to read.

A few years ago, İlke interviewed a handful of Turkish body donors. They had either been registered for a long time or had come to Istanbul University to do the paperwork to donate their bodies. Like other researchers around the world, İlke found they were fervent in their commitment to the cause. 'The individuals who donate their bodies actually consider this as a very important decision in their life and they defend it very ferociously,' he says.

Under Turkish law, a family can revoke a body donation and İlke asked the donors how they would feel if hypothetically their children, spouse or relatives stopped it from happening. Some of the donors were defensive at the thought. 'Their main idea was that "it's my decision, and they have no say in it—it's my decision". It's the final narrative in their life story and it's the final act they do as an individual, and they don't want it to be messed with by anybody else, even their loved ones.' Only a small proportion were okay about their family members stopping the donation. 'Most of them actually considered this a violation. The donation decision is very important to them and very central to their personality as I see it,' he says.

While the situation has been grim, in recent years there has been a slight rise in people signing up to donate—and they are all Muslims. For now, İlke says the anatomists and students are basically waiting for them to die.

***

So whereas powerful traditional forces make it difficult for Muslims or Zulus to donate their bodies, at the other extreme, you have the Dadhichi Body Donation Society in India or Buddhist beliefs in places like Taiwan or Thailand, which by tapping into traditional beliefs and reworking them, have developed a 'donation theology', paving the way for people to donate.

Then you have the theology of the bowel.

At the London conference, Christina Welch, who had been studying the pre-Vesalian mortuary sculptures littered in churches across Britain, had mentioned this strange idea.

I initially thought that cadaver sculptures were not especially relevant to what happened to Ruby and Julie at the University of Queensland all those years ago but there was something just so oddly alluring about them. I asked George if I should follow up on the theology of the bowel and he encouraged me to do so on the grounds that people are interested in their movements generally.

What feels like aeons after we first met at the 2019 anatomy conference, I speak to Christina over the internet. She has endured a tough British lockdown, and I start off by asking her how did she get into these sculptures in the first place? She explains she had seen the cadaver sculptures at Winchester Cathedral over the years but never really delved into them until she had a serious discussion with one of her students and it triggered an interest.

Christina could see that they were mainly sculpted during the reign of Mary and the Tudors. 'So what is the one thing that combines all of this? I'm like, well, Roman Catholicism—so that means they've got to be connected to purgatory,' she says.

Christina ended up looking into forty-one sculptures in churches around Britain and began to see what they meant. My partner was raised Catholic and said purgatory was a big deal at St Agnes primary school in the 1970s. The nuns told him it was a place for those who had sinned a bit but not so seriously that they would be forever excluded from heaven. After some time in purgatory, you could work off or repent your transgressions and get through the Pearly Gates.

For Christina, the thinking around the sculptures was 'completely bonkers' but was basically about people seeing them, and being reminded that the dead person was in purgatory and needed to be prayed for. She equates it to a points system. Basically, when you die, you take points to purgatory with you. If you have a decent number of points, you get to spend less time and experience less pain while you are there. But even though you can't pray in purgatory and keep topping up your points, people in the living world can do it for you. And you'd want people to pray for you too—measured in thousands of years, purgatory was where you hung out while your sins were purged.

High clerics, wealthy landowners and merchants commissioned these not-at-all flattering sculptures, which in their day would have looked much more lifelike—polychromed and painted with flesh-coloured skin and veins in red and green. 'They would have just looked really freaky to our eyes,' she says.

Christina has written about a few of the sculptures and I particularly love the story around Alice de la Pole, the Duchess of Suffolk and the wealthy granddaughter of the poet Geoffrey Chaucer. She had her elaborate cadaver sculpture carved before her death and it features two versions of herself, one on top of the other—in one, she looks rested and elegant and in the other, she's an anorexic, elderly mess. She died in 1475 and her sculpture is still on display at St Mary's Church in Ewelme. But Alice didn't just get people to pray at her sculpture. She and her husband also set up an almshouse where thirteen poor and respectable men lived and prayed for their benefactors. It's reminiscent of a *Monty Python* skit—a group of men sitting praying 139 Aves, sixty-nine Pater Nosters, and fifteen Creeds over a period of six daily rituals. You can imagine it got pretty boring after a while.

A wooden sculpture of an unknown cleric at the Church of St John the Baptist in Keystone is likely the oldest, dating to around 1405. It features an eviscerated man with a visible spine but no stomach or intestines and it has left Christina stumped. 'It really got me thinking why? Just why? All the rest of them—it's weird enough looking at them,' she sighs. Why would a cleric take out their bowels in their sculpture? Christina went on an odyssey trying to find out.

At the time, anything to do with the bowels was considered rotten and connected to the devil. 'It's all connected with the dark, Satanicky nasty stuff,' explains Christina. The problem is why do we have these bowels if God designed our bodies? Thomas Aquinas took up this question of resurrection and our dark, evil entrails and suggested that in Paradise we would no longer digest and or shit like we did on earth. 'The only answer I can come up with is that the cleric basically was a believer that the bowels contained stuff to do with sin and had them removed,' says Christina. She also posits that maybe he just had problems with his bowels.

She believes that whoever did the work had seen an eviscerated body, and they might have seen a hanging, drawing and quartering, which would have given them a sense of what a body actually looks like when the viscera were taken out. Christina and the forensic anatomist Wendy Birch have also been looking at paintings of saints where their bowels were taken out. 'All sorts of people had their bowels removed—it was a form of torture,' she says.

I mentioned that the sculpture of Sir Roger Rockley in Worsbrough—with his wavy intestines the wrong way around—is quite cute.

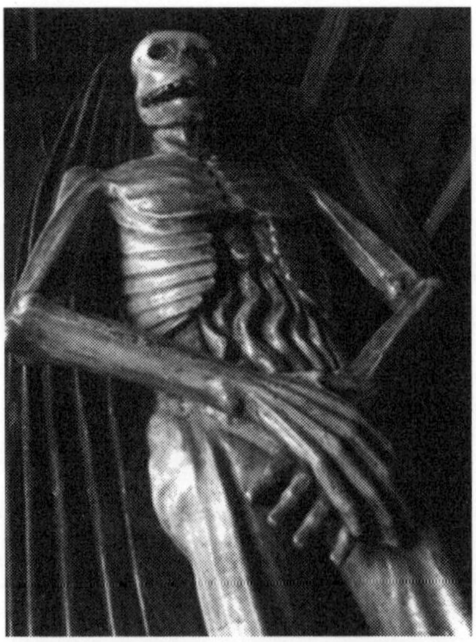

Sir Roger Rockley in St Mary's Church in Worsbrough in the UK. This sculpture dates from approximately 1524 and is one part of a double-decker tomb. Here he is shown decomposing. The other sculpture features him dressed in full armour. *Christina Welch.*

Christina mulls him over. 'Could it be that the guy at Worsbrough saw an evisceration, a hanging, drawing and quartering, and only saw the intestines in a bucket perhaps—and the sculptor thought they had that sort of wavy snake pattern? So yeah, I'm still thinking on that one. Jackie, I haven't really got an answer. All I've got is a whole load of more questions.'

***

'You can't write a book about anatomy and not have a ghost story!' he exclaimed. 'Have you got a ghost story?'

I was nearing the end of this epic quest when a technician asked me this question. He then corrected himself: 'Instead of a ghost story, I'd call it a paranormal experience.'

The technician wanted to remain anonymous. He was like another I had met, who also wanted to remain in the background, which is a shame as this person is considered a great dissector, known for their strong work ethic, speed and flawless technique.

In Melbourne, Quentin Fogg and I had discussed how hard it was getting information out of older technicians. 'They're all these old guys that are really closed books,' he'd said. 'They've grown up in a space where the academic was the deity, and you don't share "our" secrets.'

So I was a little surprised that here was a technician who was not only chatty but prodding me to put a *paranormal experience* in my book.

Anyway, as he tells it, this story happened a few years ago and it began when the body of man who died of cancer arrived at the university. Unusually, his wife had made the donation—it hadn't directly come from the man himself. It's not normal practice to accept a next-of-kin donation in Australia but it is legal in certain states and occasionally happens.

It was six o'clock at night and the funeral parlour brought the man in on a gurney. The technician was in the lab with his colleague and they were standing in front of the fridges discussing the donation. The fridge doors were not powered, and to break the seal, you needed to give them a yank. A good yank.

'Anyway, we were discussing with the undertaker how young he was and how he was donated on his wife's behalf. He was physically fit, and we could tell he was a bike rider because he had a lot of leg scarring.' But then, suddenly, as they were talking, the fridge door just opened up on its own, and began repeatedly bang, bang, bang, bang, bang, bang, banging for about three seconds. 'The undertaker goes "Aw, this is bullshit" and he took off. He got his gurney and he took off out the door. And we just stood there,' recalls the technician.

'This door banging—it was like someone was on the door handle going, "I don't want to be here." That was the first incident with this cadaver.' Strangely, his fellow technician worked the next night and reported the same thing happened at the exact same time.

The day after, the technician says he embalmed the man 'with one and a half drums' of embalming fluid and then let him sit overnight. The next day, he finished the process, and when he and a colleague were putting him in the fridge, he said to the dead man, 'I hope you are happy now.' He slammed the fridge door, and at the exact same moment, all the power in the university dropped out.

It usually takes twelve months to cure a body before dissection. One day, the technician was working when suddenly the fridge alarm started going off—it was going woo, woo, woo, and wouldn't stop. He called an engineer to come and have a look, and they didn't know what the problem was so they just reset the system. 'I said, "Hang on a minute!" I went to look at the mortuary register and it was to the day—twelve months exactly to the day. He was still in the fridge curing but it was his anniversary to the day that he came in.'

I ask the technician what he thinks happened.

'I think he didn't want to be there. That's what I think,' he says. 'I think he did not want to be donated.'

The technician says he spent the next year dissecting the man, and the strange thing is that the wife called not long after and said she wanted his body back. Under law, next of kin have full dominion over the body and the man was returned.

Chapter 33

In 1983 a letter dated 12 April arrived at our house in Makati in the Philippines, addressed to my mother. It was from the Brisbane Crematorium Limited. Now safely stored behind plastic in one of Mum's meticulous family history binders, it reads:

> Dear Mrs Dent,
>
> We are in receipt of your letter regarding disposal of ashes of the late Julie Kelly Dent.
>
> Our records show that the ashes of the late Ruby Dent were placed in single position X and the nearest available is Single position Y which is about three beds away.
>
> If this is suitable would you please complete the attached Authority form with the inscription required for the nameplate and then sign the form and return it to the office with payment.
>
> The cost involved will be $100 for the single Position, plus the cost of engraving the nameplate calculated at 30 cents per letter, figure, symbol etc, with a minimum cost of $16.25 for less than 52 letters.
>
> Yours faithfully,
> Brisbane Crematorium Limited.

Mum had obviously written to the crematorium and calculating the time it takes for letters to and from Manila, the date suggests Julie's body had been at the university for under two years, which is the same amount of time Ruby was. In 2016, Walter Wood in an interview with the ABC spoke about the end process:

> All the body parts go into one container and at the end of the year when it's decided the body is of no use and will now be cremated, the parts that are left are all put into a coffin and they are kept in the storeroom area again until the following year, when they will be disposed of en masse, usually they might get rid of forty or fifty bodies at a time.

Rohan, the former Cannon & Cripps worker, stressed to me that each donor was cremated separately in their own coffin, and their ashes then made individually available to the family. 'It was all done very respectfully,' he recalled.

Some donors' families collected their ashes, others didn't. But there was a sense that something else was needed.

***

Anatomy does have an awful past but it hasn't all been one long conga line of disrespect—there have been times when earlier anatomists and their students held rituals for the dissected, largely to allay community fears around disrupting the burial process. In 1568, a student named Lassaro Salio praised the Paduan chair of anatomy and surgery Giolamo Fabrici for his 'most honourable' burial of the remains at the end of the dissection, although he wasn't so complimentary about his teacher's actual dissection or demonstration skills.

A few years later in 1597, the transalpine student Francisco Hippolyti Hildesheim remarked that after the dissection, 'the remaining parts of the cadavers [were] carried to the Cathedral and buried' and it was attended by many students. In some instances, students in Padua were partly responsible for organising, paying for and attending the burial of the dissected, which was also seen as a way for them to ruminate on the death.

It wasn't until the 20th century that medical schools began earnestly running events for their donors. One of the first services was held in the UK in 1962. From there, they spread to the US in the 1970s and are now held in medical schools across the world—in China, Korea, New Zealand, the US, Germany, the Netherlands and many other countries. As no two anatomy labs are the same, neither are any two services. Whatever the ritual, Yale's John Harley Warner, a medical historian, and Lawrence Rizzolo, a professor of surgery, think these memorial services signified the end of the 'detached concern' period.

In Walter Wood's ABC interview, he tellingly says part of the reason the University of Queensland started putting on ceremonies in the early 1990s was that families started asking questions. 'It was very hard for the family. I mean from the time the body disappeared into the department to the time when they received notice the ashes were available—there was no communication at all between really the university and the families of the donors,' he says.

'I became very aware of it because I was not only dealing with the students who were having problems dealing with dissection, and trying to help them through it, but I was also dealing with the families and relatives as well as the donors. And I was getting feedback that they just didn't know what was going on there—[they were] all the time worried and concerned that their loved one wasn't being treated respectfully. They heard all these rumours, innuendos about what goes on.

'It ran rife and I'd felt that we'd done a lot for the medical students through the seventies and eighties trying to help them prepare them for the dissection classes and that but we still didn't have them aware of the families that were there. I thought that a thanksgiving service would be the best way of bringing both students, families, and relatives together. And the students could thank them face to face and say look, we've gained from this.'

Thus the first University of Queensland service was held in 1992, years after Ruby and Julie had been there. However, my dad says he's never heard from the university nor did he know that there was this new tradition of honouring what his parents had done. I suggested we go to the next one together.

***

Another lockdown. More time at home, more time digging around my handbag or pocket looking for a mask. With the Queensland border still closed—will it ever open again?—I'm in front of a computer in Mum's all-purpose room waiting to watch the University of Queensland's annual thanksgiving ceremony for body donors. My parents were initially not interested in it as they thought it was going to be religious, an issue that plagued the early days of holding services.

Walter Wood had told the ABC that when it first started, it was Christian-based but included a Jewish rabbi, a Muslim imam, and a Bahá'í chaplain. Indigenous groups were invited but had refused to attend because of past handling of Aboriginal remains.

At first, Walter said it was wonderfully received but as they wandered through the guests afterwards, they started getting complaints. 'I'll never forget one family that came up to me and they said, "Oh, so and so he would have been rolling over in his grave to hear all that . . . can't you just water it down a bit?"' he recalled. 'And over the years, they have tried to make it more acceptable to people that are not religious in any way. And they have even changed the name from thanksgiving service to a thanksgiving ceremony.'

I'd assured my parents a few times it wouldn't be religious but I wasn't 100 per cent sure. Either way, it must've worked as near the start time of 5.30 pm, Mum settles down next to me in front of the desktop and Dad lies on a nearby bed. Soon, the camera lets us into the River Room at Customs House, a function centre on Brisbane's riverside. The setting is a darkened room with an altar covered in purple and orange flowers, and two large books with *Book of Remembrance* written across their covers. There appear to be candles. It looks crowded—well, at least the front seats are taken up.

My parents are wriggly and talkative, so I don't expect them to be able to sit quietly through the hour-long service. At various points, Mum wanders off to check on my six-year-old son, who is watching 'the pad' in another room. She returns. Her computer crashes twice and I quickly log into my laptop. Dad asks if my son is watching ABC Me and why does Mum have the door open? Mum and Dad both wander off when my older brother randomly shows up. Mum returns with a glass of wine. Dad lies back on the bed.

I stay watching. Various dignitaries give considered and gentle speeches, acknowledging that the ceremony might be very hard for people, reigniting feelings of loss and grief. As Professor Deborah Terry, the vice-chancellor of the university, puts it: 'I particularly thank next of kin or close friends for attending tonight, whether in person or online. We value this opportunity to show our appreciation to you all for honouring loved ones' wishes in circumstances we know can be very, very difficult ... Our deep appreciation of the selfless decisions made by your loved ones is rooted in the knowledge that they are contributing ... to the advancement of science.'

Dad is lying back on the bed with his eyes closed. He looks asleep but I think he's listening.

Professor Mark Midwinter asks whether we really need bodies any more in the sophisticated tech era and says yes we do, arguing that 3D imaging often simplifies structures, idealises the body and leaves out variations.

Mum sighs when a chaplain offers a prayer. 'I knew they'd do this,' she murmurs. 'This praying is all clap-trap as far as I'm concerned but it's important to some.'

When a string quartet strikes up, Mum discusses how some people in the audience would've lost someone in recent years.

'Dad would probably be the oldest if he was there,' I say.

'Fifty years,' he calls out from the bed. 'Where is this? At Queensland University?'

'It's at Customs House,' I say.

The next part of the ceremony is made up of students thoughtfully talking about what the donors mean to them. 'My experience with the body donor program was really something that I have never really experienced before,' says one young woman. 'It really made anatomy my favourite subject and I just could not seem to comprehend how amazing it was of these donors to provide their bodies for my education. It really was something that I will greatly treasure and will definitely remember for the rest of my life.' All the students seem genuinely moved.

'Actually when you think about it—it is amazing,' says Mum. 'You never stop to think about that.'

Dad goes downstairs to talk to my brother again.

'But you know what's interesting? Dad and Maurie just accepted it and said that's it. But if you were religious and donated your body your family would probably be more emotionally involved.'

I ask Mum if Dad is okay.

'He's fine. He probably started to think about Little Mother (Dad's nickname for Ruby),' says Mum. 'They were very, very close, the two of them.'

Dad eventually returns and lies back on the bed.

The students start talking about how they were curious about who the donors were. 'In class, when looking at a brain or a heart, it's hard to not wonder who this body belonged to, how much they loved or laughed, and what kind of life they lived,' says one student. Another discusses how while studying the brain was tough—knowing it supported life, and contained memories—it motivated him to learn. 'There are heroes in our anatomy building,' he says. 'At times I wished I knew your names.' There it is again: objectivity and subjectivity, specimen and person wrestling it out in the anatomy lab.

The ceremony is winding up.

Mum says it wasn't what she thought it would be. 'I thought it was going to be too religious and emotional, too sentimentalised or something. It was good,' she says. 'I suppose they have this for the relatives. It's that terrible word—it's "closure" for a lot of people.'

'How many years has it been going?' asks Dad.

'Since the nineties?' I guess.

'Really?' he says.

'Julie died in 1981,' remarks Mum.

'How come they didn't invite us then? They must've sent a lot of letters to Megalong Street,' says Dad. Megalong Street is where Ruby and Julie used to live.

'I don't think they started it until a while after Julie was done. I'll find out what date it started. I think it's because families kept asking questions,' I say.

Mum says a lot of families probably didn't agree with their relatives wanting to do it. 'We weren't worried but some people said: "Oh gosh!"'

'The Catholics wouldn't have allowed it,' remarks Dad.

'It's actually a nice idea,' says Mum. 'It's almost like a funeral service.'

I ask Dad what he thinks about it.

'It's good marketing,' he says.

'Besides being a cynical comment Des—it's quite well done,' says Mum.

Dad replies: 'It's always been a closed shop and now all of a sudden, they've opened it up. If you went to the university in the past and asked anything they'd tell you to bugger off, which is a typical university approach. The body went and that was the end of it.' Fair enough. Walter Wood said they knew there was an issue with families.

Perhaps he's remembering Ruby. I thought he looked a bit glassy-eyed at one point but maybe I'm being over-analytical. He wouldn't say it but perhaps he appreciated the ceremony.

Obviously, each generation has its differences but it strikes me that the older doctors I spoke to bring up that people didn't question authority the way they do now. They didn't ask where the bodies or the skeletons came from. They just 'got on with things'. This is possibly why my dad never asked any questions about what happened to his parents.

***

Somebody on the radio is talking about it being Mother's Day the next day and I'm reluctantly driving to Leo's house. It's his birthday and I feel like he may want to be doing other things like watching sport with his friends or heading to church. Perhaps the house will feel particularly empty today without his wife. I tried to give him an out but he said for me to come over anyway. Also, I'm having this moment of wondering what am I doing hanging around with this retired technician trying to find out about my grandparents' dissection.

When I arrive at his house, he's wearing a navy-blue polo t-shirt with 'Vanuatu South Pacific Paradise' embroidered on it in small letters. I say, 'Happy birthday' and he says thank you, and then straight-up suggests we visit my grandparents at Albany Creek Memorial Park in North Brisbane.

'Oh wow,' I say. This is a genuinely a good idea as I'd never been to their graves.

Leo dons a red baseball cap and 1970s-style aviators, which give him a slightly cop feel. As we drive through Brisbane's traffic, Leo reminisces about his trip to Vanuatu, and then how at one point in the 1970s, there was talk of building a columbarium for the anatomised on the grounds of the university.

'Why were you going to do that? Were there a lot of ashes?' I ask.

'Oh yes but it just gave people a sense of belonging. They'd given their body to the university so they were in the university. It meant something to the families but management didn't see that,' he replied. Later on, a plot was found at a crematorium near the Gold Coast for donors whose ashes hadn't been collected.

We pull into the graveyard at Albany Creek. According to their website, it opened in 1964, and while it doesn't have the romance of Brisbane's spectacular and enormous Toowong Cemetery, which is filled with towering stone angels and vine-encrusted urns, this place has a rural, spacious and daggy-in-a-good-way feel. There's a small waterfall, a tiered water fountain and a large stone Book of Remembrance.

The Google reviews are a positive 4.1 out of 5, although a few people left one-star reviews after technical hitches during services a few years ago. Tech—the bane of any event. One man left a curious four-star review: 'Yeah...my grandparents are there's...didn't like them as they were toxic but they lived within the forest area.'

Leo and I go into the office to get a map to help us find Ruby's and Julie's spots, which according to Mum's letter are in two separate 'beds'. I need to go to the bathroom and Leo offers to start looking for them but I ask him if I can do it—I feel like I need to, that I should lead this strange charge. Mum, Dad and I have over the years looked for relatives in various graveyards, and it's a small thrill pacing past the tombstones and urgently reading the often-withered text. There is often an excitement that goes with finding the long-lost relative—you'd think they were alive.

Leo and I walk past a series of brick columbariums to find their 'section', which is made up of large rectangle-shaped garden beds, bordered by little bronze plaques engraved with the names of the dead. I record myself commentating on my phone.

'It is up here?' I ask myself, patrolling, passing a bouquet with a card for Mother's Day. After about five quiet minutes, I eventually find Julie's plain but to-the-point plaque:

JULIE KELLY DENT

1903—1981

I go looking for Ruby's bed, passing more little bronze plates.

In loving memory of our dear mother.
In memory of Russell.
In loving memory of Mildred, passed away at Caloundra.
Passed away, passed away, passed away.
In loving memory of, in loving memory of.

All these people who passed away and are in loving memory were put here in 1972. And then I can see that where Ruby's plate should be is a gap, and I sigh, feeling forlorn. I sit down on a bench, looking at the large bed she shares with so many other people, which is very dry, and has a sign saying if you leave plastic flowers they will be taken away and only fresh flowers are allowed here.

I make a sound tinged with disappointment, a bit whimpery about Ruby's gap. I watch a lady tend to a nearby grave and the traffic whizzing past outside, a gentle breeze and the currawongs squawking in the trees. It's a perfect Brisbane day, and I close my eyes, content at where I am, in a self-conscious, unsure-what-to-feel way. Whatever, I *feel* the gold and the timber, and the brain fever and the quiet of Yarraman, and the table tennis matches and when Ruby had to say goodbye to her school that final day.

Leo walks over.

'Are you okay?' he asks.

'Yeah,' I reply, making that odd feeble sound again. 'I was thinking I might go ask in the shop about putting a plaque there for her. Are you happy to hang here or do you want to come in?'

'I'll come in,' he says.

'How are you feeling? Are you all right?' I ask.

'I'm fine.'

'I suppose tomorrow being Mother's Day—do those days make you extra sad? Or it just comes in waves?'

'I do remember things. It's always remembering.'

I get up from the bench and we walk towards the front reception, passing the waterfall. At first I found the place a little daggy but it seems okay now.

'Well, this is a nice place to end up,' I say, gesturing to the fountain. I've always been a fan of water features.

We go to the office and I explain that I'd like to find out how much it costs to get a plaque, and we are steered into a nondescript holding room which has samples of plaques, pink teddies and other grave items. An administration worker advises that it will cost around $638 for a plaque with a seven-line inscription, and then leaves for a spell. She returns with Ruby's paperwork and declares that there was a plate but it has obviously come loose, and they can replace it with no charge to the family. The original inscription was plain and simple—like Julie's—and the lady advises that we can upgrade our lines but my dad would need to approve it. I quite like the minimalist plaque.

Later, at lunch, Leo doesn't say much, probably mulling over the small car crash we'd just had after we'd left the graveyard. Nothing serious—just an older woman smashing into the back of us, my body thrown forward in my seat, she flustered as they exchanged details, telling us she was on her way to see her sister in her nursing home. He remarks he's never visited the graves of body donors before. 'I've never followed through,' he says. I think how it was a first for me too—going to the graveyard with a technician who worked in the anatomy laboratory where my grandparents were body donors.

***

Klaas van Linschoten had been a prosector at the University Medical Center Groningen (UMCG) in Holland since 1982, when he was given extra secretarial work in the anatomy department, which included answering phone calls. He began speaking to potential body donors and their grieving relatives. As Sophie Bolt, put it: 'For the very first time, the bodies on the dissecting table were no longer anonymous to him.'

He began wondering why Dutch anatomists were not engaging with the relatives so after some research, discovered the global phenomenon of holding memorials and building monuments. He told Sophie he wasn't into the idea of a yearly obligatory service but liked the idea of a monument. After a 'long bureaucratic process to get the proper finances and a licence to build', they created the first Dutch monument to body donors at the Yarden Crematorium in Groningen in 2007.

The first example I could find of a physical memorial to donors dates from 1998, when the Southern Illinois University School of Medicine in the US purchased a mausoleum at a local graveyard and held a ceremony to bury body donor cremains. Since then, all sorts of monuments have popped up. The 'Forest of Life' at the University of Basque in Bilbao is made up of twenty wooden pillars where donor's ashes are stored. At its entrance it reads: 'This is a place of peace. Here lie the ashes of those who generously donated their body to science. Here death rejoices in helping life. Rest in peace.' The eminent sculptor Heather B. Swann created a cocoon-like chair on the grounds of the University of Melbourne—her mother and grandmother both donated their bodies to the anatomy department.

***

The day is moody, grey and pissing down rain in Sydney and I'm standing at a body donor memorial in Rookwood Cemetery. It's set on a landscaped lawn, surrounded by hedges, and my initial reaction is that it's very pleasant. There are flowers and bushes everywhere, and benches to sit on. Five very small plinths sit at the entrance. One says: 'In remembrance of the men and women who have made a unique contribution to the advancement of medicine and science by donating their bodies to the University of Technology Sydney.'

I'd recalled that the scientists at AFTER had mentioned there was a body donor memorial and even though the forensically studied donors generally stay on site, other donors go the university's Surgical and

Anatomical Science Facility, and it is here that they are honoured. I felt it was worth paying a visit in homage but I was also sketching a vague creative fantasy of meeting a donor's family member out there. I was yet to meet any.

The garden also features a very large copper doughnut-looking sculpture and a series of four large copper screens patterned in a way that reminds me of retro 1970s wallpaper. As I walk slowly around the garden path, the rain pitter-pattering on my umbrella, I suddenly notice it is shaped as an infinity symbol. There are no ashes here—or so I think. There are no names. There are no bunches of flowers or cards with ink smudged from the elements. I sit on a bench and envision family members of the donors coming to the site, how they feel, if it moves them, if it feels right.

It might seem like a black hole, where we see and hear nothing, but there exists a realm of prosections, corpses, teaching, the smell of formaldehyde, the sounds of the saws and yes—grieving families. This is the backstage of medicine.

As I sit here, I see this sculpture not only as a space for family members to visit, but as the anatomists wearing their hearts on their sleeves. And the sculptures aren't just communicating to the world, 'Hey, we care about the dead'—they are also telling us that what happens to the dead isn't an emotionless business for them. That some of them feel something when they do it, that it isn't an objective pursuit, that the people on the table aren't objects.

When Sophie Bolt was in the early days of her research on Dutch body donors, she saw first-hand how the Department of Anatomy at the UMCG came to the decision to create a monument for donors on the grounds of a local crematorium. 'It was really like the anatomists thinking well, it's not only a body, it's also a person, and maybe they have family, and maybe their family is mourning, and we should also express our gratitude,' Sophie told me.

But on the other side, all this time I thought that the donors were making a huge sacrifice by doing it but seems they aren't. Not at all.

Danish researchers Klaus Hoeyer and Maria Olejaz spent twelve years studying body donors and came to realise that donors actually *liked the idea*. The pair had studied body and/or organ donation between 2007 and 2019, and over that time interviewed forty-eight people on the topic. Some of the subjects were signed up as donors, some were unsure and others were a firm NO.

Over time, the social scientists came to realise that 'most interviewees expressed remarkable veneration for cadaver usage', and that it was their clear preference that their dead body be used in this way.

For the donors, it was a desire, not a sacrifice, and as the researchers pointed out, we live in a new era. Where 18th-century criminals feared the exclusion from the community that dissection represented, a new generation saw it as a useful death, one of 'post-vital productivity and meaning'.

As I walk around the site and the rain stops momentarily, my friend Anna arrives. A designer, artist and creative producer, I thought she'd be open to a graveyard visit, particularly as we'd worked on a project together where I collected ghost stories for her in Albury and Nowra which fed into her installations.

I'm keen to hear Anna's interpretation. She's quiet as she wanders around.

'It's much smaller than I expected,' she says.

'It's much bigger than I expected. They are a pretty obscure lot—the body donors. There aren't really that many of them,' I say.

We discuss the symbolism of the elements. I think the doughnut represents wholeness. Anna wonders if it's the iris of an eye, and then remarks that the flowers beneath it are edible, and bends down and eats some. 'I put these in salad.' I join her in eating them. We analyse the metal screens: it that a bird? Is that an abstract angel?

'It's the gates to heaven,' exclaims Anna.

It could indeed be the gates of heaven, but I've heard a lot of effort has gone into making body donor ceremonies and memorials not too religious. 'I think purposely with these things they make them non-religious as people who aren't religious get upset at the religion.'

She nods.

We wander around infinity a bit longer, and I'm still keen to hear more of her analysis but she's not saying much. I eat more flowers. (Not having found out until later that there were ashes underground.) My flower app says they are called sweet alyssum.

Anna proposes we look at other memorials and find three over the next few hours as we walk in the rain: one for the millennium of Christianity in Russia 988 to 1988 and St Nicholas Cathedral in Harbin destroyed in 1966 in China, another for dead babies, and a third memorial for the Holocaust. The babies' memorial is a distinctive U-shaped white statue, the shapes of a mother and child morphed into one, and they are about to give each other a kiss. It was built for the 20,000 or so babies who were found in unmarked graves during a mapping exercise of the graveyard. The babies were buried some time between the mid-1920s and the mid-1970s. The gate to the Holocaust memorial is closed but we can see the walls are engraved with the names of different extermination camps.

Anna and I talk about getting buried, where to put ashes and the like as we walk around. We are youngish so haven't planned where we will technically end up. Does anybody know what to do any more? The people in my social world seem to be throwing the ashes of their beloved parents over cliffs, into rivers, into the sea, into the bush. The rain is tumbling down so hard we decide to say our farewells.

I go back to the chair next to the body donor memorial and sit on the bench under the thundering sky, hoping by some random chance a donor relative will stop by. No one comes.

***

I do not know anyone else with a relative who donated their body to science. All these years, it's not something that erupts in conversation with anybody, anywhere at anytime. There is nothing I can see online.

I've never seen body donors or their families hosting a stall at a festival. I've not seen their flyers stuck to a lamppost. But one afternoon, at a friend's birthday party, I randomly and somewhat astonishingly discover her stepmother's parents both donated their bodies to the University of Sydney. It's not the environment to have a proper chat so we arrange to speak another time.

When we eventually meet again, she tells me the story of body donation in her family but doesn't want me to use her name.

C is in her seventies.

She says that since we spoke, she remembered it wasn't just her parents who donated but her grandfather had as well. He had been a veterinarian who graduated from the University of Sydney. 'I think he was a bit eccentric. I didn't know him very well as he died when I was fairly young but according to Mum, he spent all the family money. He donated his body to the university because he said that, having come through the university—even though he did veterinary science—he could see that the medical people needed cadavers to actually do the learning on.' He died in the 1950s, which makes him a very early donor.

A few years later, C's mother declared that she too was going to donate her body to the University of Sydney and when she died in 2005, she was accepted. Even though her parents were divorced, her father also donated his body to the same university in 2014. Her intergenerational story fits a well-known pattern—body donation becoming a family tradition.

'Well, I guess people can see there's nothing wrong with it. You mourn your normal way, and eventually you get the body back—well, I elected to have both my parents back in ashes,' she says. 'Some people think it's a bit icky but to me, it was sort of a natural thing. I'll probably do the same. I haven't even actually thought about that, which I should do.'

I ask her how she felt about it when her mother told her she was going to donate. 'I didn't really think either way. I think I was fairly young.

She explained that this is what Grandfather did, and she explained why—because of the university connection, and she thought it was a good thing, and that's what she was going to do. It was always just set up that way.'

Her mother was very religious and C held a memorial service for her in a church. 'I thought that's what she would have liked to do,' she says.

I ask: 'Did you have intrusive thoughts? Or were you thinking about what might have happened to her when she was there?'

'No, it didn't worry me at all. My daughter started university doing a science degree, and she did anatomy for a semester. They had body bits that they were dissecting. So, you know, I knew what happened. No—once you've died, you've died. The soul's gone, the body's there. That's my belief anyway.'

Her father only told her he was going to donate much later in life after he'd moved into a nursing home. C thinks he was partly motivated by the fact that he thought people may find his body interesting. 'He had some sort of spinal disorder. I forget what it was now. And he thought, "Oh, they will find this interesting" because all the doctors used to sort of "oooh" and "aaah" over him. They'd say, "Oh you had that when you're in your thirties and came through it." I think these days, it's probably something that's fixed by spinal fusion.' He used a wheelchair later in life.

He also told C body donation was convenient. 'He said, "Look it won't cost you much,"' she laughs. 'He sincerely believed that once you're gone, you're gone.' She says after he died, she went through his papers and found a whole lot of material on Buddha. 'He'd obviously researched a lot on the different religions but it was not something he spoke to me about.'

I ask her how much money played into it but she says it didn't. 'My mother wasn't at all well off, but that wouldn't have been an issue. When she died and when my father died, I could have easily afforded to put on a funeral for them.'

'My mother's was definitely an altruistic decision but my father—I was never ever quite sure. I just thought, "Hmmm, I wonder why he's doing this,"' she says.

C says that as we're speaking, she's wondering if it's something that she will do. 'Do I do the same? I have to think about it.'

Chapter 34

Before Britain's Anatomy Act was introduced in 1832, there were all sorts of proposals put forward as to where to get bodies from. Something had to be done about the grave robbing and the lurking by the gallows—but whose bodies? The list included people who killed themselves, those who died in duels, horse thieves and prisoners.

Other clever schemes included the Royal College setting up a register where people were paid a sum during their lifetime to donate, or abolishing death taxes for donors. At one point, it was thought that if the King donated his body, it would set an example and help destigmatise dissection. But in the end, the elites of Britain decided it would be the poor who would be legally dissected.

I became quite consumed by putting together the social, political and cultural forces at play that led people to start donating their bodies in the 20th century. How did it shift from shame and stigma to something acceptable, where even today in some countries like France people pay a fee to donate? Reams have been written about dissection for the past 2000 years but once you hit the 20th and 21st centuries, the story trails off. Perhaps body donors are a bit dull compared to crusty men digging up graves and stuffing bodies in barrels.

It made sense that the slow dismantling of religious faith in the West made people more likely to donate. But what else was going on? There were little clues all over the place.

In 1950s New Zealand, anatomists at the University of Otago, a small university in Dunedin, were in need of bodies and came up with the savvy idea of sending information leaflets to solicitors. Within seven years, more bequests were appearing in wills. In Germany, at the Dr Senckenbergische Anatomie, an anatomical institute in Frankfurt, the rise in body donation was attributed to a 1963 *Readers Digest* article, which explored the 'piety, sobriety and sincerity of the anatomical business'.

But what about Australia?

I'd spent probably a year asking anyone in this space what happened here and nobody had a firm answer. One day, sensing I was missing something, I randomly changed my search terms from 'body donation' to 'body bequest'.

Voila.

I had found my own Tutankhamun.

People were donating their bodies in the early part of the 20th century, but it was considered unconventional and strange. But things began shifting around the 1940s.

In 1944 A.N. Burkitt, a Professor of Anatomy at the University of Sydney, known for his courtliness of manner and shyness, gave an upbeat interview to *The Daily Telegraph* about the rise in body donation. 'More bodies are being bequeathed to us, but most people stipulate that the bequest must not be made public,' he said. Not all donations were kept quiet though—the story mentioned that 'Rufe' Naylor, a 'well-known sporting figure and investor', had bequeathed his body in 1939.

But just two years later, the professor's tone had shifted: there was a shortage of bodies, it was impacting on the medical school and 'it was necessary to awaken the public conscience in this matter'. *The Sun* was reporting that while a few 'specimens' came to the university through people bequeathing their corpses, more were needed as there were nearly double the number of students doing medicine. The Student Representative Council's medical faculty delegate Ray Dan said as many as eight students at a time were dissecting one limb. 'They are particularly concerned that they rarely have an opportunity of dissecting female cadavers. This is necessarily a serious gap in their training,' he said.

It wasn't just the University of Sydney facing problems. In 1947 Dr Medley, the vice-chancellor of the University of Melbourne, travelled to Canberra to lobby John Dedman, the minister for post-war reconstruction, to do something about the shortage of corpses in Australian universities. At the time, the University of Melbourne was only getting seventy of the 120 corpses it needed each year.

Where were all the bodies? It seems the passing of the 1943 Invalid and Old Age Pensions Bill, which gave pensioners a lump sum grant of 10 pounds to help pay for their funerals, had emptied the dissecting rooms. The Federal government said they understood there were problems with the bill but was unsure of what to do to correct it. Within a year, the shortage was so dire that universities were reportedly going to start importing bodies.

The heat remained on Professor Burkitt at Sydney. While other parts of his life were going well—he loved racing cars and at one point owned five, including a Bugatti—the situation at the medical school was dire. He told a staff correspondent at *The Sydney Morning Herald* that they needed 120 bodies but only had forty a year. 'More people are in a financial position to make provision for their own burial or have relatives who can pay for burial. Fewer men and women in old people's homes die friendless and without relatives,' he said. 'The only way to remedy this situation is by educating people to realise that they can make a valuable contribution to medical science by bequeathing their bodies to the university.'

He also cleared up a number of misconceptions, which give an insight into the particular fears about dissection at the time. He assured that all dissected bodies were given a 'Christian burial' or similar rites, and that body parts were not thrown away. He also stressed that the medical school never paid for bodies.

The story also featured Dr Neville Goodman's research into the history of dissection, which found improved social conditions in Britain had reduced the supply, and full employment and high wages since Second World War had led to the 'almost complete disappearance of the "casual" class'. Even old people dying in institutions were managing to leave behind some estate—enough for their relatives to claim them.

The story ended on a call out for 'enlightened people' to come the aid of medical students.

Throughout the 1950s, Australian anatomists continued to implore the public to donate. But soon the 10 pounds towards the pensioner funeral was not enough as by 1954, the poor were donating to the university to save on funeral costs or to avoid being buried as a pauper.

Pensioner William Stirling, who served with the Royal Inniskilling Fusiliers, was living in a hostel and signed up for it. 'The pension is not enough to provide for funeral expenses. I have made all arrangements for the Anatomy School to pick up my body,' he said in the *Barrier Miner*. William is the first reference I can find to people donating to save on funeral costs.

Shortages persisted up until the 1960s. Anatomy Professor D.C. Sinclair from the University of Western Australia's anatomy department was inundated with offers after making a public call-out for donors. In one week, he had sixty inquiries and nine people officially signed up. He pitched it that donors would not only help medicine but would be spared all funeral expenses.

During this time, Professor Michael Blunt at the University of New South Wales was also struggling to get bodies so sent requests to solicitors in Sydney asking if they could get their clients to bequeath their bodies. He was inundated: approximately 3000 letters of bequests came in over the next six months.

But still. How did Ruby hear about it? The University of Queensland never advertised. It must've been through word of mouth but how? I asked Mum so many times I think she was getting annoyed at me.

***

Dad had sent me a text ages ago telling me I should speak to his cousin Dennis, who had been an anaesthetist, and had apparently done '500 autopsies' at the University of Queensland. I wasn't sure what he meant by autopsies. I'm also not sure why it took me so long to call Dennis but when I finally got around to it—he's now retired on the north Queensland coast—aside from effusive and dramatic tales of University of Queensland surgeons who went on Second World War bombing raids, anaesthetics in Darwin in the 1960s and much more—he finally answered a riddle which had been taunting me since those Christmas drinks, which felt like years ago.

Dennis began medical school in 1959 and by 1960, was dissecting in the old US army huts, which were surrounded by the expansive Victoria Park golf course. The setting meant that golf balls often landed near the huts and rolled under. 'All the golf balls that were hit off the fairways that went under the anatomy school—no one picked them up. And golf balls were *incredibly expensive*! They were *incredibly expensive* compared with today,' he exclaims. The balls didn't go to waste. Dennis and his friends used to collect them from under the hut and with cheap golf sticks they'd managed to find, sneak around the course for an illegal game. 'Oh God!' he laughs at the memory.

The golfers too scared to collect their balls—no matter how expensive they were—reminded me of the magic of the dead. Or in this case perhaps it was the pollution? The type that prompted the funerary rituals on the island of Cos in 500 BC and fear for the people of Woollahra in Sydney who didn't want a funeral parlour on the street.

Dennis wasn't aware that Ruby and Julie—his aunt and uncle—donated their bodies to science. He also can't recall remember much about the man he dissected with five other students. But he can remember, quite distinctly, someone else who was being dissected in the hut.

'Just three dissection things away from me was a body of a young man—thirty-two years of age. He'd been a prominent senior government bureaucrat, and he donated his body to medicine, and there he was, and he only had half a body because he had malignant melanoma. That was my introduction to the widespread effects of this terrible disease,' he says. 'I saw somebody in the flesh *every day*—what was left of him—with the devastating effects of a malignant melanoma in a human body.' I clutched the phone. This was the first time that an older doctor mentioned coming across someone they knew who was a body donor. It was also the first time I'd spoken to someone who knew so much about the dead person on the table.

While the illegal golf might have been fun, Dennis' life at medical school was otherwise a period of enormous stress. Much of what he says mirrors what others recalled so vividly—that half the cohort failed at the end of first year. It's for this reason he didn't have time to really think about where the bodies came from. He was too focused on studying and passing anatomy. When I mention that he was more than likely dissecting someone who had come from the mental asylum, his reply is one that I encountered before.

As he puts it: 'I, honestly, as a student, I did everything that I was told to do. I knew that bright people had organised the course. I never questioned anything. And I did it. And the pressure was so high! There was always one or two attempted suicides. I don't know how many died by the time we'd graduated! I know one woman had six goes, and she finally committed suicide in our final year.'

While he was focused on his studies, he and friends did muse about the skeletons they all had to have. 'The skeleton that we had came from India! It was even suggested that they were body snatched, sometimes when they might have been alive! And then they just turned them into bones to make money to sell them overseas,' he says. 'I didn't know. But that was the sort of stories that we heard.'

Ruby and Kate—Dennis' mother—were close. I remember as a little girl visiting Aunt Kate—she was soft and kindly, and we ate cake on the porch of her Brisbane home. Dennis doesn't remember much about Ruby and Julie except that Ruby had a stronger personality than her sisters, and that Julie wasn't around much. He recalls his mother saying 'Poor Ruby' and that she felt sorry for her but didn't go into details. 'That was the impression but as you can imagine as children we didn't pay much attention,' he says.

But he fills in other small details of Ruby's childhood, mentioning that his mother Kate told him that when she was a little girl in Boulder, the Wongatha people used to have corroborees at the end of the street, and she found it frightening. Ruby must've seen that too, and it chimes with another random story I'd heard about Eleanor pulling a gun on Aboriginal people who had come near the family home.

Dennis also recalls that Eleanor had terrible varicose veins—the ones that Ruby had written about in her diary, and left her in fear every night in Yarraman. 'When she stood up there were all these blue streaks all the way up to her hips almost—it was just amazing, and she had to have them all bandaged up,' says Dennis.

But most unexpected was a story he told me about my dad and his friends, who helped out a fellow engineering student at the University of Queensland who was gifted and autistic. 'He was brilliant and by the time he had graduated, the university had made him a lecturer—he was just stunning at maths but his social interactions, as they are with people who are on the spectrum, were very poor,' recalls Dennis. 'And they befriended him. And they tried to help him. And he did very well.'

Dennis and I spoke for ages about his career and life in medicine all over Australia. He said one thing he found difficult was keeping a patient alive who was about to have their organs harvested.

***

That night I wake up, and lying in the dark, my brain marauding here and there as it does at 2 or 3 am, something *clicks*.

I could never quite work out how Ruby heard about body donation, especially as the technician Leo Brown had mentioned that they never advertised. The general sense was that it was a word-of-mouth, in-the-family sort of thing to do, and I'd hypothesised that Ruby might have heard about it through one of the parents at her primary school or one of her netball friends.

Dennis was the first and only doctor I'd spoken to who knew all these details about someone in the dissecting hall—a thirty-two-year-old senior bureaucrat *who had donated his body*. He and his friends were clearly moved by someone so close to them in age dying from such an awful disease, and they somehow saw themselves in him. This donor wasn't old like so many other people in the dissecting room. He had died too young.

Dennis doesn't remember if he told his mother about this young body donor but it's likely he did, especially as it's one of the first things he tells me nearly sixty years later. He was living at home while he was a medical student and perhaps Ruby was there one afternoon, having a cup of tea, hearing him talk about his life in the dissecting halls. *Oh, can you donate your body to the university? What's it like there?*

Chapter 35

When I walk around my house pottering and playing with the indoor plants, a spike of excitement and joy strikes whenever I see a little shoot of a new baby green leaf coming through. It's the anima. It's life. It's the spark. It also means I'm not overwatering them and they are basking in the right amount of light.

In the early 1900s there was an argument that anatomy was epistemologically dead. That's it, game over, we've identified everything, let's move on from the body. In 2022 this perception persists. On top of it, some surgeons worry about the fate of the next generation of doctors as deep anatomical knowledge wanes.

But no. Little green shoots are still popping up everywhere.

Anatomists still find new stories in the human body. In the clinical wing of anatomy, even though it's rare, actual physical discoveries are still being made and when it happens, it is often excitedly reported in the mainstream press. In 2022 a number of donors helped reveal to scientists at the University of Basel a new deep third layer of the masseter muscle, which raises the lower jaw. It's been officially named 'coronoid part of the masseter'.

But the 'big news' findings aren't always through the dead. Surgical specimens taken during twelve operations found a previously unknown tissue part called *interstitium*, a macroscopic, collagen-bound, fluid-filled space between cells. The CT scans of 106 people's knees showed the *fabella*, a little bone behind the knee, was now 3.5 more times likely to show up today than it did in 1918.

The #Anatomy hashtag on Twitter gives a sense of the contemporary profession—images of cross-sections of brains, anatomy teaching tips, artistic drawings, how Covid-19 has changed the way they teach and job ads. Every so often, debates erupt and probably the biggest discoveries and shifts in anatomy are coming about because of social forces.

The passionate anatomist Jenny Hayes, who set up the body donor memorial service at the University of Melbourne and commissioned the body donor sculpture on the campus grounds, has found new inspiration in researching and doing a PhD on labiaplasty, a cosmetic procedure which is on the rise. The labia are the 'lips' at the entrance to the vagina and women are getting theirs reduced or reshaped in the quest to be so-called 'normal'.

'I could not find an anatomist's voice anywhere in labiaplasty,' she says. 'So there's all of this work internationally being done by feminists, sociologists, psychologists, historians, anthropologists, surgeons, cosmetic surgeons, but not one anatomist! When the whole topic of discussion is around "What is normal anatomy?"'

By looking at ten population-based studies that recorded labial dimensions, she found significant variation in labial length and width, and that a protruding *labia minora* was more common than not. 'They can be long or short, dark or light, wrinkled or smooth. Protruding is more common than not ... they change with age,' she says.

'And more importantly, they've got a function—they're involved in sexual pleasure, they stream urine, the flow of urine, they protect the vaginal urethral opening. And for all of that, they need to be at least a centimetre in length.'

Jenny says she's not judging people who have labiaplasty. 'I just don't want them to have it because they think they're not normal.'

She says her pitch to anatomy is that it is 'not immutable'.

'Everyone thinks that the body—we know it and all we've got to do is teach it. But it's changing because it's changing in terms of the sociopolitical context we're teaching into. And that is our student population—they've got the lived experience of that so we have to stay in touch with them.

'We have to contemporise, we have to talk about what they want. And then they won't glaze over and go, "Anatomy is hard and just tell me

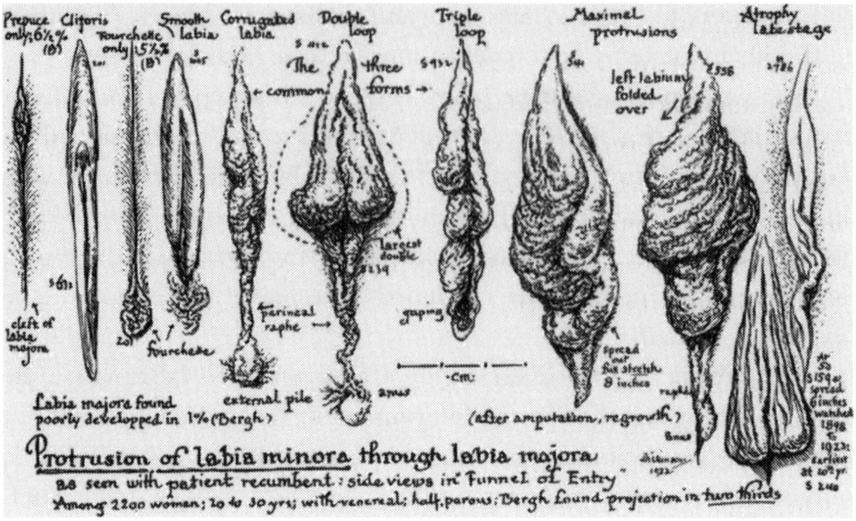

Gynecologist, medical illustrator and sex researcher Robert Latou Dickinson's 1949 drawing depicts the range of variation in the size and morphology of the labia minora. *Atlas of Human Sex Anatomy.*

what's on the exam, and I'll memorise it."' More importantly, as Jenny points out, these medical students will now know about the variations of women's labia and take this to frontline consultations, as this is what patients will be asking about.

'It looks like an improbable leap from spending so much time getting students to think about the donors and the body donor program to labiaplasty but in fact, it isn't, because it's all still about appreciating the enormous variation in human form and celebrating it rather than reducing it to one version.'

This notion of diversity has also exploded into the broader anatomical world, and the profession seems to be waking up to wider social and political movements, much of it being discussed and debated on Twitter.

In January 2021 Heather F. Smith—an anatomist, paleontologist and physical anthropologist—was made the first female editor-in-chief of *The Anatomical Record* in its 100-year history, and the first woman to lead any of the American Association of Anatomy's journals.

A year later, a special issue of the *Record* declared it was doing something it had never done before: it was discussing elements of its dark history and troubled ethics, as well as questions of diversity, equality and inclusion. Everything was on the table: structural racism in the American Association of Anatomy; eugenics; antisemitism and sexism in the profession; the ethics of Black skeletons, embryos and foetuses in collections; dissection under the Nazis; decolonising the curriculum; gender diversity; and transgender and non-binary anatomical language.

Anatomists from all over the world tuned into an Anatomy Festival in late 2021 along the theme of 'Inclusive, Diverse and Accessible'. An ever-smiling Nalini Pather co-hosted the International Federation of Associations of Anatomists event alongside Claire Smith, whose online backdrop consisted of four full-sized skeletons mounted on stands in an anatomy lab.

Nalini kicked off by exploring how anatomy textbooks largely present the human body as young, white and male. To make her point, she spoke over images of anatomised male figures who looked like they had been to the gym. Nalini said while the last three to five years had seen different types of bodies in the textbooks, she lamented that anatomy software was taking a few steps backwards, with much of the representation dominated by traditional male stereotypes. 'This highlights that the importance of inclusive representation has not really made its way into the thinking of our discipline, across the spectrum and globally,' she said.

Continuing this theme, Dr Claudia Krebs, an anatomist from the University of British Colombia, demonstrated the various ways her department had updated their collection of illustrations. Mr White Buff had been replaced with all sorts of grey-scaled characters in the anatomical position. One had a gut. One was skinny. One had thick thighs. Another page told the story of fetal circulation and featured a woman who had just had a baby. Not only was she Black, but Claudia said a decision was made to draw her with stretch marks and a bit of a belly.

Weary of systemic racism, Dr Melissa A. Carroll, an associate professor of anatomy and cell biology at George Washington University, started the not-for-profit Black in Anatomy in 2020, symbolised by a very cool-looking skull with an afro and a Black Power skeleton fist. Melissa discussed wanting to raise awareness about Black contributions to the science. 'Where were the people that looked like me in anatomy?' she asked her fellow anatomists, 'especially when we consider the bodies like mine were unceremoniously brutalized over years, decades and centuries for anatomical investigation.'

Some of the ethical issues stumped me. Dr Brendon Billings from Wits University in South Africa pondered what it meant for diversity that his medical school had gone from dissecting mainly black unclaimed bodies to now exclusively working on white donors.

'My question is do we need a diverse representation of population groups within our dissection walls that reflects our general population? I don't know. But for me personally, I definitely think I do. I'd like to see my own,' he said. 'However, is it acceptable to use unclaimed remains to achieve this diversity? And that's really the conundrum that I'd like to pitch you this evening. Do we follow an ethical platform with a lack of diversity or do we depend on unclaimed remains to ensure diversity?' (I later mentioned this conundrum to one anatomist who remarked that it didn't matter, as once you took the skin off a person, we're all the same.)

As anatomists continue to push boundaries and ask questions, some also push back into its dark past, which includes exploring what their predecessors did under the Nazis. The German anatomist Eduard Pernkopf and a team of artists first published the *Pernkopf Topographic Anatomy of Man* in 1937. Filled with 800 watercolours, it is based on the bodies of hundreds of people killed by the Nazis, many of them political prisoners, and in recent years has been considered too tainted and unethical to use. Many other German anatomists were involved in dissecting and studying the executed during the Third Reich, and clinical anatomists such as Dr Sabine Hildebrandt have attempted to document the many victims and restore their humanity by telling their stories.

I checked in with Andreas Winkelmann to see what was happening with the body donor map—which is slowly being updated—but also to ask him about his ongoing research into anatomists under the Nazis, in particular the Berliner Hermann Stieve. I asked Andreas how he felt about engaging with such terrible material.

'I was always interested in this question—when are you allowed to use bodies? And what is the context and what is the ethics behind it? And it was obvious that in the 1930s and 40s, there was no objection to take a body from somebody who was executed and give it to the anatomy department,' he says.

'There was not much debate about it—it was something traditional. Anatomists would be allowed to have the bodies of the executed. It was not against the law.' He says one has to ask if it was okay to benefit from that.

I told Andreas I found it interesting that anatomists were bringing the dissected to life, as they tended to be so 'objective' in their work. He says as these Nazi victims were treated like objects and not like mortal remains, 'one way to counteract it was by going back and giving them an identity'.

In his latest paper, Andreas reconstructed the stories of fifteen people whose names appeared on histological slides that belonged to Stieve—all executed between 1937 and 1945 for often small crimes. Arnold Hackbarth worked at a Berlin post office and was condemned to death for 'stealing parcels for cigarettes'. Margarete Jucksch, thirty-eight, and Erna Margarete Francke, forty-seven, were executed for criticising Hitler.

When he first began researching the Nazi anatomist Stieve, Andreas said he had a tendency to defend what the anatomists at the time did. But then he began thinking about it from the perspective of the victims, and the families. 'It was awful that anatomists just used the bodies and negotiated with the justice system to have the bodies directly after death,' he says. It was then he began to see that what happens to the body is part of people's biography.

'You're not dealing with the people any more, and you can't interact with them, but you will as an anatomist, if you dissect somebody, you will become part of a biography of someone. Because what happens to their remains is part of them in a way. I still know where my grandmother is buried because for me, that's part of what I know about my grandmother.'

***

There are different ways that we just don't want to know—I don't want to know about rugby league or non-fungible tokens or most PowerPoint presentations. Then there is a vehemently don't want to know—it's too painful, like a news story about a child killed by their shitty parents or a poor baby animal born in an evil zoo. There are lots of ways of wanting to know too—I can stay up all night reading a book or grip the phone as a friend tells a story about a bizarre date they had or spend days searching academic papers for answers to a historical fact. I went through a hall of mirrors of emotions of wanting to know and not wanting to know what happened to Ruby and Julie and all the other dissected people.

At one point, Sven had asked me outright: 'Do you really want to know what happened to them?' I didn't know how to answer, especially as it was a week where I was wavering—I felt like I was dishonouring them in some way or that I would upset someone or I didn't have the steel for the details. I now *sort of* know what happened to Ruby and Julie, which at times meant I had to walk away from an interview transcript, go outside and look at the sky for a break. I began to see myself as a dissector, ghoulish, disrespectful as I picked away at a past that was best left dormant.

All this time there have been things about anatomy that have burned away inside me about Ruby and Julie, and all the other dissected people—that they were just objects. I started to see why it could happen too. The deeper I got into it, I too began draping myself in an emotionally detached concern to get on with it. But I found a way back to them because ultimately, I knew this was part of their biography, and what an incredibly rich story it was.

But what settled me in the end was finally talking to people who have signed up for body donation, as well as stumbling across interviews where they talked directly about it. I see Ruby and Julie in these interviews, sitting across the kitchen table in their small Holland Park home with a cup of tea and cake.

***

Decades ago, David Jellie stood watching the undertaker come to collect an in-law who had died—it was an old aunt, and she had willed her body to the University of Melbourne. It was all very unexpected as she'd never discussed it with the family, and they only found out at the very last moment.

'It was all done with dignity,' he recalls of her body being taken away. He wasn't thinking much about his own death at the time but what she had done stuck in his head and about a decade ago, he decided to donate his body.

David is an old family friend and has known my parents since the 1960s, when they were all young Australians hanging out in London. I only found out he was a body donor after deliberating with Mum that I couldn't seem to find any—they weren't forming online groups, and the anatomists I'd spoken to seemed reluctant to connect me with them. 'Mr Jellie is a body donor,' remarked Mum casually. I pounced.

A physically big man with a big, warm personality, I knew he'd *talk* about it, that he wasn't likely to answer questions with a one-word 'yes' or 'no'.

Being a body donor makes sense to David. 'I've always been one who's participated in medical trials,' he says. He'd done one on the efficacy of taking an aspirin every day and when we spoke on the phone, he was involved with one on controlling cholesterol in the blood. 'I've always been susceptible to these sorts of things,' he jokes.

He says the other thing is he's not religious. 'I'm an atheist and I think when you're dead, you're dead,' he says. 'You're just put in the ground, and the worms will get at you or you'll just rot away to nothing. I don't believe in any hereafter or any spirits or godliness, or anything like that. So I think I've got a fairly well—not an unusual aspect about this, but death is final, and I think if my body can contribute to the learning and to improvements in medical science or improving the efficiency of surgeons so be it. And I think that was probably the main motivation for me taking it on.'

I tell him that even though I'm an atheist, I keep thinking about what would happen to my body if it were dissected.

'To me, death is finality.'

With the signed body donor forms attached to his will, he's ready to go. I ask how the family feels about it.

'My kids were quite sanguine about it. They understand. And I don't think they care much. They don't care that I'm giving my body away.' He also has no interest in a funeral. 'I suppose there's one very practical aspect of this too is there's no need for a funeral. And, you know, I don't even want to attend my own funeral. They might have a sort of a wake for me or something like that. But I don't want any official church funeral, overseen by a minister or some other appointed person. So there's also that practical side of it. I'm saving the kids probably $10,000.'

So much of what he says is a mixture of what Mum, Dad and Lindy said—it's done to help people, to save money and to avoid the bother of a funeral.

I ask him how much saving on a funeral plays into it. 'It's a peripheral thing,' he says. 'I'd have to say my consideration was not saving money. It was I think, if this can help in just a minute way—research and the development of skills, train surgeons and so forth, then, so be it.'

A trip to India got him thinking about the different ways people approach death. 'In the Hindu society, of course, burning the bodies was part of their culture. In fact, in Nepal and Bhutan, they leave the bodies out in the mountains for the vultures to pick at. And that seems to me to be the normal process,' he says. 'Really, that's not much different to giving a body to science and having research carried out.' He has a fair point: there is some symmetry between medical students and surgeons picking at a corpse like a vulture would.

***

When Hans was just eight years old, he, his mother, and his aunt wandered the streets of the small town of Wuppertal in north-western Germany looking for their relatives but all they saw were bodies, everywhere, all burned by the napalm bombs dropped during allied air raids in 1943.

Some 6000 people were killed in the town, which was targeted as it was home to a Bayer factory that made chemicals. 'All the old buildings which dated back two hundred years were partly made of wood, and it was an inferno,' he says. 'We saw the dead bodies in the rubble and the streets, and they were burned to death.'

He says this childhood experience gave him different ideas about bodies.

Hans is now eighty-seven and lives in Sydney with his wife Irme, who is originally from Czechoslovakia. The pair arrived in Sydney in 1960, and over the ensuing years he held various jobs: builder's labourer, lab technician at the University of New South Wales, and as a scientist at the Atomic Energy Commission and then the CSIRO.

During his time at the university, he worked as a biotechnology laboratory technician and his building was at a right angle to the medical school. He occasionally worked in their electron microscopy department and it was here that he saw medical students cutting up human bodies. He recalls students started out by first practising on green capsicums—they had tweezers and carefully plucked out the seeds. 'I was not involved in it—I had nothing to do with the medical school but I was interested in how they did it,' he says.

He was only in his thirties but he and Irme decided to sign up as body donors, largely because as they couldn't have children, they didn't want to bother friends or relatives with what to do with their bodies when they died. 'Nobody looks after your grave,' he chuckles. 'If you've been buried at Sutherland cemetery, there's nobody there. We decided it's just a body—why not give it to the university?'

He thinks he signed up in 1970, not long after he'd seen the dissections. At one point about thirty years ago, the couple got a letter from the university saying they had too many bodies and asked if they would be comfortable sending their bodies to a Pacific Island medical school. 'We didn't mind. If we are dead, we are dead.' He hasn't heard from the university recently.

He sounds pragmatic about dissection. 'I've never had nightmares about it or anything,' he chuckles again. Hans adds that it's a chance for the students to learn. 'Maybe they have to reset your arm or do an operation on your knee—they can have a go at my knee. They can find out how to get the cartilage out or whatever.'

***

In 2016 researchers Maria Olejaz and Klaus Hoeyer sat down with thirteen body donors and, like other researchers in this space, wanted to go beyond the 'altruism' paradigm. They found there wasn't one particular motivation—it was a mix and melding of life's events and beliefs that led them there.

For one eighty-year-old lady, after years of suffering from a rare form of arthritis, she hoped 'the students could enjoy my deformed hands that have been operated on eleven times and have had swanson plastic put in instead of bones'. Karen, seventy-seven, was equally pragmatic. 'Well, they lack such objects to practise on. On a purely cultural level I can't see any idea in burying a worn overcoat, because that is after all what our body is when we die, and I fully and firmly believe that the soul leaves the body and I am also partial to the outlook that we don't make do with living [only] one life and the universe is so infinitely big, so it might be that we get a one-way ticket to another planet, who knows.'

After hearing that Maria had interviewed donors, medical students often asked if the donors understood that they were going to be cut up. The answer? Yes. They all knew and were not frightened by the idea or how the students might treat their bodies. These donors—for all their varying reasons—wanted to be dissected.

***

Buried in Ruby's red book, I think there is a glimpse of her future path into the anatomy lab as a great body teacher to train doctors. The book is of course written at a terrible time for her—for years she had looked after her strange, slightly depressed mother both emotionally and financially, only to be deceived by her and then estranged from her sisters. But still Ruby had a sense of herself—that she was a good person:

> My sons have been talented. I've denied myself many things to ensure they're making a place for themselves in the world but then, I guess I'm no different from any other mother doing the best she can for her children. Much more could be written of my many kindnesses and yet I have been branded otherwise. I haven't lived all these years to change my nature now and it has been and still is a great happiness to be able to give to help people. One can't change their nature.

Postscript

My Uncle Maurie died when I was writing this book. Movie star looks. Into his sport and punting on the races. My dad says he was always above pettiness. I'd hoped to go and see him with Mum and Dad on Bribie Island but it just didn't happen. The Virus. The closed borders.

It's the day after his funeral and I'm lying in bed, tired and melancholy, the dregs of a Covid-19 infection in my bloodstream, thinking that as I'm back in Brisbane, I should try get in touch with the University of Queensland anatomists one more time or at least go and stand outside the anatomy school, get a sense of where Ruby and Julie ended up, where Robert stood and re-enacted *Monty Python* skits, where Frank listened to the Cassius Clay fight, where Leo spent all that time, where Juliet begrudgingly watched people smoke cigarettes.

But that part of my grandparents' story has ended.

Instead, I catch the bus to Holland Park, and stand outside Ruby and Julie's old house. It is about 8.30 am and the light is so bright I almost can't see anything. A strange, sparkling brilliance. I'm not sure what I am doing there either but I feel impelled to go. In a street filled with renovations, their house is physically the same, a bit how I remembered it all those years ago—a bit groovy, still looking a bit *Jetsons* with its unusual driveway. It's a bit rundown. A sign on the fence says 'Beware of the Dogs' and sitting in the driveway is indeed a dog to beware of, as well as another smaller one sunning itself in the bushes. I look at the retro fabric awnings on the side and they look very old, as if they could've possibly been there from my grandparents' time. What am I looking for? I could knock on the door but Ruby and Julie aren't there, and they are who I've come for.

I head out to Norman Park Public School across town, which is where Ruby taught for so many years, and where my dad studied as a child. Again, I'm not sure what I am doing but have a sense that I need to go. Emblazoned on one side of the school building is its motto *'Onwards and upwards'*.

It is school holidays. I spot a caretaker and introduce myself, explaining that my grandmother had taught at the school decades ago, and ask if it is okay if I have a quick look around? I explain I am writing a book. He says that should be all right.

It's a lovely old school with an unusual design. On the ground level is a bricked area with vaulted archways and benches and coolers for the kids to hang out. Above, on the first floor, are the classrooms—old wooden spaces with towering high ceilings. A divine breeze whooshes through the space, perfect for summer but I imagine freezing in winter, and from one end of the school, there is an expansive view out on to the city, which Ruby would've looked out on each day. She was here. I walk past the classrooms, the kids' scraggly little drawings stuck to the glass. She was here. Miss Ruby.

I find the caretaker again and thank him for letting me have a quick look around, and he asks me what the book is about. After all this time, I still don't know what to say as people aren't expecting what I will say. *It's about dissection. It's about my grandparents donating their bodies to science, and what happened, and anatomy. I find it amazing.* The caretaker is immediately interested, and begins telling me that his daughter's friend was about to start dissecting at university, and that she was feeling nervous about it. Ah, dissection. How you keep popping up in my life.

I walk back to look out at the view of the city and walk down the stairs, and look back up again at the old school, imagining my grandmother Ruby doing this, and suddenly choke up, struck by a sadness that I'm going to miss being with her and where she has taken me, and that this is the end of my time with my grandparents.

Acknowledgments

This book could not have been written with the support of my partner George. I cannot imagine anybody but him being by my side during this wonderful odyssey—a thinker, reader, proofreader, true book lover, drinker of unusual teas and interesting commentator on all things. Whenever I felt guilty about having to choose writing over family time, he would reply: 'Books don't write themselves!' Thank you! Deep love also goes to my dear son Ambrose, whose cheerfulness and vibrant mind sparked my world as I lay in bed tapping away.

Many anatomists, doctors, dentists, surgeons, technicians, biologists, scientists, artists, medical students and other characters connected to anatomy and whole-body donation spoke to me on and off the record for this book. To all of you—thank you! I'm honoured that I've captured your stories before they were lost to time. A particular thanks goes to a family friend who told me about what was at happening at her surgical centre at Christmas drinks, and Goran Štrkalj for opening that first door the led me into anatomy.

I send a crate of champagne to Pippa Masson, my agent at Curtis Brown, who has supported me for so many years. Massive thanks goes to all the staff at Ultimo Press. I feel particularly lucky to have worked with publisher Robert Watkins, who was equally fun and strict, and into wearing exciting-coloured clothes.

I send love to friends who listened to me going on about dissection, and who offered advice, cheerleading, and chats along the way: Jodi Thiessen, Anna Watts, Brigid Delaney, Mel Mackenzie, Jen Fleming, Jo Dunlop, Justin Ellis, Gregor Salmon, Steve Cannane, Saskia Kohnen, Tamara Dean, Diana Vidovic, Mike Bell and Antonia Leigh. I am also enormously grateful to Anna Whitfeld and colleagues at Late Night Live for their kindness and support. A special shout-out goes to my dear friend Bronwyn Geddes for her relaxing company and West End back porch when I was in Brisbane on research trips. And big love goes to my posse!

Waves of appreciation also go to those who assisted me in researching St Chiara of Montefalco. Angelo Mazzaferro and his mother Maria Cecilia Mazzaferro translated an obscure video of a contemporary nun discussing Chiara's holy organs, which are still in the church today. I couldn't believe my luck when Robyn Alexander, the Library Manager at the Augustinian Province Library in Brookvale said she indeed had a rare copy of Berengario's biography of Chiara in their collection.

I want to mention author, teacher and biologist Tom Cheetham. His imagination classes—held with Kimberly Christensen—have had an enormous impact on my thinking and I hope to fully deploy the teachings some day.

I'd also like to thank whoever programs SBS Chill. I found it an interesting station to listen to as I beavered away on the book.

Much appreciation goes to Aunt Lindy and Dennis Fitzsimmons for insights into the family, and cousin Kelly for her support. I also send love to my brothers Chris and Andrew for always being there for me.

Lest we forget Maurie Dent—rest in peace.

This story would not have happened without my father Desmond, with whom there is never a dull moment. Who would've known after all these years and adventures that there was such a big story at Dent HQ? Thank you for letting me tell it.

And finally, massive love must go to my unique, clever, fun and wonderful mother Elizabeth. Her years of research into the family tree—as well as her broad interest in history, graveyards, medicine and the world really—have influenced me and come to life in the most unexpected way.

I'd like to end with honouring all the great dead body teachers—known, unknown or otherwise. Where would we be without you?

Notes

Preface

The noble lie: reams has been written on this concept. For a basic working definition see Smith, R.M. (2022). *Lies: The science behind deception.* Greenwood.

'from death and dismemberment come life and order': Corristine, S. (2014). Dismemberment: A historical perspective. In S. Black (Ed.). *Criminal Dismemberment: Forensic and investigative analysis.* Crc Press.

Mother Marge story: Z'graggen, J.A. (2012). The Myth of Mother Marge: Self-sacrifice in Papuan mythology. *Anthropos.*

Sedna Sea Goddess: can be sourced from many spots, including in Shane McCorristine (2014).

Chinese dissection history: Zhang, Y. (2021). Introduction of Human Anatomy Before Modern China: The preface of anatomical education in mainland China. *Anatomical Record, 304*(11), 2632–2640.

Polly Chapman story: Richardson, R. (1987). *Death, Dissection, and the Destitute.* Routledge & Kegan Paul.

Chapter 1

'We know only too well that dissection is an abomination to the popular mind': quoted in Warner, J.H., & Rizzolo, L.J. (2006). Anatomical Instruction and Training for Professionalism from the 19th to the 21st Centuries. *Clinical Anatomy, 19*(5), 403–14.

Chapter 2

Samuel Edgerly visiting dissection rooms: Sappol, M. (2018). *A Traffic of Dead Bodies: Anatomy and embodied social identity in nineteenth-century America.* Princeton University Press.

Public lectures in Vienna: Buklijas, T. (2010). Public Anatomies in Fin-de-Siècle Vienna. *Medicine Studies, 2*(1), 71–92.

Paris morgue visits: Cain, T. (2015). Paris Morgue and a public spectacle of death. Wellcome collection. wellcomecollection.org/articles/W-RTBBEAAO5mfQ3M

Melbourne morgue visits, including head of a poor young girl: Jones, R.L. (2016). Cadavers and the Social Dimension of Dissection. In S. Wilde (Ed.), *The Body Divided: Human beings and human 'material' in modern medical history.* Routledge.

Albert Carter III: quoted from Carter, A. (1998). *First Cut: A season in the anatomy lab.* Picador.

Goran's paper: Alexander, M., Marten, M., Stewart, E., Serafin, S., Štrkalj, G. (2014). Attitudes of Australian Chiropractic Students Toward Whole Body Donation: A cross-sectional study. *Anatomical Sciences Education, 7*(2),117–123.

Global body acquisition: Štrkalj, G., El-Haddad J., Hulme A. (2020). A Global Geography of Body Acquisition for Anatomy Education: Issues, challenges and prospects. In L.K. Chan & W. Pawlina (Eds.), *Teaching Anatomy: A practical guide* (223–235). Springer, Springer Nature.

Global body donor map: Habicht, J.L., Kiessling, C., Winkelmann, A. (2018). Bodies for Anatomy Education in Medical Schools: An overview of the sources of cadavers worldwide. *Academic Medicine, 93*(9), 1293–1300.

Clementine ditty: Wilson, H. (1986). *Medicine Without Tears: Humanity and humour in the early medical school, Queensland.* Boolarong Publications.

The old anatomy is dead: Reidenberg, J.S. & Latiman, J.T. (2002). The New Face of Gross Anatomy. *The Anatomical Record, 269*(2), 81–88.

Chapter 3

Bentham's motivations: quoted in Marmoy, C.F.A. (1958). The 'Auto-Icon' of Jeremy Bentham at University College, London. *Medical History, 2*(2), 77–86.

All Gray's anatomy text found in Gray, H. (1977). *Grays Anatomy: The classic collector's edition.* Bounty Books.

General Gray's history: Richardson, R. (2008). *The Making of Mr Gray's Anatomy: Bodies, books fortune, fame.* Oxford University Press.

Carter's name as big as Gray's: statement in Elsevier Health Education (2021). The History of Gray's Anatomy with Professor Susan Standring [Video]. YouTube. https://www.youtube.com/watch?v=CDZryt3r3Kk

Anatomy being 'the most beautiful hymn': quoted page 225 in Richardson, R. (2008). *The Making of Mr Gray's Anatomy: Bodies, books fortune, fame.* Oxford University Press.

Chapter 4

Notes of an Anatomist: González-Crussi, F. (1985). *Notes of an Anatomist.* Harcourt.

Leonardo's search for the soul: Del Maestro, R.F. (1998). Leonardo da Vinci: 'The search for the soul'. *Journal of Neurosurgery, 89*(5):874-87.

Chapter 5

Boulder history: life patched together from various newspaper articles from the period, including no byline, Boulder City. (25 December 1900), *Kalgoorlie Western Argus* (WA: 1896–1916), p. 35.

Haricot bean soup recipe: 'Woman's World', (19 September 1903), *The Evening Star* (Boulder, WA: 1898–1921), p. 1.

Henry the VIII edict and gallows scuffles: Magee, R. (2001). Art Macabre: Resurrectionists and anatomists. *ANZ Journal of Surgery, 71*(6), 377–380; and Linebaugh, P. (1975). The Tyburn Riot Against the Surgeons. In D. Hay, P. Linebaugh, J.G. Rule, E.P. Thompson, C. Winstow, (Eds.), *Albion's Fatal Tree: Crime and society in eighteenth century England* (65–117). Penguin.

Bribing the hangman and giving money to condemned men, murder top up for dissection: Ward, R. (2015). The Criminal Corpse, Anatomists and the Criminal Law: Parliamentary attempts to extend the dissection of offenders in late eighteenth-century England. *Journal of British Studies, 54*(1), 63–87.

Andreas Vesalius' digging up the dead: quote from Park, K. (1994). The Criminal and the Saintly Body: Autopsy and dissection in renaissance Italy. *Renaissance Quarterly, 47*(1), 1–33.

John Bishop story: Anonymous. (1832). *The History of the London Burkers.* Accessed via Project Gutenberg; and Richardson, R. (1987). *Death, Dissection, and the Destitute.* Routledge & Kegan Paul.

Grave robbing in 19th century England: Richardson, R. (1987). *Death, Dissection, and the Destitute.* Routledge & Kegan Paul.

Bodies of US slaves used for dissection: Halperin, E.C. (2007). The Poor, the Black, and the Marginalized as the Source of Cadavers in United States Anatomical Education. *Clinical Anatomy, 20*(5), 489–95.

Structural violence: Nystrom, K.C. (2014). The Bioarchaeology of Structural Violence and Dissection in the 19th-Century United States: Structural violence and dissection. *American Anthropologist, 116*(4), 765–779.

Sydney dissection at the Mint, dog food story: Starr, F. (2017). The 'Sidney Slaughter House': Convict experience of medical care at the general 'rum' hospital, Sydney, 1816–1848, *Health and History, 19*(2), 60–89.

1876 law: 'a most significant amendment was made to the Medical Practitioners Statute 1865 Part IV that enabled all unclaimed asylum bodies, the bodies of prisoners and those who died in public institutions to be used for dissection by medical staff teaching anatomy at the University of Melbourne' quoted in MacKinnon D. (2016). Bodies of Evidence: Dissecting madness in colonial Victoria. In S. Wilde & S. Ferber (Eds.), *The Body Divided: Human beings and human 'material' in modern medical history.* Routledge.

Unclaimed bodies sent for dissection in Australia until the 1980s: Ross Jones in chapter 'Cadavers and the Social Dimension of Dissection' writes: 'From 1951 until 1983 under direction from the Chief Secretary, the Department of Mental Hygiene supplied bodies from its institutions to the university for the purpose of dissection. See Public Record Office of Victoria series VPRS 7688 "Record of Subjects sent to School of Anatomy, University of Melbourne".' In S. Wilde &

S. Ferber (Eds.), *The Body Divided: Human beings and human 'material' in modern medical history*. Routledge.

Nazi dissection statistics: Hildebrandt, S. (2022). Books, Bones and Bodies: The relevance of the history of anatomy in Nazi Germany for medical education today. *Anatomical Record, 305*(4), 886–901.

Hermann Stieve: Seidelman, W. (2000). The Legacy of Academic Medicine and Human Exploitation in the Third Reich. *Perspectives in Biology and Medicine, 43*(3), 325–334.

Chapter 6

'A dog can be an animal, a pet, a friend, a police officer, or something soft.': Contreras Kallens, P.A., Dale, R., & Smaldino, P.E. (2018). Cultural Evolution of Categorization. *Cognitive Systems Research, 52*, 765–774.

Sir John Knill biographical information: Anonymous. (1853, November) Correspondence of Sylvanus Urbanus. *The Gentleman's magazine, Volume 40 and* Baring-Gould, S. (1909). *Cornish Characters and Strange Events.* J. Lane.

Sir John Knill will found by Elizabeth Dent (Mum) at: All England & Wales Prerogative Court of Canterbury Wills Prob11 Will Register 1811—1814 Piece 1521 Quire159-213 (1811) Seen online at Ancestry.

Fact John Knill wasn't dissected: Anonymous. (1845, November). A letter by a 'near relative of John Knill'. *The Gentleman's Magazine.* Volume 40, page 482.

Bentham possible autism diagnosis: Lucas, P., & Sheeran, A. (2006). Asperger's Syndrome and the Eccentricity and Genius of Jeremy Bentham. *Journal of Bentham Studies, 08*, 1–37.

Bentham reading Latin: UCL, (2018). *About Jeremy Bentham.* www.ucl.ac.uk/bentham-project/about-jeremy-bentham

Bentham seeing dissection at Oxford: Bentham, J. (2017). In T. Sprigge (Ed.), *The Correspondence of Jeremy Bentham, Volume 1: 1752–76.* UCL Press.

'Use of the Dead to the Living': Southwood Smith, T. (1827). *Use of the Dead to the Living: From the Westminster Review.* Websters and Skinners.

Bentham writing Anatomy Act: Richardson, R., & Hurwitz, B. (1987). Jeremy Bentham's Self Image: An exemplary bequest for dissection. *BMJ (Clinical Research Ed.), 295*(6591), 195–198.

Bentham hair paintings: Marmoy, C. (1958). The 'Auto-Icon' of Jeremy Bentham at University College, London. *Medical History, 2*(2), 77–86.

Description of Bentham's 'dissection': see above.

Can you look on the sweetness?: Southwood Smith, T. (1832). A Lecture Delivered Over the Remains of Jeremy Bentham, Esq. Accessed via Wellcome Collection. https://wellcomecollection.org/works/bjf39kvb

John Stuart Mill on Bentham: Lucas, P., & Sheeran, A. (2006). Asperger's Syndrome and the Eccentricity and Genius of Jeremy Bentham. *Journal of Bentham Studies.*

86–1955. *Journal of the History of Medicine and Allied Sciences, 72*(2),193–218.
ilson, J.A. (2006). Anatomical Nomenclature of Fossil Vertebrates: Standardized
·ms or 'Lingua Franca'? *Journal of Vertebrate Paleontology, 26*(3), 511–18.
ative eponyms: Buttner, R., Lee, J., & Cadogan, M. (2020). De-eponymizing
atomical Terminology. *Emergency Medicine News, 42*(10), 29–30.
n Draper and pudendum: Draper, A. (2021). The History of the Term
dendum: Opening the discussion on anatomical sex inequality. *Clinical Anatomy,*
(2), 315–319; and Gross, R. (2021, Sept 21). Taking the 'Shame Part' Out of
male Anatomy. *The New York Times.* https://www.nytimes.com/2021/09/21/
ence/pudendum-women-anatomy.html
mical position development: Wilson, J.A. (2006). Anatomical Nomenclature
Fossil Vertebrates: Standardized terms or 'Lingua Franca'? *Journal of Vertebrate*
leontology, 26(3), 511–18.
ford anatomists and the anatomical position: Greulich, W.W., Bacon, R.L.,
ssett, D.L., Danforth, C.H., Gray, D.J., Kirkman, H., & Turner, R.S. (1945).
rms of Position and Direction in the NK-INA revision of the Basle Nomina
atomica. *The Anatomical Record, 92(*4), 359–362.
ups between Mammal and Avian: again Jeffrey Wilson.

ter 8

uis de Sade private dissection room: Ariès, P. (1981). *The Hour of our Death.*
fred A. Knopf.
as W. Laqueur quote: Laqueur, T.W. (2015). *The Work of the Dead: A cultural*
story of mortal remains. Princeton: Princeton University Press.
bodies as a source of pollution: von Staden, H. (1992). The Discovery of
e Body: human dissection and its cultural contexts in ancient Greece. *The Yale*
rnal of biology and medicine, 65(3), 223–241.
Charles II drinking skull drops and Dr Christian Friedrich Garmann's
onders of the corpse: The brilliant Ariès, P. (1981). *The Hour of Our Death.*
fred A. Knopf. References on 357–358.
es about funeral parlour in Woollahra: Taylor, A. (2021, July 4). Dining
xt to death: Residents object to funeral home neighbouring restaurant. *Sydney*
orning Herald. https://www.smh.com.au/national/nsw/dining-next-to-death-
sidents-object-to-funeral-home-neighbouring-restaurant-20210701-p585zq.html
into Guidetti rejected at coffeehouses: Märker, A. (2006). The Anatomical
odels of La Specola: production, uses, and reception. *Nuncius, 21*(2), 295–321.
s for funeral directors and anatomical prosectors: Checked on Seek.com in
ay 2022.
ction videos on YouTube: Anatomy Innsbruck. (2021, Feb.11). How to
ssect Muscles and Fascia [Video]. YouTube. https://www.youtube.com/
atch?v=LrRSXZQu8xI

Society of Mutal Autopsy: Hecht, J. (2005). *The End of the S*
atheism, and anthropology in France. Columbia University P

Miss Elizabeth R. Branson's body to science: Anonymous.
her body to science. *Warwick Examiner and Times*. http://n
article82114646

Arthur Polkinghorne body to science: Anonymous. (1931, J
journalist Mr. A. Polkinghorne Passes Body to Science. *T*
Darling Downs Gazette. http://nla.gov.au/nla.news-article2

Frederick James body to science: Anonymous. (1910, July 1
suicide bequeaths his body to science. *The Age*. http://nla.g
article191344789

Seraphin Desire Casile: Anonymous. (1938, Jan 7). Offers B
Wiluna Miner. http://nla.gov.au/nla.news-article25806925

The young man in the Royal Botanical Gardens: Anonym
22). Disgusted with Mankind. *The Newcastle Sun*. http://nl
article163177116

Vienna letters, Anna Astl-Leonhard 'I was never hysterica
(2010.) Public Anatomies in Fin-de-Siècle Vienna. *Medici*

Thai professor donating his body: Winkelmann, A., & Güld
Cadavers as Teachers: The dissecting room experience in
Research Ed.), 329(7480), 1455–1457.

The poetess: Anonymous. (1953, April 9.) Will in Handbag 7
The Sun. http://nla.gov.au/nla.news-article229733824

Chapter 7

For general early dissection history: See Persaud, T.V.N, L
S.R. (2014). *A History of Human Anatomy*. Charles C. Thor
Ghosh, S.K. (2015). Human Cadaveric Dissection: A hist
ancient Greece to the modern era. *Anatomy & Cell Biology*

Mondino de Luzzi: Mavrodi, A., & Paraskevas, G. (2014). M
A luminous figure in the darkness of the Middle Ages. *Cro*

1405 regulations: Ferrari, G. (1987). Public Anatomy Lesson
The anatomy theatre of Bologna. *Past & Present, 117*(1), 5

Vesalius putting naked woman on cover quote: Park, K. (20
Gender, Generation, and the Origins of Human Dissection. Zon
Extraordinary work!

Details about Vesalius' Fabrica: Case Western Reserve Univ
The Body in the Book: The Fabrica and the Epitome (1543). [V
https://www.youtube.com/watch?v=v2IA-eIxG4o

Cleaning up anatomical nomenclature and development o
The Science and Politics of Naming: Reforming anatomic

1886–1955. *Journal of the History of Medicine and Allied Sciences, 72*(2),193–218.
Wilson, J.A. (2006). Anatomical Nomenclature of Fossil Vertebrates: Standardized terms or 'Lingua Franca'? *Journal of Vertebrate Paleontology, 26*(3), 511–18.

Alternative eponyms: Buttner, R., Lee, J., & Cadogan, M. (2020). De-eponymizing Anatomical Terminology. *Emergency Medicine News, 42*(10), 29–30.

Allison Draper and pudendum: Draper, A. (2021). The History of the Term Pudendum: Opening the discussion on anatomical sex inequality. *Clinical Anatomy,* 34(2), 315–319; and Gross, R. (2021, Sept 21). Taking the 'Shame Part' Out of Female Anatomy. *The New York Times.* https://www.nytimes.com/2021/09/21/science/pudendum-women-anatomy.html

Anatomical position development: Wilson, J.A. (2006). Anatomical Nomenclature of Fossil Vertebrates: Standardized terms or 'Lingua Franca'? *Journal of Vertebrate Paleontology, 26*(3), 511–18.

Standford anatomists and the anatomical position: Greulich, W.W., Bacon, R.L., Bassett, D.L., Danforth, C.H., Gray, D.J., Kirkman, H., & Turner, R.S. (1945). Terms of Position and Direction in the NK-INA revision of the Basle Nomina Anatomica. *The Anatomical Record, 92(*4), 359–362.

Breakups between Mammal and Avian: again Jeffrey Wilson.

Chapter 8

Marquis de Sade private dissection room: Ariès, P. (1981). *The Hour of our Death.* Alfred A. Knopf.

Thomas W. Laqueur quote: Laqueur, T.W. (2015). *The Work of the Dead: A cultural history of mortal remains.* Princeton: Princeton University Press.

Dead bodies as a source of pollution: von Staden, H. (1992). The Discovery of the Body: human dissection and its cultural contexts in ancient Greece. *The Yale journal of biology and medicine, 65*(3), 223–241.

King Charles II drinking skull drops and Dr Christian Friedrich Garmann's wonders of the corpse: The brilliant Ariès, P. (1981). *The Hour of Our Death.* Alfred A. Knopf. References on 357–358.

Worries about funeral parlour in Woollahra: Taylor, A. (2021, July 4). Dining next to death: Residents object to funeral home neighbouring restaurant. *Sydney Morning Herald.* https://www.smh.com.au/national/nsw/dining-next-to-death-residents-object-to-funeral-home-neighbouring-restaurant-20210701-p585zq.html

Giancinto Guidetti rejected at coffeehouses: Märker, A. (2006). The Anatomical Models of La Specola: production, uses, and reception. *Nuncius, 21*(2), 295–321.

Wages for funeral directors and anatomical prosectors: Checked on Seek.com in May 2022.

Dissection videos on YouTube: Anatomy Innsbruck. (2021, Feb.11). How to Dissect Muscles and Fascia [Video]. YouTube. https://www.youtube.com/watch?v=LrRSXZQu8xI

Society of Mutal Autopsy: Hecht, J. (2005). *The End of the Soul: Scientific modernity, atheism, and anthropology in France*. Columbia University Press.

Miss Elizabeth R. Branson's body to science: Anonymous. (1879, March 22.) Gave her body to science. *Warwick Examiner and Times*. http://nla.gov.au/nla.news-article82114646

Arthur Polkinghorne body to science: Anonymous. (1931, July 25). Brisbane journalist Mr. A. Polkinghorne Passes Body to Science. *Toowoomba Chronicle and Darling Downs Gazette*. http://nla.gov.au/nla.news-article254210941

Frederick James body to science: Anonymous. (1910, July 1.) Intending suicide bequeaths his body to science. *The Age*. http://nla.gov.au/nla.news-article191344789

Seraphin Desire Casile: Anonymous. (1938, Jan 7). Offers Body for Science. *The Wiluna Miner*. http://nla.gov.au/nla.news-article258069257

The young man in the Royal Botanical Gardens: Anonymous. (1923, Oct 22). Disgusted with Mankind. *The Newcastle Sun*. http://nla.gov.au/nla.news-article163177116

Vienna letters, Anna Astl-Leonhard 'I was never hysterical': quoted in Buklijas, T. (2010.) Public Anatomies in Fin-de-Siècle Vienna. *Medicine Studies*. *2*(1), 71–92.

Thai professor donating his body: Winkelmann, A., & Güldner, F.H. (2004). Cadavers as Teachers: The dissecting room experience in Thailand. *BMJ (Clinical Research Ed.)*, *329*(7480), 1455–1457.

The poetess: Anonymous. (1953, April 9.) Will in Handbag 7 years. (1953, April 19). *The Sun*. http://nla.gov.au/nla.news-article229733824

Chapter 7

For general early dissection history: See Persaud, T.V.N, Loukas, M., & Tubbs, S.R. (2014). *A History of Human Anatomy*. Charles C. Thomas. Also check out Ghosh, S.K. (2015). Human Cadaveric Dissection: A historical account from ancient Greece to the modern era. *Anatomy & Cell Biology*, *48*(3), 153–69.

Mondino de Luzzi: Mavrodi, A., & Paraskevas, G. (2014). Mondino de Luzzi: A luminous figure in the darkness of the Middle Ages. *Croat Med J*, *55*(1), 50–3.

1405 regulations: Ferrari, G. (1987). Public Anatomy Lessons and the Carnival: The anatomy theatre of Bologna. *Past & Present*, *117*(1), 50–106.

Vesalius putting naked woman on cover quote: Park, K. (2006). *Secrets of Women: Gender, Generation, and the Origins of Human Dissection*. Zone Books. Extraordinary work!

Details about Vesalius' Fabrica: Case Western Reserve University. (2015, April). *The Body in the Book: The Fabrica and the Epitome (1543)*. [Video]. YouTube. https://www.youtube.com/watch?v=v2IA-eIxG4o

Cleaning up anatomical nomenclature and development of TA: Buklijas, T. (2017). The Science and Politics of Naming: Reforming anatomical nomenclature, ca.

Sanyal, S. (2018, Aug.10). Exenterated Eyeball 1—Conjunctival Dissection with Clinical Aspects – Sanjoy Sanyal.

Anatomy Made Easy (2019, Mar 3). Dissection—Removal of Brain.

Bodies R Us: Champney, T.H., Hildebrandt, S., Jones, G.D., & Winkelmann, A. (2019). BODIES R US: Ethical views on the commercialization of the dead in medical education and research. *Anatomical Scientific Education, 12*(3), 317–325.

Chapter 9

Tzu Chi University in Hualien Lin, S.C., Hsu, J., & Fan, V. (2009). 'Silent Virtuous Teachers': Anatomical dissection in Taiwan. *BMJ (Clinical Research Ed.) 339* (December): b5001.

Master Cheng Yen background: Huang, C. J. (2009). *Charisma and Compassion: Cheng Yen and the Buddhist Tzu Chi movement.* Harvard University Press.

Dr Angelina Whalley: Chambless, R. (2008). The Leonardo podcast.

LEEC Anatomical Sciences stall: LEEC stands for Laboratory, Electrical, Engineering Company. https://www.leec.co.uk/about-us/

Showman/pushing the boundaries of embalming: Morbid Anatomy. (2021). Lecture by Dr John. Troyer, Centre for Death and Society, University of Bath. Bodies Embalmed by Us NEVER TURN BLACK!: A Brief History of the Hyperstimulated Human Corpse.

Why did Joseph Jernigan donate?: Rothman, D. (1996). *NetWorld: What people are really doing on the Internet, and what it means to you.* Murderpedia.org https://murderpedia.org/male.J/j1/jernigan-joseph-paul.htm

Details of Jernigan's scanning: Spitzer, V., Ackerman, M. J., Scherzinger, A. L., & Whitlock, D. (1996). The Visible Human Male: A technical report. *Journal of the American Medical Informatics Association, 3*(2), 118–130.

Team liaising with death row: Ackerman, M. J. (2022). The Visible Human Project. *Information Services and Use, 42*(1), 129–136.

Chapter 10

Walter Wood interview: Fidler, R. (Host). (2016, April). Walter Wood: dignifying body donation [Audio podcast episode]. In *Conversations with Richard Fidler.* Australian Broadcasting Corporation. https://www.abc.net.au/local/stories/2016/04/14/4443060.htm

Details about cervical cancer: Löwy, I. (2011). *A Woman's Disease: The history of cervical cancer.* Oxford University Press.

Details about brain fever: Peterson, A.C. (1976). Brain Fever in Nineteenth-Century Literature: Fact and fiction. *Victorian Studies, 19*(4), 445–64.

Chapter 11

First ever body donor study: Fennell, S., & Jones, D. G. (1992). The Bequest of Human Bodies for Dissection: A case study in the Otago Medical School. *The New Zealand Medical Journal, 105*(946), 472–74.

Peking Union Medical College research: Zhang, C. et al (2022). Analysis of Population Representation Among Willed Whole-Body Donors to Facilitate the Construction of a Body Donation Program in China: From the perspective of medical students and anatomists. *Omega: Journal of Death and Dying*, *84*(4), 1146–1159.

Brazil body donor profile: da Rocha, A.O. et al (2017). Using Body Donor Demographics to Assist the Implementation of Donation Programs in Brazil. *Anatomical Sciences Education*, *10*(5), 475–486.

Thailand's body donors: Techataweewan, N. et al (2018). Human Body Donation in Thailand: Donors at Khon Kaen University. *Annals of Anatomy*, *216*, 142–151.

Turkey research: Gürses, Ertaş, A. et al (2019). Profile and Motivations of Registered Whole Body Donors in Turkey: Istanbul University experience. *Anatomical Sciences Education*, *12*(4), 370–385.

Hong Kong studies: Chiu, H. Y et al (2012). Voices of Donors: Case reports of body donation in Hong Kong. *Anatomical Sciences Education, 5*(5), 295–300.

Dutch research: Bolt, S. et al (2010). Motivation for Body Donation to Science: More than an altruistic act. *Annals of Anatomy – Anatomischer Anzeiger, 192*(2), 70–74.

Chapter 13

Picture of first person to be dissected at UQ in 1927: Image in Doherty, R.L. (1986). *A Medical School for Queensland.* Boolarong Publications.

Goodna mental hospital statistics: Finnane, M. (2008). Wolston Park Hospital 1865–2001: A retrospect. *Queensland Review*, *15*(2), 39–58.

Goodna escapee: Goodna Asylum Escapee. (1927, January 18). *The Brisbane Courier (Qld. : 1864–1933)*, p. 9, from http://nla.gov.au/nla.news-article21107487

Goodna strike: Low Wages in Asylums Unfair to Patients. 1927, March 25. *Daily Standard (Brisbane, Qld. : 1912–1936)*, p. 1 (SECOND EDITION-3 p.m.) from http://nla.gov.au/nla.news-article185453755

QLD cabinet approves bodies from Goodna and Diamantina Hospital, Ernie Bagnall applies for job at school: Doherty, R.L. (1986). *A Medical School for Queensland.* Boolarong Publications.

Chapter 14

Gandhi on dissection: Copeman, J. (2006). Cadaver Donation as Ascetic Practice in India. *Social Analysis*, *50*(1), 103–126.

Alok Kumar back story: Kumar, A. Patron's message. *Dadhichi Deh Dan Samiti.* https://dehdan.org/president_message.html

Jyoti Basu dissection details: Mandal, S. & Banerjee, T. (2010, January 28). Basu Brain Preserved. *The Telegraph.* https://www.telegraphindia.com/india/basu-brain-preserved/cid/555972

Basu obituary: Bhushan Rawat, V. (2010, 18 January). Remembering Jyoti Basu. *Countercurrents.* https://www.countercurrents.org/rawat180110.htm

Greek body donation: Papagaroufali, E. (1999.) Donation of Human Organs or Bodies after Death: A cultural phenomenology of 'flesh' in the Greek context. *Ethos, 27*(3), 283–314.

Body donor funerals: Bolt, S., & Venbrux, E. (2010). Funerals Without a Corpse: Awkwardness in mortuary rituals for body donors. In A. Michaels (Ed.) *Ritual Dynamics and the Science of Ritual: Body, performance, and experience*. Harrassowitz.

Chapter 16

Mouldy bodies at USYD in 1883: The University of Sydney. (2008). *A Slice of Life: The development of anatomy and dissection at the Faculty of Medicine.* (Exhibition booklet).

Chapter 17

History of the word 'section', rise of 'anatomy' in book titles: Sugg, R. (2007). *Murder After Death: Literature and anatomy in early modern England.* Cornell University Press.

Cambridge University study with medical students apologising to bodies: Douglas-Jones, R. (2020). 'Silent mentors': Donation, education, and bodies in Taiwan. *Medicine Anthropology Theory, 4*(4), 69–98.

Med students group photos, Renée Fox and 'sufficiently detached': Warner, J.H. & Rizzolo, L.J. (2006). Anatomical Instruction and Training for Professionalism from the 19th to the 21st Centuries. *Clinical Anatomy 19*(5), 403–14.

'Cadavers are persons and things': Prentice, R. (2012). *Bodies in Formation: An ethnography of anatomy and surgery education.* Duke University Press.

Chapter 18

Formaldehyde discovery: Fox, C.H. et al (1985). Formaldehyde Fixation. *Journal of Histochemistry & Cytochemistry, 33*(8), 845–53.

Frederik Ruysch using clotted pig's blood, Berlin blue and mercury oxide: Brenner, E. (2014). Human Body Preservation—Old and New Techniques. *Journal of Anatomy, 224*(3), 316–44.

Thiel background: Denis-Rodríguez, E., & Aguirre-Gutiérrez, A.A. (2018). Thiel Soft-Fix Method for Long Term Preservation Review Article. *Rev mex Med Forense, 3*(2), 91–98.

Friedrich Anderhuber, Dr Thiel's assistant: Cain, P. (2013, June 15). The Living

Dead: New embalming method aids surgical training. *British Broadcasting Corporation*. https://www.bbc.com/news/health-22908661

Erich Brenner paper on embalming, University of Sydney mixes: Brenner, E. (2014). Human Body Preservation—Old and New Techniques. *Journal of Anatomy. 224*(3), 316–44.

How to plastinate: Body Worlds. Plastination. *Körperwelten*. https://bodyworlds.com/plastination/plastination-technique/

Chapter 19

Calcutta skeleton trade: Stephan, C. et al (2017). Complexities and Remedies of Unknown-provenance Osteology. In G. Štrkalj and N. Pather (Eds.), *Commemorations and Memorials: Exploring the human face of anatomy*. World Scientific.

Chapter 21

Maclise and homoerotic work: Sappol, M. (2021). Mr Joseph Maclise and the Epistemology of the Anatomical Closet. *British Art Studies*.

Maclise edition different in the US: interesting discussion between Ludmilla Jordanova and William Schupbach c/o Paul Mellon Centre for Studies in British Art. (2021, July 21). *Joseph Maclise's Anatomical Atlases: His Works and Influences*. [Video]. YouTube. https://www.youtube.com/watch?v=Bma7VvPat-Y

The dead used by Clemente for his works, body numbers, Susini bitching about cemetery worker: Märker, A. (2006). The Anatomical Models of La Specola: Production, uses, and reception. *Nuncius, 21*(2), 295–321

'Little Venus' cause of death: Mazzotti, F. et al. (2010). The Diagnosis of the Cause of the Death of Venerina. *Journal of Anatomy, 216*(2), 271–274.

John Bell quote: Dream Anatomy Gallery National Institute of Health. Engravings of the bones, muscles, and joints, illustrating the first volume of the Anatomy of the Human Body. 2d ed. *US National library of medicine*. https://sites.nlm.nih.gov/exhibition/dreamanatomy/da_g_II-B-6.html

Scientists creating facts: Latour, B., & Woolgar, S. (2013). In J. Salk (Ed.), *Laboratory Life: The construction of scientific facts*. Princeton University Press.

Head sawing video: Anatomy Made Easy (2019, Mar 3). *Dissection–Removal of Brain*. [Video]. YouTube. https://www.youtube.com/watch?v=bqGzvuG6CVU&t=407s

Chapter 23

Fahrer and R Tubiana palmaris longus: Fahrer, M., & Tubiana, R. (1976). Palmaris Longus, Anteductor of the Thumb: An experimental study. *The Hand, 8*(3), 287–289.

Abductor digiti minimi paper: Fahrer, M., & Millroy, J. (1981). Ulnar Compression Neuropathy Due to an Anomalous Abductor Digiti Minimi—Clinical and Anatomic Study. *The Journal of Hand Surgery, 6*(3), 266–268.

J Littler on spira mirabilis: Littler, J.W. (1973). On the Adaptability of Man's Hand. *The Hand, 5*(187).

Fahrer egg paper from 1973: Fahrer, M. (1973). Fingers Toes, Palmar and Plantar Arches. Presented at *XIII Biennial Congress of the Australian Physiotherapy Association,* published 1974 *Australian Journal of Physiotherapy, 20*(4), 166–168.

Hand paper that freaked me out: Fahrer, M. (1980). The Proximal End of the Palmar Aponeurosis. *The Hand, 12*(1), 33–38.

Fahrer obituary: Chapuis, P., Obituary of Marius Fahrer. *Royal Australasian College of Surgeons.* https://www.surgeons.org/en/about-racs/about-the-college-of-surgeons/in-memoriam/obituaries/marius-fahrer

Anatomy seen as epistemologically exhausted and Dr Carl Hamann describing it as 'fixed and unchangeable': quoted in Warner, J.H. & Rizzolo, L.J. (2006). Anatomical Instruction and Training for Professionalism from the 19th to the 21st Centuries. *Clinical Anatomy, 19*(5), 403–14.

Quentin's dissection series: BBC Studios. (2015). Dissecting A Human Foot, 'Hands and Feet' [Video]. YouTube. https://www.youtube.com/watch?v=8Bkxyy5g0g0

Sawday and Renaissance dissection: Sawday, J. (1995). *The Body Emblazoned: dissection and the human body in Renaissance culture.* Routledge.

Chapter 24

Sue Black on body farms: Black, S. (2017). Body Farms. *Forensic Science, Medicine, and Pathology, 13*(4), 475–476.

Total body score: Megyesi, M.S., Nawrocki, S.P., & Haskell, N.H. (2005). Using Accumulated Degree-days to Estimate the Postmortem Interval from Decomposed Human Remains. *Journal of Forensic Sciences, 50*(3), 618–626.

Maiken interview: Katsnelson, A. (2021, October 3). Forensic chemist Maiken Ueland examines emissions from human remains. *Chemical and Engineering News.* https://cen.acs.org/analytical-chemistry/forensic-science/Forensic-chemist-Maiken-Ueland-examines/99/i36

Maiken research: Ueland, M., Harris, S., & Forbes, S.L. (2021). Detecting Volatile Organic Compounds to Locate Human Remains in a Simulated Collapsed Building. *Forensic Science International (Online), 323.*

Vesalius 'know oursleves': Sawday, J. (2015). The Fabrica Remade: A new translation of the De Humani Corporis Fabrica Libri Septem (1543, 1555) of Andreas Vesalius. *Isis, 106*(3), 677–683.

Maiken and the tusks: Ueland, M. et al. (2020). Profiling Volatilomes: A novel forensic method for identification of confiscated illegal wildlife items. *Separations, 7*(1), 5.

Val Plumwood: Plumwood, V. (1993). *Feminism and the Mastery of Nature.* Routledge, London.

Chapter 25

Zoroastrians and the universe in the body: Shoja, M.M., & Tubbs, R.S. (2007). The History of Anatomy in Persia. *Journal of Anatomy*, *210*(4), 359–378.

Information about Integrated Pathology Learning Centre: School of Biomedical Sciences. Integrated Pathology Learning Centre—History. *University of Queensland.* https://biomedical-sciences.uq.edu.au/facilities/integrated-pathology-learning-centre

Jessica Mitford part of 20th rise in body donation: Garment, A., Lederer, S., Rogers, N., & Boult, L. (2007). Let the Dead Teach the Living: The rise of body bequeathal in 20th-century America. *Academic Medicine*, *82*(10),1000–1005.

The Murray Black and Berry collections: Victorian Aboriginal Heritage Council. An historical overview of the desecration of Aboriginal burial places and repatriation of Ancestors back to Country. https://www.aboriginalheritagecouncil.vic.gov.au/historical-overview

History of dissection talk: Collection of Historical Scientific Instruments. (2015, March). *500 Years of Human Dissection.* [Video]. YouTube. https://www.youtube.com/watch?v=R1HoeKDPO6Q

Book about Vrolik: Rooy L., et al (2009). *Forces of Form.* Netherlands: Amsterdam University Press.

Chapter 26

Maurice Twomey court case and documents admitting to asylum: all researched by Elizabeth Dent. Maurice at times listed as Morris Twomey in Asylum records. See Public Records Office of North Melbourne, Victoria: Medical Certificates & a Statement from wife Sarah before Admission to Kew Asylum Admission Reg of Patients Kew Asylum 1817–1919, VPRS 7680 P1 / Nominal Reg of Patients at Kew Asylum 1871–1906, Discharge To Beechworth Asylum VPRS 7425/ P1 CVA 2840 / Case books of Male Patients Beechworth Asylum VPRS 7395 P1 / Inquest & Coronial Inquiry Morris Twomey Beechworth 1906 VPRS 24/P0000/800 1906/1151.

ANCESTRY online—Kew Asylum Male Case books 1871–1912, VPRS 7398 P1/ Vol13 P163. Birth Death Marriage Register Victoria—Death Certificate of Morris Twomey 1906.

Postmortems on asylum patients between 1850 and 1900 and general details: Mackinnon, D. (2012). Bodies of Evidence: Dissecting madness in colonial Victoria (Australia) *The Body Divided: Human beings and human 'material' in modern medical history*. Routledge.

Chapter 27

Material on ancient Egyptian life and Herophilus patched together from: Von Staden, H. (1989). *Herophilus: The art of medicine in early Alexandria: Edition, translation, and essays*. Cambridge University Press.

Harris, W.V., & Ruffini, G. (2004). Ancient Alexandria between Egypt and Greece. BRILL.

Loon, A.J. van (2014). Law and Order in Ancient Egypt. The Development of Criminal Justice from the Pharaonic New Kingdom until the Roman Dominate, [Masters thesis, Leiden university], Student repository.

Erskine, A. (2002). Life after Death: Alexandria and the body of Alexander. *Greece and Rome, 49*(2), 163–179. Jackson, R. (1988). *Doctors and Diseases in the Roman Empire.* British Museum Press. Marie, M. (2020, Dec 6). The Ancient Egyptians rigorously fought corruption. *Egypt Today.* https://www.egypttoday.com/Article/4/95029/The-Ancient-Egyptians-rigorously-fought-corruption

'he was to be taken from his cell and laid open while still alive, and while still breathing, the doctors': this line is from Celsus' first century tome *De Medicina,* republished in Jackson, R. (1988). *Doctors and Diseases in the Roman Empire.* British Museum Press.

Wang Sun-Qing and Ou Xi-Fan dissected: Schnorrenberger, C.C. (2013) Anatomical Roots of Acupuncture and Chinese Medicine. *Swiss Journal of Integrative Medicine, 25*(2), 110–118.

Cotula and Sancta dissected: French, R. (1999). *Dissection and Vivisection in the European Renaissance*. Ashgate.

Lazaro the glass eater: Moes, R.J., & O'Malley, C.D. (1960). Realdo Colombo: 'On those things rarely found in anatomy'. An Annotated Translation From the 'De Re Anatomica' (1559*). Bulletin of the History of Medicine, 34*(6), 508–528.

Vesalius' dissected: Biesbrouck, M., & Steeno, O. (2014). Andreas Vesalius' Corpses. *Acta Medico-historica Adriatica, 12*(1), 9–26.

Bartolomea Rinieri dissection: Park, K. (1994). The Criminal and the Saintly Body: Autopsy and dissection in renaissance Italy. *Renaissance Quarterly, 47*(1), 1–33.

Young women dissected: Hurren, E. (2012). Dying for Victorian Medicine English Anatomy and its Trade in the Dead Poor, c.1834–1929. Palgrave Macmillan UK.

Early anatomies, including Chiara: Park, K. (2006). *Secrets of Women: Gender, generation, and the origins of human dissection.* Zone Books. Extraordinary work!

Details of Chiara's life and dissection: Berengario, O'Connell, M. J., & Rotelle, J.E. (1999). *Life of Saint Clare of Montefalco*. Augustinian Press. Klotz, M. (2001). Clare of Montefalco (1268–1308), the life of the soul is the love of God, [Thesis, University of Toronto], Tspace.

Susrata: See Persaud, T.V.N, Loukas, M., & Tubbs, S.R. (2014). *A History of Human Anatomy.* Charles C Thomas.

Lloyd and Ganz take on vivisection: Ganz, J. (2014). Herophilus and Vivisection: A re-appraisal. *History of Medicine, 4*(4).

Mihaly Csikszentmihalyi and flow: Csikszentmihalyi, M. (1991). *Flow: The psychology of optimal experience.* HarperCollins.

Chapter 29

Australian medical education: Geffen, L. (2014). A Brief History of Medical Education and Training in Australia. *Medical Journal of Australia, 201*(S1), S19–S22.

Is anatomy necessary: Fahrer, M. (2001). Art Macabre: Is anatomy necessary? *ANZ Journal of Surgery, 71*(6), 333–334.

Chapter 30

Cooper comments: The House of Commons. (22 July 1828). *Report from the Select Committee on Anatomy.*

Chapter 31

UQP statement: McMillan, A. (2016, December). *Statement from UQP regarding 'Skeleton School', December 2016.* [Statement on website].

Professor Claire Smith: Smith, C. (2018). *The Silent Teacher: The Gift of Body Donation*, Anatomically Correct.

Smith, C. and Farsides, T. (2020). Proceedings of the 19th International Federation of Associations of Anatomists Congress, 9th–11th August 2019, London, UK. *Journal of Anatomy, 236*(1), 1–364.

Smith, C. et al. (2022). Understanding Beliefs, Preferences and Actions Amongst Potential Body donors. *Anatomical Sciences Education.*

Chapter 32

Avicenna: Shoja, M.M., & Tubbs, R.S. (2007). The Disorder of Love in the Canon of Avicenna (A.D. 980–1037). *The American Journal of Psychiatry, 164*(2), 228–229.

Otago soul studies: Martyn, H., Barrett, A., & Nicholson, H.D. (2014). A Belief in the Soul May Contribute to the Stress Experienced in the Dissecting Room. *Journal of anatomy, 224*(3), 345–351.

Martyn, H., Barrett, A., & Nicholson, H. (2012). Medical Students' Responses to the Dissection of the Heart and Brain: A dialogue on the seat of the soul. *Clinical Anatomy, 25*(3), 407–413.

Anatomists donating: Arráez-Aybar, L.A., Bueno-López, J.L., & Moxham, B.J. (2014). Anatomists' Views on Human Body Dissection and Donation: An international survey. *Annals of Anatomy, 196*(6), 376–386.

Zulu donation: De Gama, B., Jones, D.G., Bhengu, T.T., & Satyapal, K.S. (2020). Cultural Practices of the Zulu Ethnic Group on the Body and Their Influence on Body Donation. *Anatomical Sciences Education, 13*(6), 721–731.

Body donation in Turkey: Gürses Ertaş, A et al. (2019). Profile and Motivations of Registered Whole Body Donors in Turkey: Istanbul University experience. *Anatomical Sciences Education, 12*(4), 370–385.

The beloved theology of the bowel: Welch, C. (2020). The Imagined Emaciated Body in Late-Medieval English Memorial Sculpture. In C. Mounsey & S. Booth (Eds.), *Bodies of Information*. Routledge.

Alice de Pole: Welch, C. (2019). Exploring Alice: the Theological, Socio-Historical, and Anatomical Context of the De La Pole Cadaver Sculpture. In Z. Murat (Ed.), *English Alabaster Carvings and their Cultural Contexts*. Boydell & Brewer.

Chapter 33

16th century burials of the dissected: Klestinec, C. (2011). *Theaters of Anatomy: Students, teachers, and traditions of dissection in renaissance Venice*. Johns Hopkins University Press.

Walter Wood: see above.

UMCG memorial: Bolt, S. (2012). Dead Bodies Matter: Gift giving and the unveiling of body donor monuments in the Netherlands. *Medical Anthropology Quarterly*, *26*(4), 613–634.

Donors liking idea of dissection: Hoeyer, K., & Olejaz, M. (2019). Desire, Duty and Medical Gifting: How it became possible to long for a useful death. *Mortality*, 25, 1–15.

Chapter 34

Alternative plans to find bodies: Richardson, R. (1991). 'Trading assassins' and the Licensing of Anatomy. In R. French, & A. Wear (Eds.), *British Medicine in an Age of Reform (1st ed.)*. Routledge.

Chapter 35

Coronoid part of the masseter: Mezey, S. et al (2021). The Human Masseter Muscle Revisited: First description of its coronoid part. *Annals of Anatomy*, 240.

Interstitium: Benias, P.C., et al (2018). Structure and Distribution of an Unrecognized Interstitium in Human Tissues. *Scientific Reports*, *8*(1), 4947–4948.

Fabella: Berthaume, M.A. et al (2019). Fabella Prevalence Rate Increases over 150 Years, and Rates of Other Sesamoid Bones Remain Constant: A systematic review. *Journal of Anatomy*, *235*(1), 67–79.

Diversity talks: IFAA. (2021) *Anatomy Education Symposia Recordings: The Anatomy Festival 2021*. https://ifaa.net/anatomyfestival/

Nazi dissection: Winkelmann, A. (2021). Traces of Nazi Victims in Hermann Stieve's Histological Collection. *Annals of Anatomy = Anatomischer Anzeiger: Official organ of the Anatomische Gesellschaft*, *237*, 151720.

Donor interviews: Olejaz, M., & Hoeyer, K. (2016). Meet the Donors: A qualitative analysis of what donation means to Danish whole body donors. *European Journal of Anatomy*, 20, 19–29.

Contact your local university if you are interested in donating your body. If you would like to specifically donate to AFTER, get in touch with the University of Technology Sydney body donor program.

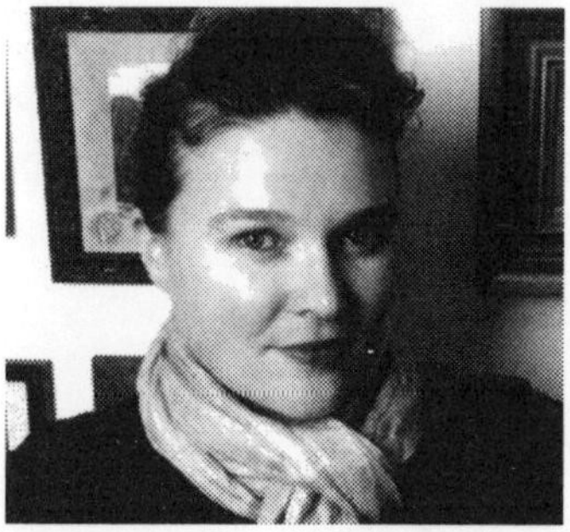

Jackie Dent is a journalist who has worked for major media outlets including *The Sydney Morning Herald*, *The Guardian*, *Monocle*, *The New York Times*, *Reuters*, *Strewth!* and others. Her career has included stints with the United Nations in Afghanistan, Pakistan, North Ossetia and South Sudan. She has also produced radio for The Australian Broadcasting Corporation and curated talks for Tedx Sydney, the Ethics Centre and Clear Spot Club. She lives in Sydney.

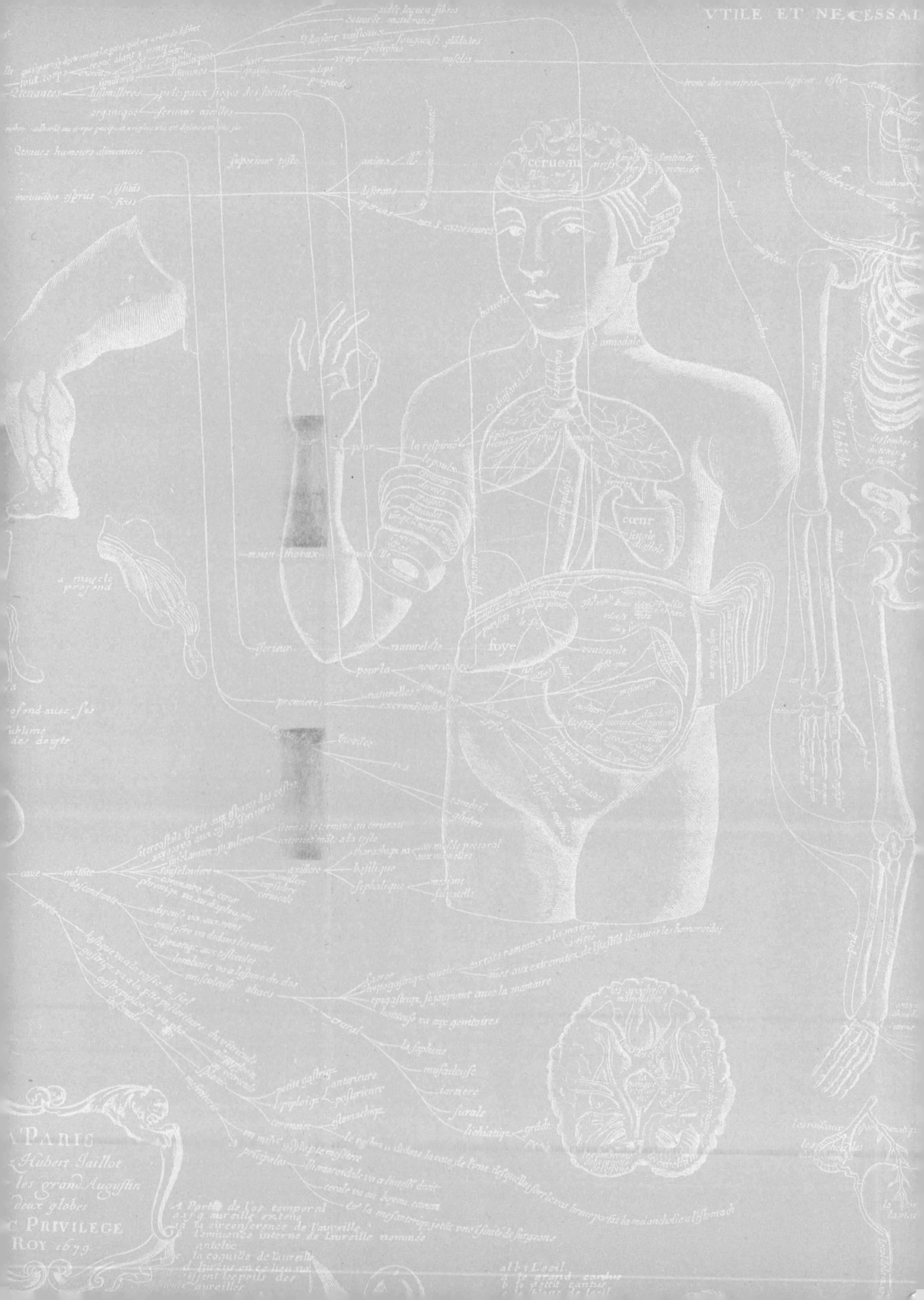

VTILE ET NECESSAI
cerueau
cœur
foye
premieres
naturelles
pour la
Paris
Hubert Iaillot
les grand Augustin
deux globes
c Privilege
Roy 1679